Patents eBook Series
"Topics in Anti-Cancer Research"

(Volume 6)

Edited by

Atta-ur-Rahman, *FRS*
Kings College University of Cambridge, Cambridge, UK

&

Khurshid Zaman
Bentham Science Publishers, USA

Topics in Anti-Cancer Research

Volume # 6

Editors: Atta-ur-Rahman, *FRS* and Khurshid Zaman

ISSN (Print): 2468-5860

ISSN (Online): 2213-3585

ISBN (Online): 978-1-68108-455-8

ISBN (Print): 978-1-68108-456-5

General:

1. Any dispute or claim arising out of or in connection with this License Agreement or the Work (including non-contractual disputes or claims) will be governed by and construed in accordance with the laws of the U.A.E. as applied in the Emirate of Dubai. Each party agrees that the courts of the Emirate of Dubai shall have exclusive jurisdiction to settle any dispute or claim arising out of or in connection with this License Agreement or the Work (including non-contractual disputes or claims).
2. Your rights under this License Agreement will automatically terminate without notice and without the need for a court order if at any point you breach any terms of this License Agreement. In no event will any delay or failure by Bentham Science Publishers in enforcing your compliance with this License Agreement constitute a waiver of any of its rights.
3. You acknowledge that you have read this License Agreement, and agree to be bound by its terms and conditions. To the extent that any other terms and conditions presented on any website of Bentham Science Publishers conflict with, or are inconsistent with, the terms and conditions set out in this License Agreement, you acknowledge that the terms and conditions set out in this License Agreement shall prevail.

Bentham Science Publishers Ltd.
Executive Suite Y - 2
PO Box 7917, Saif Zone
Sharjah, U.A.E.
Email: subscriptions@benthamscience.org

BENTHAM SCIENCE

CONTENTS

FOREWORD

The sixth volume of Topics in Anti-Cancer Research presents some exciting contributions in frontier areas of anti-cancer research. These include the role of microtubules for the treatment of various cancers, novel chemoimmunotherapy drug combinations & methods in clinical studies/trial and current studies in targeting polyunsaturated fatty acids (PUFAs) in the treatment of colorectal cancer. Natural and synthetic chalcones and their derivatives that have shown potent anticancer activity against a number of cancer cell lines and murine tumor models are discussed. The discovery of selective small-molecule hLDH-A inhibitors and LDH-based approaches in the progress of anticancer therapy are also presented. Recent advances in microRNA-based cancer therapeutics for the treatment of cancer are presented. The role of inflammation in chemotherapy-induced neuromuscular effects and the side effects and recent relevant patents for beneficial approaches to improve heart failure cases due to inflammation, mitochondria and energy metabolism in cancer cachexia are also covered. It is hoped that the present volume will be found useful by a large number of scientists working in this field.

The editors are thankful to the authors for their excellent contributions and to the reviewers for their in -depth comprehensive comments for the improvement of chapters. We are also grateful to Mr. Mahmood Alam, Mrs. Rafia Rehan and other colleagues for their support and assistance in the finalization of this volume.

Atta-ur-Rahman, *FRS*
International Center for Chemical and Biological Sciences
University of Karachi
Karachi 75270
Pakistan

Khurshid Zaman
Honorary Editor
Bentham Science Publishers

INTRODUCTION

Topics in Anti-Cancer Research covers important advances on both experimental (preclinical) and clinical cancer research in drug development. The book series offers readers an insight into current and future therapeutic approaches for the prevention of different types of cancers, synthesizing new anti-cancer agents, new patented compounds, targets and agents for cancer therapy as well as recent molecular and gene therapy research.

The comprehensive range of themes covered in each volume will be beneficial to clinicians, immunologists, and R&D experts looking for new anti-cancer targets and patents for the treatment of neoplasms, as well as varied approaches for cancer therapy.

The topics covered in the sixth volume of this series include:

- The role of microtubules for the cure of various untreated cancers
- Novel chemoimmunotherapeutic drug combinations & methods in clinical studies/trials
- Targeting polyunsaturated fatty acids (PUFAs) in the treatment of colorectal cancer
- Anti-cancer activity of natural and synthetic chalcones and their derivatives
- Recent advances in microRNA-based cancer therapeutics
- Treatment of heart failure due to inflammation, mitochondria and energy metabolism in cancer cachexia
- Regulation/inhibition of human lactate dehydrogenase A for discovering anti-cancer drugs

List of Contributors

Ali, Amjad	Atta-ur-Rahman School of Applied Biosciences (ASAB), National University of Sciences and Technology (NUST), H-12 Islamabad, Pakistan Email: amjaduni@gmail.com; amjad.ali@asab.nust.edu.pk
Ashraf, Shifa T.	Atta-ur-Rahman School of Applied Biosciences (ASAB), National University of Sciences and Technology (NUST), H-12 Islamabad, Pakistan Email: stariq.asab@gmail.com
Awan, Faryal M.	Atta-ur-Rahman School of Applied Biosciences (ASAB), National University of Sciences and Technology (NUST), H-12 Islamabad, Pakistan Email: faryal_mehwish@yahoo.com
Bagban, Needa N.	Department of Biotechnology, St. Xavier's College (Autonomous), Mumbai-400001, India Email: neebagban@gmail.com
Bhavsar, Riddhi I.	Department of Biotechnology, St. Xavier's College (Autonomous), Mumbai-400001, India Email: riddhibhavsar2@gmail.com
Chatterji, Biswa P.	Department of Biotechnology, St. Xavier's College (Autonomous), Mumbai-400001, India Email: biswaprasun@gmail.com
Fichna, Jakub	Department of Biochemistry, Faculty of Medicine, Medical University of Lodz, Lodz, Poland Email: jakub.fichna@umed.lodz.pl
Muzammal, Hussain	Institutes of Biomedicine and Health, Chinese Academy of Sciences, 190 Kaiyuan Avenue, Science Park, Guangzhou, 510530, P.R. China Email: muzammal@gibh.ac.cn
Ikonomidis, Thomas G.	Mechanisms of Disease and Translational Research Group, Department of Pathology, School of Medical Sciences, University of New South Wales, Sydney 2052, Australia Email: thomasikono@gmail.com
Ikram, Aqsa	Atta-ur-Rahman School of Applied Biosciences (ASAB), National University of Sciences and Technology (NUST), H-12 Islamabad, Pakistan Email: aqsa_ikram@yahoo.com
Kumar, Vinit	Amity Institute of Molecular Medicine and Stem Cell Research, Amity University, Noida 201313, India Email: vkumar25@amity.edu
Kumar, Atul	Amity Institute of Engineering & Technology, Amity University, Greater Noida 201313, India Email: atul206@gmail.com
Luqman, Suaib	CSIR-Central Institute of Medicinal and Aromatic Plants, Lucknow-226015, Uttar Pradesh, India Email: s.luqman@cimap.res.in

Michalak, Arkadiusz	Department of Biochemistry, Faculty of Medicine, Medical University of Lodz, Lodz, Poland Email: arkadiusz.michalak.lek@gmail.com
Mosińska, Paula	Department of Biochemistry, Faculty of Medicine, Medical University of Lodz, Lodz, Poland Email: paula.mosinska@gmail.com
Polly, Patsie	Mechanisms of Disease and Translational Research Group, Department of Pathology, School of Medical Sciences, University of New South Wales, Sydney 2052, Australia Email: patsie.polly@unsw.edu.au
Rani, Reshma	Amity Institute of Biotechnology, Amity University, Noida 201313, India Email: reshudcy@gmail.com; rrani@amity.edu
Tan, Timothy C.	Western Clinical School and Westmead Hospital, Westmead, New South Wales, Australia Email: timothy.tan9@gmail.com
Wani, Zahoor A.	National Postdoctoral Fellow at CSIR-Central Institute of Medicinal and Aromatic Plants, Lucknow-226015, Uttar Pradesh, India Email: zahoorwani5@gmail.com
Zhang, Jiancun	Institutes of Biomedicine and Health, Chinese Academy of Sciences, 190 Kaiyuan Avenue, Science Park, Guangzhou, 510530, P.R. China Email: zhang_jiancun@gibh.ac.cn

CHAPTER 1

Targeting Polyunsaturated Fatty Acid Metabolism in Colorectal Cancer Therapy: A Review of Recent Patents

Arkadiusz Michalak[#], **Paula Mosińska**[*,#] and **Jakub Fichna**

Department of Biochemistry, Faculty of Medicine, Medical University of Lodz, Lodz, Poland

Abstract: In the recent years, fatty acids (FAs) have been acknowledged not only as building materials for lipid membranes and carbon source for β-oxidation, but also as important signaling molecules. In this field, polyunsaturated fatty acids (PUFAs) have received special attention as modulators of inflammation. The enzymes that process PUFAs into bioactive metabolites (cyclooxygenases, lipoxygenases) have already been targeted by pharmaceutical agents. Given the fact that intense synthesis of FAs is a metabolic hallmark of cancer, it is expected that FAs play an important role in cancer development, progression and invasion, and could be targeted by modern therapies. In this chapter, we will discuss the possible use of FAs and drugs affecting their metabolism against colorectal cancer (CRC), which is strongly associated with environmental factors such as high-fat, high caloric diet and obesity. We will cover the role of n-3 PUFAs as dietary supplements in primary prevention of CRC based on the results obtained from clinical trials, and elaborate on the latest patents designed to improve the bioavailability of PUFAs concentrates as nutritional treatments for patients with CRC. We will also discuss the enzymes processing PUFAs and their role in tumorigenesis with focus on their potential as markers for "molecular staging" (fatty acid synthases and elongases) and targets in therapy (cyclooxygenase 2 and lipoxygenase 5). Finally, we will examine new drug formulations (e.g. liposomes) and their utility in CRC therapy. The chapter is based on the review of literature (PubMed Database) and patent documents.

Keywords: Adjuvant therapy, chemotherapy, colorectal cancer, cyclooxygenase, dietary supplementation, docosahexaenoic acid, eicosapentaenoic acid, fatty acids, gastrointestinal cancer, inflammation, lipoxygenase, liposomes, nutritional treatment, polyunsaturated fatty acids, prevention, patents.

[*] **Corresponding author Paula Mosińska:** Department of Biochemistry, Faculty of Medicine, Medical University of Lodz, Mazowiecka 6/8, 92-215 Lodz, Poland Tel: ++48 42 272 57 07; Fax: ++48 42 272 56 94;
E-mail: paula.mosinska@gmail.com
[#] Equal contribution

Atta-ur-Rahman and Khurshid Zaman (Eds.)

1. INTRODUCTION

Colorectal cancer (CRC) is the second most common cancer in women and third in men, responsible for 600,000 deaths annually worldwide [1 - 3]. It is the fourth cause of oncological deaths, which creates a substantial global burden [4]. Up to 50% of CRC risk is lifestyle-related - most prominent risk factors include obesity, sedentary behavior, alcohol consumption, tobacco smoking, high-meat / high-calorie intake, as well as fat-rich and fiber-deficient diet [5]. All of these disturb the metabolic balance and add to CRC development. A cause-effect relation has been proven for alcohol (which promotes folate deficiency and thus leads to DNA instability and carcinogenesis) and tobacco smoking (which spreads carcinogens from cigarettes to colorectal mucosa, stimulating carcinogenesis) [5]. In turn, dietary habits and sedentary lifestyle not only cause obesity but also lead to the development of metabolic syndrome highlighted by a range of abnormalities encompassing impaired glucose tolerance, elevated blood pressure and dyslipidemia. These metabolic disorders tip the cytokine balance toward chronic low-grade inflammation and further disturb the levels of adipokines e.g. adiponectin and leptin, and insulin growth factors which all affect cellular proliferation, adhesion and migration [6 - 8]. Moreover, unbalanced diet can directly promote carcinogenesis by modifying the intestinal microbiome and making alterations in the complexity of the colorectal mucosa - for details see [6].

Alterations in lifestyle patterns through higher intake of fish and fish oils, dietary fiber, vitamin D and calcium, regular use of aspirin and habitual physical exercise modulate the course of CRC, especially at the initial stage of its development, and improve the quality of life of patients [5]. The protective role of fish and fish oils is mainly attributed to the high content of polyunsaturated fatty acids (PUFAs). The fact that aspirin also acts on the metabolism of PUFAs further suggests that these fatty acids may play a significant role in CRC development and possible prevention.

PUFAs are organic acids comprising of a carbohydrate chain with more than one double (C=C) bond in their structure. Long-chain PUFAs are divided into n-6 PUFAs (first double bond at C6, counting from the methyl C) and n-3 PUFAs (first unsaturated bond at C3). The main representatives of these groups are linoleic acid (LA, 18:2) for n-6 PUFAs and α-linolenic acid (ALA, 18:3) for n-3 PUFAs, together called essential fatty acids (FAs). The term "essential" emphasizes their importance in maintaining the optimal health of humans and other animals, as they cannot be synthesized de novo but have to be supplemented in the diet. These FAs provide the carbon chain necessary for the synthesis of longer FAs: n-6 arachidonic acid (AA, 20:4), and n-3 eicosapentaenoic acid (EPA, 19:5) and docosahexaenoic acid (DHA, 22:6) in the reactions catalyzed by elongases and desaturases. In humans, the efficacy of transforming ALA to longer n-3 PUFAs is low and personally variable [9] and thus its derivatives should also be supplemented in diet. Animal-derived products (meat, eggs, dairy) are the most common source of LA and its derivative AA, whereas fish, particularly salmon, provides mainly n-3 PUFAs.

This chapter will briefly describe the fundamental knowledge of PUFAs and their metabolism. A detailed section is devoted to reports from the *in vitro* and *in vivo* studies investigating links between PUFAs and CRC. The main body covers various ways in which PUFAs could be utilized to prevent or treat cancer, especially CRC, based on the already established patents and promising reports from the literature.

The review is based on literature search conducted in the following databases: PubMed (for original papers and reviews), ClinicalTrials.gov, EU Clinical Trials Register and UMIM (for clinical trials), and WIPO (for pertaining to patents). The keywords used to search for patents included: adjuvant therapy, chemotherapy, colorectal cancer, dietary supplementation, docosahexaenoic acid, eicosapentaenoic acid, endocannabinoids, fish oil, liposomes, polyunsaturated fatty acids and resolvins. The literature was searched in relation to relevant patents. Non-English articles were not included in the review. All patents and clinical trials mentioned in this paper are summarized in Tables **1** and **2**, respectively.

2. PUFAS AND THEIR METABOLITES

PUFAs are important elements of cellular lipid membranes released into circulation by phospholipase A2. By undergoing various enzymatic and non-enzymatic pathways, PUFAs are converted into biologically active lipid metabolites and mediators (Fig. **1**). The most prominent enzymes participating in the formation of bioactive metabolites of n-3 and n-6 PUFAs include:

- Cyclooxygenases (COXs) that produce prostaglandins (PGs), thromboxanes (TXs) and prostacyclins;
- Lipoxygenases (LOXs) which process AA into lipoxins (LXs) and leukotrienes (LTx), and n-3 PUFA into protectins, marensins and resolvins;
- Cytochrome 450 (Cyp 450) which converts PUFAs into hydroxyeicosatetraenoic acids (HETEs).

Table 1. Summary of Patent Applications Mentioned Throughout the Main Text.

Patent Number	Inventor	Title	Comment
US20130115618	Swinnen, J.	Phospholipid profiling and cancer	Prognostic and predictive methods and kits for determining the lipogenicity of a tumor in a subject by making use of phospholipid profiling
WO2013144325		Fatty acid elongation enzymes as targets for cancer diagnostics and therapeutics	Methods for identifying and categorizing cancers on the basis of their expression and activity of enzymes of the fatty acyl chain elongation pathway; lipid compositions with potential for detecting, monitoring and predicting the tumor response to anti-cancer treatment
WO2016046347	Munoz, G., Morse, M.	Pharmaceutical product, medical food or dietary supplement for preventing cancer and inflammatory diseases	Invention relates to the composition of a pharmaceutical, medical food or dietary supplement comprising the combination of the following three active ingredients: hydroxytyrosol, fish oil EPA/DHA and curcumin
WO2016046347	Diaz, C.M.P., Munoz, F.G., Morse, G.	Pharmaceutical product, medical food or dietary supplement for preventing cancer and inflammatory diseases	Invention relates to cancer therapy based on administering specific dietary compensation. Composition comprises of the combination of the following three active ingredients: hydroxytyrosol, fish oil EPA/DHA and curcumin
US20160106696	Diaz, C.M.P., Munoz, F.G., Morse, G.	Pharmaceutical product, medical food or dietary supplement for preventing cancer and inflammatory diseases	The invention relates to the composition of a pharmaceutical, medical food or dietary supplement composition comprising the combination of the following three active ingredients: hydroxytyrosol, fish oil EPA/DHA and curcumin
WO2015176780	Coulter, I., Mcdonald, BF., Aversa, V	Celecoxib formulations useful for treating colorectal cancer	The invention provides (amongst other things) a liquid comprising water, solubilised celecoxib, a polyethoxylated non-ionic surfactant and a hydrogel-forming polymer, and the dried liquid in the form of minibeads. The formulation may be used for treating colorectal cancer
WO2001076588	Collin, P., Yang, P., Newman, R.	Method to inhibit lipoxygenase and cancer cell proliferation	Disclosed for prevention and/or treatment of diseases in which 5- and 12-lipoxygenase activity contributes to the pathological condition, by administration of 12-methyltetradecanoic acids alone and in conjunction with other therapeutic compounds

(Table 1) contd.....

Patent Number	Inventor	Title	Comment
US9328060	Van Dross, R.T., Ladin, D.A., Burns, C.S., Danell, A.S.	J-Series prostaglandin-ethanolamides as novel therapeutics	The present invention relates to novel therapeutics and pharmaceutical compositions including J-series prostaglandin-ethanolamides, or a derivative thereof, and salts thereof, and a pharmaceutical carrier
US20130172407	Kuo, Y.H., Tang, F.Y., Lin, H.Y.	Inhibition of cancer cell proliferation using oleoylethanolamide	Disclosed is a pharmaceutical composition including an OEA to inhibit tumor/cancer cell proliferation
WO2009039157	Kothamasu, S.S., Sah, A., Asapu, U.S., Arumalla, M.R.	Orlistat pharmaceutical formulations	The invention relates to pharmaceutical compositions comprising orlistat, including its salts, solvates, polymorphs, racemic mixtures, enantiomers, and mixtures thereof
US20120289570; US20140363522	Lengyel, E., Nieman, K., Kenny, H.	Compositions and methods for treating and/or preventing cancer by inhibiting fatty acid binding proteins	The present invention concerns methods and compositions for the inhibition or reduction of the primary tumor and metastasis by inhibition of fatty acid binding proteins
WO2015107244	Moreno Egea, F., Cerdan Garcia Esteller, S., Calle Hernandez, D.	Compositions containing liposomes, long-chain Omega-3 polyunsaturated fatty acids and superparamagnetic nanoparticles, and the use thereof in the treatment of malignant tumours	The invention relates to preparation, characterization and evaluation *in vivo* of compositions containing liposomes, long-chain ω-3 polyunsaturated fatty acids and superparamagnetic nanoparticles, in the treatment of malignant tumors
WO2015107244	Moreno Egea, F., Cerdan Garcia Esteller, S., Calle Hernandez, D.	Composiciones que contienen liposomas, ácidos grasos poliinsaturados Omega-3 de cadena larga y nanopartículas superparamagnéticas y su uso en el tratamiento de tumores malignos	The invention relates to preparation, characterization and evaluation *in vivo* of compositions containing liposomes, long-chain ω-3 polyunsaturated fatty acids and superparamagnetic nanoparticles, in the treatment of malignant tumors
US20160067202; WO2014175748	Mathisen, J.S.	Use of a composition comprising fish oil and juice for the treatment and/or post treatment of cancer	Disclosed is a composition including a fish oil and a juice in an oil-in-water emulsion for the use in treatment and post-treatment of cancer

(Table 1) contd.....

Patent Number	Inventor	Title	Comment
WO2010033424	Schiffrin, E., Burke Miller, K., Brassart, D.	Nutritional support of the immune system during anti-cancer treatment	The present invention relates to methods and immunonutritional compositions that can transiently augment or enhance the immunocompetence of an immune cell and the immunogenecity of a tumor cell of a patient undergoing anti-cancer therapy to preserve the innate and adaptive immune functions and normal physiology of the immune cell, which, in turn, lead to (i) better tolerance and increased efficacy to anti-cancer therapy; (ii) transient augmentation or enhancement of immunocompetence of the immune cell and immunogenecity of the tumor cell; and (iii) optimization of the effects of an increase of immunocompetence of the immune cell weakened by anti-cancer therapy
US20150297549; EP2425833	Schlotzer, W., Krampitz, B., Suchner, U.	Composition comprising a combination of DHA and EPA for administration prior to commencement of chemotherapy	The invention relates to a composition comprising a combination of the Omega-3 fatty acids EPA and DHA. The composition can be used for enhancing the activity of chemotherapy or radiotherapy and/or in the prevention or reduction of side effects caused by the chemotherapy or radiotherapy in a cancer patient
US20160015666	Burattin, L.	Mixture of fatty acids for use in the treatment of inflammatory pathologies	This invention relates to a mixture of at least three fatty acids selected from palmitic acid, oleic acid, stearic acid, linoleic acid, alpha-linolenic acid, gamma-linolenic acid, EPA, DHA, azelaic acid and myristic acid. This invention also relates to the use of the aforesaid mixture in the treatment of inflammatory pathologies
US9034389	Driscoll, D.F.	Omega-3 enriched fish oil-in-water parenteral nutrition emulsions	The present disclosure relates to an emulsion and a composition containing at least Omega-3 acid triglycerides and a medium-chain triglyceride. The emulsion can be an oil-in-water emulsion. The emulsion and composition can be used, for example, in parenteral administration

(Table 1) contd.....

Patent Number	Inventor	Title	Comment
WO2006067498	Courtney, E.D.J., Leicester, R., Bennett, A.	Eicosapentaenoic acid for the treatment of cancer	The use of an Omega-3 fatty acid composition, containing eicosapentaenoic acid in the free acid form in an amount of 80 or more per cent (w/w) of the total amount of omega- 3 fatty acids present in said composition, in the manufacture of a medicament for the treatment or prophylaxis of cancer
US20130046020; WO2012109539	Liang, S.C., Orlandi, R.D.	Eicosapentaenoic acid concentrate	This invention pertains to an Omega-3 oil concentrate comprising the long-chain polyunsaturated fatty acid cis-5,8,11,14,17-EPA and, more particularly, to an EPA concentrate comprising at least 70 weight percent of EPA, measured as a weight percent of oil, and substantially free of cis-4,7,10,13,16,19-DHA

EPA: Eicosapentaenoic Acid; DHA: Docosahexaenoic Acid; OEA: Oleoylethanolamide

Table 2. Overview of Current Trials in Europe Investigating the Use of FAs in the Treatment or Prevention of Gastrointestinal Cancers.

Trial Number	Title	Trial Design	Subjects	Intervention	Primary End-Points	Status
2009-009470-27	Phase II trial of the effect of gemcitabine with intravenous omega 3 fish oil infusion in patients with unresectable pancreatic adenocarcinoma	Therapeutic exploratory (Phase II) trial, single arm	Patients with histologically or cytologically confirmed unresectable pancreatic adenocarcinoma	Lipidem 200mg/ml, iv in addition to standard 4-week gemcitabine protocol	Objective response rate (complete + partial response)	Ongoing
2011-001477-14	Phase 3 prospective randomized, blinded and controlled investigation of Hepasphere/Quadrasphere microspheres for delivery of doxorubicin for the treatment of hepatocellular cancer	Phase 3 prospective blinded RCT	Patients with hepatocellular cancer (Stage Child-Pugh B 7, Recurrent HCC, Performance status ECOG 1) not suitable for resection or percutaneous ablation at time of study entry	TACE procedure using HepaSphere/QuadraSphere Microspheres loaded with doxorubicin vs. conventional TACE procedure using PVA, lipiodol and doxorubicin	Median overall survival	Ongoing
2013-003664-32	Effect of omega-3 fatty acids on the perioperative immune response and erythrocyte function	Open RCT	Patients (male or female) undergoing elective laparoscopic surgery for colon cancer	Parenteral nutrition supplemented with n-3 PUFAs (Omegaven-Fresenius, iv.) vs. NaCl 0,9% 2ml/kg body weight iv	*Ex vivo* production of pro-inflammatory cytokine IL-6 in LPS stimulated whole blood cells	Ongoing
2006-000044-71	Randomized controlled trial of the effects of fish oil emulsion in total parenteral nutrition upon tumor vascularity in patients with hepatic colorectal metastases	Double-blind RCT	Patients with resectable hepatic colorectal metastases	Total parenteral nutrition supplemented (Lipidem) or not (Lipofundin MCT/LCT 20%) with n-3 PUFAs for 3 days before surgery	Ongoing tumor vascularity measured by change in gadolinium chelate enhancement on Dynamic Contrast Enhanced Magnetic Resonance Imaging between study entry and exit	

(Table 2) contd.....

Trial Number	Title	Trial Design	Subjects	Intervention	Primary End-Points	Status
2010-020943-10	A randomized controlled trial of eicosapentaenoic acid (EPA) and/or aspirin for colorectal adenoma (or polyp) prevention during colonoscopic surveillance in the NHS Bowel Cancer Screening Programme: The seAFOod (Systematic Evaluation of Aspirin and Fish Oil) polyp prevention trial	Therapeutic confirmatory (Phase III) double-blind RCT	60-73 year-old NHS Bowel Cancer Screening Programme patients identified as 'high risk'	EPA-FFA 1 g twice daily + aspirin 300 mg once; EPA-FFA 1 g twice daily + aspirin placebo once daily; EPA placebo twice daily plus aspirin 300 mg once daily; EPA placebo twice daily plus aspirin placebo once daily for 12 months	The number of 'high risk' participants with one or more adenomas detected at the first surveillance colonoscopy	

EPA: Eicosapentaenoic Acid; FFA: Free Fatty Acid; HCC: Hepatocellular Cancer; iv: Intravenous; LPS: Lipopolysaccharide; MCT/LCT: Medium/Long Chain Triglycerides; PUFAs: Polyunsaturated Fatty Acids; PVA: Polyvinyl Alcohol; RCT: Randomized Clinical Trial; TACE: Transcatether Artherial Embolisation.

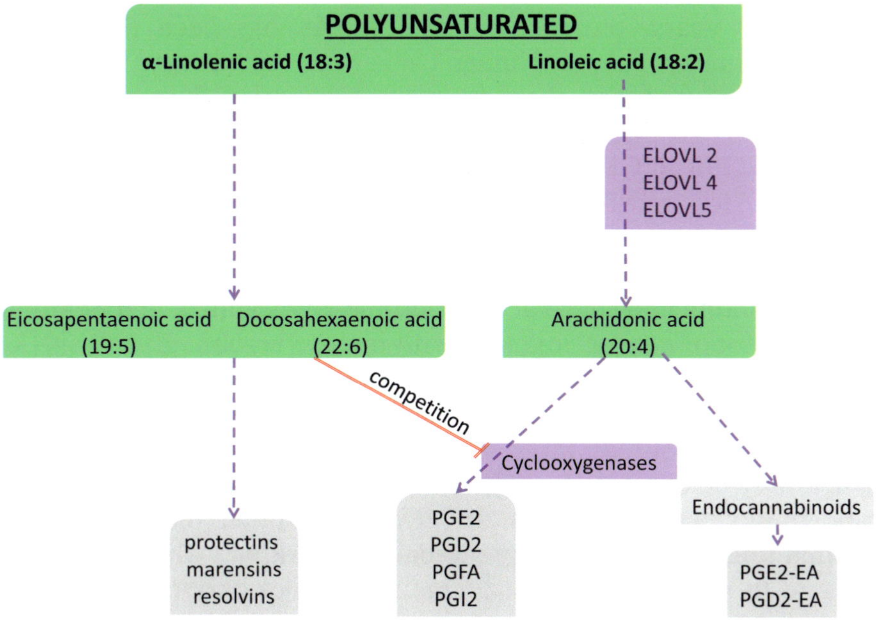

Fig. (1). Polyunsaturated fatty acids and selected enzymes participating in the formation of their bioactive metabolites.

ELOVL2: Fatty Acid Elongase 2; ELOVL4: Fatty Acid Elongase 4; ELOVL5: Fatty Acid Elongase 5; PGD2: Prostaglandin D2; PGE2: Prostaglandin E2; PGD2-EA: Prostaglandin D2 Ethanolamide; PGE2-EA: Prostaglandin E2-Ethanolamide; PGFA: Prostaglandin F; PGI2: Prostaglandin I2.

PGs are a family of AA metabolites produced from a common precursor prostaglandin H2 (PGH2). Among all PGs, prostaglandin E2 (PGE2) is the most potent pro-inflammatory lipid compound secreted by macrophages and neutrophils that induce fever, increase vascular permeability, cause vasodilation and sensitize cells to other inflammatory factors, such as histamine and bradykinin. In contrast, prostaglandin D2 (PGD2) presents purely anti-inflammatory features. Other important PGs include prostaglandin F2 (PGFA2) - involved in parturition in uterus, water absorption in kidneys and vasoconstriction - and prostaglandin I2 (PGI2), which plays a role in platelet inhibition, vasodilation and regulation of renal flow.

Other AA derivatives include thromboxane A2 (TXA2), leukotriene B4 (LTB4) and LXs. The main role of TXA2 is to promote platelet aggregation and vasoconstriction. LTB4 is a pro-inflammatory chemokine which attracts neutrophils and causes vascular leakage, whereas LXs are considered pro-resolution mediators as they reduce leukocyte infiltration.

Over the last 20 years, the metabolism of FAs has been recognized as an important part of tumor biology. Human cancer cells need vast amounts of FAs to grow but instead of capturing them from the circulation they tend to synthesize them on their own. To this end, cancer cells rely on various growth factors and their receptors (EGFR, KGF, HER2) to stimulate intracellular signaling pathways (MAPKs, PI3K-AKT and JNK), and activate transcription factors (e.g. SREBP-1). This leads to overexpression of mRNA for lipogenic enzymes such as fatty acid synthase (FAS) [10]. This intensified lipid synthesis is viewed as a mechanism promoting cell survival in anaerobic environment and highlighted as a metabolic hallmark of cancer, together with intense aerobic glycolysis (known as Warburg effect) and increased protein and DNA synthesis [11]. Of note, the expression of FAS also rises in response to acidic microenvironment and boosts tumor resistance to cellular injuries caused by e.g. chemotherapy [11]. This phenomenon may be explained by the fact that FAS synthesizes mostly saturated or at most monounsaturated FAs. In effect, saturated phospholipids tend to arrange within lipid bilayer into microdomains (or "rafts") which remain insoluble after exposure to various detergents. This affects not only the structure of lipid membrane but also its functionality, as rafts are physiologically involved in signal transduction, intracellular trafficking and cell migration [12]. These changes may decrease the efficiency of chemotherapeutic agents. Moreover, increased FA synthesis may also promote acylation of proteins and - among others - change their intracellular destination by targeting to rafts [10]. Another observation that may explain the role of FAS in tumor chemoresistance comes from studies on breast cancer cell lines. It has been reported that FAS overexpression coupled with hyperglycaemic growth conditions induces resistance to standard chemotherapeutics (5-fluorouracil, doxorubicin and paclitaxel) in MCF-7 and T47D cell lines. This may be explained by the impact of intensive endogenous synthesis of palmitate on cell homeostasis. In normal conditions, palmitate is a precursor for synthesis of ceramide, which is involved in intracellular signaling and mediates the apoptotic effects of ionizing radiation, chemotherapeutics or ischemia/reperfusion process. Increased FAS activity leads to intense synthesis of palmitate and then ceramide. Accumulation of ceramide is suspected to increase resistance to chemotherapeutics, which in non-accustomed cells stimulate apoptosis [13].

Currently, there are no reliable markers for identifying increased lipogenicity in a tumor, however, one method has been designed and patented by Swinnen (US20130115618) [14]. It utilizes electrospray ionization mass spectrometry tandem mass spectrometry (ESI-MS/MS) to compare the composition of a cancer cell membrane with healthy tissue. The phospholipids are identified by the intensity of ionized species expressed as the % of total intensity of all measured phospholipids. A shift toward monounsaturated phospholipids indicates a more resistant and aggressive lipogenic cancer phenotype. In detail, an increase in monounsaturated and decrease in polyunsaturated phospholipid species has been found to correlate with increased FAS gene expression and indicates an increased tumor resistance to lipid peroxidation and apoptosis, oxidative stress and chemotherapeutics [15]. Both the tumor and reference samples can be obtained from tissues, cells as well as cell extracts. For non-invasive samples authors suggest: urine, serum, whole blood or plasma concentrate, a precipitation from blood/plasma/urine (e.g. exosomes). The flexibility of the method enables to create a personalized model of treatment depending on patient's condition and the type of tumor. It provides an insight into molecular profile of cancer, which may complement the clinical staging. Authors suggest this invention may also help monitor the effects of cancer therapy.

Fatty acid elongases (EVOVLs) participate in lipid metabolism. These endoplasmatic enzymes catalyze a four-step reaction of extending FAs into very long chain FAs [16]. So far, 7 different EVOVLs have been identified; ELOVL1, ELOVL3, and ELOVL6 act on saturated and monounsaturated FAs, whereas ELOVL 2, ELOVL 4, and ELOVL5 elongate PUFAs. Some of these enzymes have been studied in relation to breast (ELOVL2 and 5) and prostate (ELOVL7) cancer. Analysis of EVOVLs profile may be therefore utilized in diagnostics and profiling of various cancers (WO2013144325) [17]. In detail, the patent discloses the methods for measuring, in a biological sample, the expression of genes involved in fatty acid synthesis and elongation and comparing their expression with a reference genes in the same sample or with expression of genes in a reference sample. The analyzed set includes genes for FAS, various elongases, fatty acid desaturases, acetyl-CoA carboxylase and malonyl-CoA decarboxylase, as well as for protein-tyrosine phosphatase-like proteins, estradiol 17-beta-dehydrogenase 12 and sterol regulatory element-binding proteins 1c. This method may help diagnose cancer in a particular sample and more importantly, can determine the lipid phenotype of the cancer.

3. PRIMARY PREVENTION

CRC develops over the years and gradually transforms from normal epithelium through adenomatous pre-cancerous lesions to a full-blown tumor. Due to its growth dynamics, it is a suitable candidate for primary prevention. In this field, FAs have been studied as potential supplements that may delay or prevent CRC development. The most promising candidates so far are n-3 PUFAs, which show great tolerability profile and exhibit anti-inflammatory effects [18, 19]. However, despite theoretical background from basic science and promising epidemiological studies, intervention trials yielded mixed results and metaanalyses have failed to definitely support or overthrow their usefulness in CRC therapy [20, 21].

However, there are naturally occurring substances that may enhance n-3 PUFAs anti-cancer properties. Curcumin, a polyphenol derived from *Curcuma longa,* could play such a role. It displays pleiotropic biological effects both *in vitro* and *in vivo* i.e. it exerts anti-inflammatory, hypoglycemic, antioxidant, wound-healing, antimicrobial and anti-cancerous activity [22, 23]. This variety of actions is explained by a wide range of its molecular targets described *in vitro* - curcumin acts on a range of transcription factors (e.g. NF-κB, AP-1, and STAT-3), PGE2 and other inflammatory mediators, enzymes, growth factors, protein kinases, and cell-cycle regulatory proteins [24]. The safety, tolerability and nontoxicity of curcumin have already been proven in human clinical trials; however, its pharmacological efficiency (demonstrated by decrease in the level of the oxidative DNA adduct 3-(2-deoxy-β-di-erythro-pentafuranosyl)-pyr(1,2-α)-purin-10(3H) one (M1G)) has only been confirmed in surgical CRA samples taken from patients.

Curcumin holds promise as a primary prevention drug in high risk groups (e.g. smokers) as it reduces the formation of aberrant crypt foci, the precursors of colorectal polyps. In patients with familial adenomatous polyposis (FAP) who are a high risk group for CRC, treatment with combination of curcumin (480mg) and quercetin (20mg) orally decreased the number and size of polyps, without any reported toxicity [22]. However, due to small numbers of patients enrolled in the trials and varying methodology, the so-far reported results are inconsistent. Large RCTs are needed to determine its beneficial effects.

Halder *et al.* [25] studied the suspected synergy of curcumin and two n-3 PUFA formulations *in vitro* - a standard marine oil and a "smartfish" formulation enhanced with naturally occurring anti-oxidants. The agents in various combinations were incubated with MP2 cells and the cytotoxic effect was assessed by measuring caspase-3 expression, a mediator of programmed cell death. The experiment showed that high dose of curcumin successfully induced apoptosis in co-administration with marine oil n3-PUFA, whereas by adding anti-oxidants to the mixture the effect was potentiated. The study also verified the interactions between curcumin, "smartfish" n-3 PUFAs and NK cells-induced cytotoxicity. While "smartfish" oil partially induced NK-related cytotoxicity, adding curcuminoids significantly enhanced the effect. Unfortunately, the same study simultaneously showed that curcuminoids inhibit IFN-y production (an important anti-tumor cytokine) by NK cells, which may put obstacles in the way of its clinical utilization [25]. It is necessary to verify whether this ambivalent interaction between curcumin and cancer cells translates to in vivo models and, in the long term, to clinical trials.

Nevertheless, a new medical food and dietary supplement have already been developed and claimed in patents, for example fish oil, curcumin and hydroxytyrosol, and the combination of those components (WO2016046347, WO2016046347, US20160106696) [26 - 28]. Its clinical value in preventing cancer remains to be assessed.

4. TREATMENT

PUFAs give rise to various active metabolites, which display a wide range of biological actions. Thus, key enzymes of PUFAs metabolism represent another target to modulate tumor biology. A prime example of this strategy is the use of low-dose aspirin, which demonstrated (both in observational studies and RCTs) a protective effect in CRC prevention [29]. At first, this effect was attributed to the suppression of COXs, including COX-2 isoenzyme, whose expression is increased in 50% of colorectal adenomas and 85% of adenocarcinomas [29]. COX-2-derived PGs were proved to boost cell proliferation rate, promote angiogenesis and metastasis and suppress apoptosis [30]. However, many reports suggest that the doses of aspirin used in general population or in most RCTs are not high enough to effectively suppress COX-2. On the other hand, low-dose aspirin is perfectly capable of inhibiting COX-1 in platelets, which has been showed to induce COX-2 expression [29]. It is therefore possible that permanent COX-1 inactivation in platelets protects cells in intestinal mucosa from overexpression of COX-2.

Moreover, platelets can interact directly with cancer cells [31]. When cocultured with HT29 cells, human thrombocytes stimulate CRC cells toward more malignant gene expression phenotype. In turn, such "primed" CRC cells injected in mice can increase PGE2 systemic synthesis and platelet synthesis of TXA2. Importantly, aspirin administration counteracted these changes, either when used to pretreat platelets before coculturing with CRC cells, or when administered to mice injected with already primed HT29 [31]. Finally, it is possible that the action of aspirin on CRC cells is independent of COX-inhibition and interaction with platelets. This is supported by the observation that aspirin regulates sirtuin-1 expression and can modulate phosphatidylinositol 3-kinase-related intracellular signaling pathways [29]. However, extensive studies are needed to determine which mechanism is the most important in aspirin action.

Despite these ambiguities, aspirin is now officially recommended for CRC chemoprevention even though its usage confers significant side effects mainly associated with an increased risk of bleeding.

To solve this, selective COX-2 inhibitors (coxibs) were developed to target PGE-2 synthesis and prevent tumor-associated angiogenesis and growth. The key representant of this class, celecoxib, indeed exhibits chemoprotective effects against cancer [32]. Surprisingly enough, most of celecoxib`s anti-proliferative effects were found to be COX-independent and unique in the coxib`s family [30]. Celecoxib induces G1-phase arrest by inhibiting phosphoinositide-dependent kinase 1 (PDK-1), protein kinase B (PKB) and other cell-cycle kinases, and promotes apoptosis by decreasing the concentration of anti-apoptotic proteins Bcl-2, Bcl-xl, mcl 1 and survivin. Extrinsic apoptotic pathway (FAS-FADD) also takes part in celecoxib`s action [32]. Collectively, celecoxib affects the expression of over 1400 genes involved in, among others, immune response, inflammatory reaction, cell signaling and adhesion, response to stress, transforming growth factor-b signaling and apoptosis [30]. Given the vast pleiotropic effects of the molecule designed to affect solely AA metabolism, it might be enlightening to study the interactions between PUFA and coxib molecules, which may yield a better insight into the variety of PUFA metabolites. The beneficial properties of celecoxib have been confirmed both in vitro and in vivo, and currently the agent is approved as adjuvant treatment in FAP.

Worth mentioning, the celecoxib has low bioavailability and to induce the desired effect it must be administered at high doses, what in turn significantly increases the risk for adverse effects and undermines it as a potential chemoprevention drug. However, very recently Coulter et al. have developed a new multiple minibead formulation of celecoxib (WO2015176780) [33], which allows to lower the dosage and promises fewer adverse effects. It has already been claimed for prevention or treatment of CRC. Authors declare minibeads may be coated with polymers that ensure targeted release of celecoxib in the colon. Additionally, recent studies indicate that celecoxib might be used to break CRC resistance to chemotherapeutics like imatinib or cetuxizumab [34, 35].

Other agents that target PUFA metabolism, such as 5-LOX inhibitors, are currently under evaluation in the management of CRC. 5-LOX is reported to be overexpressed in the early stages of CRC and associated with markers of transformation of adenomatous polyps to cancer [36]. Historically, LOX inhibitors were reported to cause apoptosis of human leukemia blast cells and lung cancer cells. More recently, a new 5-LOX inhibitor, Zileuton, registered for asthma therapy, was proved to disrupt signaling in prostate cancer and induce apoptosis in pancreatic cancer cells [37 - 39], as well as to decrease proliferation in CRC cell lines and reduce the size of xenografted metastases [36]. Currently, no LOX inhibitors have been approved for cancer therapy.

One of prospective drugs is 12-methyltetradecanoic acid isolated from *Cucumaria frondosa* which inhibits 5-LOX and 12-LOX, and suppresses cancer cell proliferation *in vitro* (WO2001076588) [40]. However, it might be worthwhile to go even a step further and combine COX and LOX inhibitors to create a novel class of anti-cancer agents. Recent studies revealed that COX-2 and 5-LOX expression is tightly connected and balanced, i.e. when one of the enzymes is downregulated (e.g. by treatment or viral silencing), the other gets upregulated [41]. Thus, targeting them both may prove very efficient against CRC. There is a positive correlation between COX-2 and 5-LOX expression in CRC samples during cancer proliferation, migration and invasion [41]. Consequently, different analogues of indomethacin (COX-2 specific non-steroid anti-inflammatory drug), rofecoxib and celecoxib have been studied in search of agents displaying properties of dual inhibition. In effect, a new group of agents - di-ter-butyl phenols - has emerged, which inhibit selectively both COX-2 and 5-LOX [42]. The key representatives of this class are darbufelone, lycofelone and KME4. They all demonstrated their efficacy in *in vitro* studies [42]. Importantly, darbufelone proved to be more efficient as proliferation inhibitor than celecoxib, zileuton or their combination against LoVo CRC cells [41]. In turn, lycofelone has been studied most extensively and is the first to have reached clinical trials. *In vitro*, it triggered apoptosis in HCA-7 (human CRC cells) in a time- and dose-dependent manner, whereas *in vivo* it inhibited tumorigenesis in APC Min/+ mice [42]. More compounds are now being tested in *in vitro* studies.

Another class of agents having potential in CRC treatment are endocannabinoids. This heterogenous group of lipid mediators acts on G protein-coupled cannabinoid (CB) receptors expressed on neurons and immune cells. Their key representatives are N-arachidonoylethanolamine, named anandamide (AEA), and 2-arachidonoylglycerol (2-AG), both derived from AA. Anandamide displays promising anti-neoplastic effects in vitro in human (breast cancer, prostate cancer, cervical carcinoma, lymphoblastic cells) and animal cell lines (rat glioma, mouse lymphoblastic cells). Furthermore, it suppresses proliferation and promotes cell death in CRC cell lines via COX-2-depedent manner [43]; however its pro-apoptotic properties are less potent when compared to the AEA metabolites, prostaglandin-ethanolamine (PG-EA), such as PGE2-EA or PGD2-EA. Therefore, a composition including J-series PGs (PGJ-EAs) has been registered for treatment of non-melanoma skin cancer and CRC (US9328060) [44]. This patent offers a chance to specifically target CRC cells in which PGE2 expression is usually elevated, and at the same time to protect healthy tissues.

Other known acylethanolamides include palmitoylethanolamide (PEA) and oleoylethanolamide (OEA). In contrast to AEA, OEA has only one double bond in its structure and does not bind CB receptors (CBR), but instead activates peroxisome proliferator-activated receptor α (PPAR-α) and consequently induces satiety, inhibits weight gain and stimulates lipolysis and FA oxidation. Surprisingly, OEA also induces cell cycle arrest and apoptosis in cancer cells; nonetheless, its mechanism of action has not been elucidated yet. Thus, a pharmaceutical composition including OEA in combination with other active ingredients (e.g. vitamin A, carotenoids, ω-3 PUFA, ω-6 PUFA and/or conjugated LA), has been claimed in a patent to inhibit cell proliferation in tumors and cancers, including CRC (US20130172407) [45].

Another way to affect CRC biology is to target the key enzymes of tumor lipid metabolism. As mentioned before, cancers exhibit intense lipid turnover which is driven, among others, by their high proliferation rate [46]. Thus, excessive amounts of FAs are needed to provide the fuel for the cells, building materials for new lipid membranes and signaling molecules. This demand can be satisfied either by taking up the FAs from the bloodstream or synthesizing them *de novo*. In effect, cancer cells may use lipoprotein lipase (LPS) to degrade circulating triglycerides and take up the FAs with CD36 channel or FAS to synthesize their own [47, 48]. Although *de novo* synthesis seems to be the main source of FAs for most cancers, Kuemmerle *et al.* demonstrated that lipolytic pathway is also active in many cancer types [47]. Therefore, in order to cut down the supply of FAs for cancers, we may need to combine FAS inhibitors and lipoprotein lipase inhibitors such as Orlistat [47] (WO2009039157) [49]. This agent exhibited toxicity towards B-cell chronic lymphoblastic leukemic cells [50]. It remains to be seen if this or similar agents find their use in CRC therapy.

Fatty acid binding proteins (FABPs) are intracellular proteins, which bind and transport long chains of fatty acids between cell compartments [51]. Besides regulation of lipid trafficking, they also modulate metabolic and inflammatory pathways, and influence cellular differentiation. So far, as many as 10 FABP tissue-specific isoforms have been identified [51]. Furthermore, certain FABPs are emerging as important enzymes in CRC biology. For example, liver-FABP (L-FABP/FABP-1) is viewed as cell protector as it binds potentially toxic FAs, heme, and other molecules [52]. Moreover, it displays significant anti-oxidant properties thanks to the presence of cysteine and methionine groups in its structure, which take part in utilizing ROS in redox reactions. It is also associated with metabolic homeostasis due to its close relations with PPAR-α and PPAR-γ receptors [52]. In neoplasms, FABP-1 plays a tissue-specific role in cancer development. An increased expression of FABP-1 was reported in both primary prostate tumors and prostate cancer cell lines [53]. Similarly, elevated expression has been observed in primary liver tumors [53]. In contrast, CRC cells are characterized by FABP-1 loss of expression, both in mice and in humans, which occurs early in intestinal tumorigenesis and decreases progressively from early adenomas to poorly differentiated tumors [53, 54]. Interestingly, genetically modified mice lacking FABP1 gene were protected from CRC development, which occurred due to global changes in lipid trafficking and insufficient lipid supply for cancer uncontrolled proliferation [54]. Finally, FABP1 serves as a good prognostic factor for patients undergoing hepatic resection of CRC metastases [55]. The next FABP associated with CRC is adipocyte-specific FABP (A-FABP/ FABP4), which integrates metabolic and inflammatory signaling. In a study of differentially-expressed genes between colon tumor samples and adjacent normal mucosal tissues, FABP4 has been reported as one of the downregulated genes in CRC cells [56]. However, these findings have not proved any cause-effect relation between FABP4 expression and CRC metabolism and their findings have yet to be supported.

Another FABP possibly involved in CRC development is a bile acid transporter specific for ileal epithelium (I-FABP/ FABP6). Bile acids are known to induce apoptosis and inflammation in colonic epithelial cells as well as cause oxidative DNA damage which all lead to colon carcinogenesis [57]. In turn, bile acid exposure induces FABP6 expression in the Caco-2 colon cancer cells what suggests there is a feedback loop between bile acids, cellular FABP6 expression and cancer development. Moreover, in CRC patients FABP6 expression in adenoma or cancer cells was significantly higher than in unaffected tissue [57]. However, high FABP6 expression was also associated with smaller tumor size, what suggests FABP6 as important factor for carcinogenesis but not for cancer progression. Similarly, lymph node metastases showed no elevated expression of FABP6, and concurrently are not implicated in tumor promotion [57].

The last type of FABP studied in relation to CRC is epidermal FABP (E-FABP/ FABP5). FABP5 is overly expressed in four different CRC cell lines (HCT116,

LoVo, DLD-1 and Caco-2) compared with normal colon fibroblasts. This upregulation is particularly higher in malignant CRC lines (HCT116, LoVo, and DLD1). Moreover, a knockdown of FABP5 by siRNA in HTC116 cells significantly suppressed cell proliferation, increased the number of cells in G1/G0 phase of cell cycle and decreased the number of cells passing through the Matrigel-coated membrane (which indirectly measures cell invasiveness). These findings suggest that FABP5 may promote cell proliferation and invasive properties in CRC, what makes it a potential molecular target [58].

Vast involvement of FABPs in cancer metabolism makes them good molecular targets. One proposed approach (US20120289570, US20140363522) [59, 60] utilizes carbazole butanoic (FABP4 inhibitor) and indole (FABP5 inhibitors) derivatives to disrupt the cross-talk between cancer cells and adipocytes in surrounding tissue. This way, the invention is intended to reduce metastasis to omentum, breast and other fatty organs. Although the expression of FABP4 is low in primary ovarian tumors, its significant upregulation is observed in omental metastases. Moreover, coculturing ovarian cancer cells with adipocytes caused FABP4 overexpression in cancer cells as well as in media. In line, authors reported that FABP4 is strongly expressed solely in those cells of omental metastases of ovarian cancer that are in contact with adipocytes, but not in cells distant from the adipocytes or in the corresponding primary ovarian tumor. These findings suggest that FABP4 is a key mediator of cancer-adipocyte metabolic crosstalk and might be targeted to reduce metastases to adipose tissue. The inventors supported their outcomes in several *in vitro* and *in vivo* experiments, nevertheless, the authors base their invention on their studies of ovarian cancer and may too quickly generalize their results to breast, gastric, colon and prostate cancer which are all included in the patent. As demonstrated above, FABPs play cancer-specific roles and can be differently expressed in various types of cancers. At this point, further studies are needed to confirm if FABP4 plays a similar role in both ovarian cancer and CRC, and if it can be targeted by specific inhibitors. Similarly, despite holding great promise as anti-CRC agent, FABP5 inhibitors also require further in-depth studies.

5. NOVEL TECHNOLOGIES IN CANCER THERAPY

Novel anti-cancer agents are designed to target tumor cells specifically and preserve healthy tissues. Consequently, precise drug delivery has become an important issue to consider when developing new pharmaceutics. Among many emerging technologies, liposomes are those of particular importance as they have already proved their efficacy and usefulness in many different medical fields. Liposomes are lipid-based vesicular systems with an aqueous core contained within a double lipid layer. These drug delivery vehicles undergo constant research and improvements in surface modification, size optimization and drug encapsulation. Currently, 13 liposome-based products have been approved by Food and Drug Administration (FDA) for clinical use [61]. Importantly, 5 of them are liposome-delivered chemotherapeutics used in blood, breast, ovarian cancer and Kaposi`s sarcoma [61].

Further research has led to creation of hybrid liposomes (HLs), in which a lipid bilayer consists of more than one lipid, usually L-alpha-dimyristoyl-phosphatidylcholine with add-ons. *In vitro*, in animal models and in clinical settings in patients with lymphoma, HLs exert anti-cancer effects even when not loaded with a chemotherapeutic [62, 63]. Enriching HLs with PUFAs strengthened the inhibition of tumor cell growth even further; the effect was most potent with DHA, which increased peroxidation and further necrosis of the cell [64]. These findings were later confirmed in hepatic metastasis mouse model [65]. Most recently, Calle *et al.* prepared liposomes imbued with superparamegnetic nanoparticles and loaded with n-3 PUFA ethyl esters. In addition to their effective anti-inflammatory action, these liposomes could be visualized and tracked throughout the body [66]. This invention was later claimed in a patent (WO2015107244, WO2015107244) [67, 68].

6. SUPPLEMENTARY TREATMENT

Given the promising effects during *in vivo* studies, it is possible that n-3 PUFA may supplement already-existing protocols for CRC treatment which currently include various combinations of surgery and chemotherapy. So far, a composition of fish oil and fruit juice in the form of oil-in-water emulsion, which strongly induces apoptosis of cells is under evaluation for the treatment of cancer and post-treatment care (US20160067202, WO2014175748) [69, 70]. As suggested by the authors, the fish oil must be low-oxidated and have omega-3 content above 10%. Low oxidation is defined as totox value below 20 (calculated on the basis of peroxide and anisidine value), which corresponds with oil quality, clearness that simultaneously minimizes fishy taste. Juice is used to counteract unpleasant taste of oil and improve patients compliance. The emulsion is stabilized by emulsifiers, e.g. milk solids or proteins. In vitro, this emulsion induced caspase-3 activity in pancreatic ductal adenocarcinoma cells (PDACs), demonstrating pro-apoptotic effect of the mixture. It also moderately decreased the production of interferon γ (IFN-γ) by natural killer cells cocultured with PDAC. Anti-proliferative characteristics of the invention were measured in three different CRC cell lines - Caco-2, HT-29 and HCT-116. In all cell lines, the emulsion reduced proliferation rate, being most effective in HCT-16 cells. A study in mice with neuroblastoma xenografts showed delayed tumor progression after administration of the emulsion. These results make the emulsion a promising dietary supplement for oncological patients, although clinical trials are needed to verify if *in vitro* and animal results translate well into humans. In another way, n-3 PUFAs have also been claimed as part of nutritional support of the immune system during cancer therapy (WO2010033424) [71].

7. ADJUVANT TREATMENT IN CHEMO- OR RADIOTHERAPY

n-3 PUFAs exert a strong effect on cancer cells that depends on the differentiation stage of targeted cells and cannot be explained solely by their anti-inflammatory profile. Carlo *et al.* reported that EPA can sensitize cancer stem like cells to 5-fluorouracil (5-FU) and stimulate their differentiation, as demonstrated by the decrease in expression of CD133 [72]. A similar effect was observed in HT-29 and HCT-116 cells exposed to increasing concentrations of 5-FU and oxaliplatin which created chemoresistant cell lines. In these cells, EPA coupled with oxaliplatin and 5-fluorouracil (chemotherapeutics used widely in CRC) inhibited cell growth, formation of colonospheres and increased the sphere disintegration [73]. A similar synergy of n-3 PUFA and chemotherapeutics was also reported elsewhere [74]. Furthermore, DHA and - to a lesser extent - EPA, also improved the effects of radiotherapy in human CRC cell lines [74]. This proves that n-3 PUFAs may synergize well with standard chemo- and radio-therapy used in CRC and can be used to reduce the risk of CRC recurrence. However, the described studies used highly purified n-3 PUFAs and cannot indicate that marine-derived oils will have similar properties. In fact, Daenen *et al.* revealed that a hexadeca-4,7,10,13-tetraenoic acid (HDTA, 16:4(n-3)), which belongs to PUFA, induces resistance to platinum-based chemotherapeutics in mouse models [75]. A measurable amounts of this acid have been found in various fish and fish oils e.g. herring and mackerel fish. More importantly, when these fish were given to healthy volunteers, HDTA was rapidly taken up in the plasma [75], suggesting that such supplementation may interfere with chemotherapy. These reports do not undermine the promising studies on n-3 PUFA and chemotherapeutics synergy, yet indicate that caution is needed when translating their results into *in vivo* models and clinical trials. Fish oil supplementation, and particularly the intake of HDTA, should probably be avoided during chemotherapy in oncological patients until further data of its biological effects become available.

In line with these findings, several patents recommend to use fish oil or n-3 PUFA specifically in addition to chemo- and radiotherapy. For example, a composition of EPA and DHA can be administered enterally or parenterally to patients with cancer to enhance the effect of chemo- or radiotherapy (US20150297549, EP2425833) [76, 77]. In addition, the composition may also alleviate inflammatory-associated adverse effects of radiation. Similarly, a mixture of at least 3 FAs (selected from palmitic, oleic, stearic, linoleic, α-linolenic, gamma-linolenic, EPA, DHA, azelaic and myristic acid) has been claimed for treating inflammatory pathologies, especially in patients with anal cancer receiving the radiotherapy (US20160015666) [78].

Finally, FAs remain an important component of nutritional treatment. However, the composition of supplements may influence the patient`s nutritional state and the outcome of therapy. A study by van der Meji *et al.* [79] compared the supplements containing n-3 PUFAs with isocaloric control oral nutritional supplement without EPA and DHA but with higher content of monounsaturated fatty acids. They reported that n-3 PUFAs supplementation improved the nutritional status of patients with stage III non-small cell lung cancer during multimodal treatment [79]. Patients benefited in terms of weight maintenance, higher energy and protein intake and lower IL-6 production. Importantly, oil-i--water emulsion enriched with n-3 PUFA for parenteral administration has already been devised (US9034389) [80]. Hopefully, this emulsion will stabilize patients` nutritional and inflammatory state better than mixtures used so far.

8. FORMULATIONS OF PUFAS

Given the ongoing development in the field, PUFAs stand a good chance to become popular preventive, nutritional and adjunct agents in fighting CRC. However, the question that needs answering is in what form should they be administered?

Currently, fish and fish oils are the main sources of many PUFAs, including EPA and DHA. However, as mentioned before, in some cases an additional supplementation with fatty acids may diminish the desired effects of agents, for example HDTA and its chemotherapy- negating action, and thus affect clinical outcomes. It is therefore advised that to achieve high quality of studies and to provide best care for the patients in the future, an upcoming clinical trials should use highly purified fatty acids separately, or in controlled combinations.

Methods for obtaining highly concentrated EPA (purity close to 100% of mass) include fractional and molecular distillation, and chromatography (preferable) (WO2006067498) [81]. The purified form of EPA, when administered for three months (2g/day), significantly reduced crypt cell proliferation and induced apoptosis in patients with history of colorectal polyps (randomized trial, total number of patients 28), when compared with control individuals.

Furthermore, an alternative method has been devised for obtaining n-3 PUFA concentrate (especially EPA), other than fish oil processing, (US20130046020, WO2012109539) [82, 83]. It utilizes recombinant Yarrowia cells to produce EPA-rich microbial oil which is further extracted to produce non-concentrated

EPA. It then undergoes transesterification and enrichment to produce highly concentrated (at least 70% of weight mass) EPA-rich oil. The enrichment procedure can, according to authors, utilize various methods such as fractional distillation, urea adduct formation, short path distillation, supercritical fluid fractionation with counter current column, supercritical fluid chromatography, liquid chromatography, enzymatic separation and treatment with silver salt, simulated moving bed chromatography, and actual moving bed chromatography. This method holds great promise for production of n-3 PUFAs in industrial quantities. However, the microbial oil should be thoroughly tested for presence of unwanted fatty compounds and purification process should be made as efficient as possible.

Since the pharmacokinetics of FAs (absorption rate, distribution in the body, and clearance) depend on the molecule`s structure, different formulations may change bioavailability of n-3 PUFAs and, consequently, enhance their biological action and potential clinical utility. Usually, long chain n-3 PUFAs are administered as ethyl esters (EE) or triglycerides (TAGs). In these forms, their absorption is similar, although some studies suggest that assimilation of natural TAGs is more efficient [84]. The structure of TAG forms can be further modified chemically or enzymatically to acquire structured lipids, in which PUFAs are placed in sn-2 position. Bandarra *et al.* [84] used Golden Syrian male hamsters to compare sn-2 TAG form of DHA with commercially available fish oil rich in DHA, regardless of the sn position of TAG. The structured sn-2 position DHA-containing TAG improved the incorporation of FAs in tissues and exerted more efficient biological action as reflected by the favorable effect on total cholesterol, LDL and total lipids concentrations [84]. The obtained outcomes indicate that the anti-cancer properties of DHA could be enhanced by its administration in the sn-2 TAG form.

Lately, it has been reported that oil enriched with sn-1(3)-monoacylglycerol (MAG) provides a better carrier for n-3 long-chain PUFAs than fish oil containing TAGs [85]. Another available formulation is the free fatty acid (FFA) form, which effectively increases the bioavailability of EPA, compared with its standard EE or TAG form, by improving its absorption in the small intestine [86, 87]. This formulation is also intended for cancer-related therapy (WO2012109539) [83]. These advances may help carry out more uniform and comparable clinical trials necessary to elucidate the role of n-3 PUFAs supplementation in cancer prevention or therapy.

CURRENT & FUTURE DEVELOPMENTS

Colorectal cancer possesses an intricate network of metabolic pathways that distinguish it from healthy mucosa and promote its growth and survival in a hostile environment. Many of the said abnormalities include imbalanced lipid metabolism or signaling, which calls for new drugs targeting FAs processing enzymes or their products. Recent years brought great insight into lipid physiology. The role of FAs, their metabolism and signaling pathways has been uncovered and indicated in CRC development. The key enzymes of this lipid network have already been claimed as potential therapeutic targets or staging markers. However, the current aim is to identify the specific regulators of lipid metabolism and interactions between different pathways as well as the downstream metabolites of FAs that could be modulated by future therapies. The discovery of interconnection between COX-2 and 5-LOX-dependent n-3 PUFA metabolism is the prime example and should be investigated thoroughly.

Meanwhile, currently developed agents face another challenge. Many of them are about to or have already reached clinical trials. At this stage, they will be tested not on identical cloned cell lines nor on homogenous inbred animals - but on genetically, immunologically and environmentally diverse humans. Given the multifactorial pathogenesis of CRC, the following years will show if any of the agents yield impactful clinical results. n-3 PUFAs may become a welcome addition to optimize current radio- and chemotherapy. Moreover, the current treatment might be transformed and enhanced by introducing cancer-targeting vehicles in the form of liposomes. They can be loaded either with classic chemotherapeutics or, possibly, with n-3 PUFAs as free fatty acids.

Finally, as medical focus shifts from therapy to prevention, FAs and especially n-3 PUFAs may play an important role in CRC prevention. However, to this end, we need refined technology that will allow manufacturing and administration of high-purity, concentrated FAs in bioavailable formulations. Whether this will be done by thorough purification of fish oils or microbial oil, remains to be evaluated.

CONFLICT OF INTEREST

The authors declare no conflict of interest, financial or otherwise.

AUTHOR CONTRIBUTIONS

Arkadiusz Michalak, Paula Mosińska & Jakub Fichna provided the overall concept and framework of the chapter.

Arkadiusz Michalak & Paula Mosińska researched and identified appropriate articles, and wrote the chapter.

Paula Mosińska & Jakub Fichna revised the chapter.

All authors approved the final version of the chapter.

ACKNOWLEDGEMENTS

Supported by the Medical University of Lodz (503/1-156-04/503-11-001 to JF and 502-03/1-156-04/502-14-343 to PM) and National Science Center (2016/21/N/NZ5/01932 to PM).

LIST OF ABBREVIATIONS

2-AG	2-Arachidonoylglycerol
5-FU	5-Fluorouracil
A-FABP4/FABP4	Adipocyte Fatty Acid Binding Protein
AA	Arachidonic Acid
AEA	Anandamide
ALA	α-Linolenic Acid
CBR	Cannabinoid Receptor
COX	Cyclooxygenase
CRC	Colorectal Cancer
CYP 450	Cytochrome P-450
DHA	Docosahexaenoic Acid
EE	Ethyl Esters
EPA	Eicosapentaenoic Acid
E-FABP/FABP5	Epidermal Fatty Acid Binding Protein
ESI-MS/MS	Electrospray Ionization Mass Spectrometry Tandem Mass Spectrometry
EVOVLs	Fatty Acid Elongases
FAAH	Fatty Acid Amide Hydrolase
FABP	Fatty Acid Binding Protein
FA	Fatty Acid
FAS	Fatty Acid Synthase
FDA	Food and Drug Administration
FFA	Free Fatty Acids
HETE	Hydroxyeicosatetraenoic Acid
HLS	Hybrid Liposomes
I-FABP/FABP6	Ileal Fatty Acid Binding Protein
L-FABP/FABP1	Liver Fatty Acid Binding Protein
LA	Linoleic Acid
LOX	Lipoxygenase

LPS	Lipoprotein Lipase
LTx	Leukotrienes
LTB4	Leukotriene
LXs	Lipoxines
MAG	Monoacylglycerol
NK	Natural Killer
OEA	Oleoylethanolamide
PDAC	Pancreatic Ductal Adenocarcinoma Cells
PDK-1	Phosphoinositide-Dependent Kinase 1
PEA	Palmitoylethanolamide
PGs	Prostaglandins
PG-EA	Prostaglandin-Ethanolamine
PKB	Protein Kinase B
PPAR-α	Peroxisome Proliferator-Activated Receptor α
PUFA	Polyunsaturated Fatty Acid
RCT	Randomized Control Trials
SLCP	Solid Lipid Curcumin Particle
TGs	Triglicerides
TXs	Thromboxanes

REFERENCES

[1] Ferlay J, Soerjomataram I, Ervik M, Dikshit R, Eser S, Mathers C, *et al.* 2013.http://globocan.iarc.fr/Pages/fact_sheets_population.aspx

[2] Ferlay J, Soerjomataram I, Dikshit R, *et al.* Cancer incidence and mortality worldwide: Sources, methods and major patterns in GLOBOCAN 2012. Int J Cancer 2015; 136(5): E359-86. [http://dx.doi.org/10.1002/ijc.29210] [PMID: 25220842]

[3] Bray F, Ren J-S, Masuyer E, Ferlay J. Global estimates of cancer prevalence for 27 sites in the adult population in 2008. Int J Cancer 2013; 132(5): 1133-45. [http://dx.doi.org/10.1002/ijc.27711] [PMID: 22752881]

[4] Favoriti P, Carbone G, Greco M, Pirozzi F, Pirozzi RE, Corcione F. Worldwide burden of colorectal cancer: a review. Updates Surg 2016; 68(1): 7-11. [http://dx.doi.org/10.1007/s13304-016-0359-y] [PMID: 27067591]

[5] Marley AR, Nan H. Epidemiology of colorectal cancer. Int J Mol Epidemiol Genet 2016; 7(3): 105-14. [PMID: 27766137]

[6] Wang X, Yang Y, Huycke MM. Microbiome-driven carcinogenesis in colorectal cancer: Models and mechanisms. Free Radic Biol Med 2017; 105: 3-15. [http://dx.doi.org/10.1016/j.freeradbiomed.2016.10.504] [PMID: 27810411]

[7] Jurjus A, Eid A, Al Kattar S, *et al.* Inflammatory bowel disease, colorectal cancer and type 2 diabetes mellitus: The links. BBA Clin 2015; 5: 16-24. [http://dx.doi.org/10.1016/j.bbacli.2015.11.002] [PMID: 27051585]

[8] Michalak A, Mosińska P, Fichna J. Common links between metabolic syndrome and inflammatory bowel disease: Current overview and future perspectives. Pharmacol Rep 2016; 68(4): 837-46. [http://dx.doi.org/10.1016/j.pharep.2016.04.016] [PMID: 27238750]

[9] Glaser C, Heinrich J, Koletzko B. Role of FADS1 and FADS2 polymorphisms in polyunsaturated fatty acid metabolism. Metabolism 2010; 59(7): 993-9. [http://dx.doi.org/10.1016/j.metabol.2009.10.022] [PMID: 20045144]

[10] Swinnen JV, Brusselmans K, Verhoeven G. Increased lipogenesis in cancer cells: New players, novel targets. Curr Opin Clin Nutr Metab Care 2006; 9(4): 358-65. [http://dx.doi.org/10.1097/01.mco.0000232894.28674.30] [PMID: 16778563]

[11] Menendez JA, Lupu R. Fatty acid synthase and the lipogenic phenotype in cancer pathogenesis. Nat Rev Cancer 2007; 7(10): 763-77. [http://dx.doi.org/10.1038/nrc2222] [PMID: 17882277]

[12] Swinnen JV, Van Veldhoven PP, Timmermans L, *et al.* Fatty acid synthase drives the synthesis of phospholipids partitioning into detergent-resistant membrane microdomains. Biochem Biophys Res Commun 2003; 302(4): 898-903. [http://dx.doi.org/10.1016/S0006-291X(03)00265-1] [PMID: 12646257]

[13] Zeng L, Biernacka KM, Holly JM, *et al.* Hyperglycaemia confers resistance to chemotherapy on breast cancer cells: The role of fatty acid synthase. Endocr Relat Cancer 2010; 17(2): 539-51. [http://dx.doi.org/10.1677/ERC-09-0221] [PMID: 20356977]

[14] Swinnen J. Phospholipid profiling and cancer. US20130115618, 2013.

[15] Rysman E, Brusselmans K, Scheys K, *et al. De novo* lipogenesis protects cancer cells from free radicals and chemotherapeutics by promoting membrane lipid saturation. Cancer Res 2010; 70(20): 8117-26. [http://dx.doi.org/10.1158/0008-5472.CAN-09-3871] [PMID: 20876798]

[16] Jakobsson A, Westerberg R, Jacobsson A. Fatty acid elongases in mammals: Their regulation and roles in metabolism. Prog Lipid Res 2006; 45(3): 237-49. [http://dx.doi.org/10.1016/j.plipres.2006.01.004] [PMID: 16564093]

[17] Johannes S, Bagadi MR, Machiels J, Berkers J, Rinkon NR, Dehairs J, *et al.* Fatty acid elongation enzymes as targets for cancer diagnostics and therapeutics. WO2013144325, 2013.

[18] Park J-M, Kwon S-H, Han Y-M, Hahm K-B, Kim E-H. Omega-3 polyunsaturated fatty acids as potential chemopreventive agent for gastrointestinal cancer. J Cancer Prev 2013; 18(3): 201-8. [http://dx.doi.org/10.15430/JCP.2013.18.3.201] [PMID: 25337547]

[19] Michalak A, Mosińska P, Fichna J. Polyunsaturated fatty acids and their derivatives: Therapeutic value for inflammatory, functional gastrointestinal disorders, and colorectal cancer. Front Pharmacol 2016; 7: 459. [http://dx.doi.org/10.3389/fphar.2016.00459] [PMID: 27990120]

[20] Bordeleau L, Yakubovich N, Dagenais GR, *et al.* The association of basal insulin glargine and/or n-3 fatty acids with incident cancers in patients with dysglycemia. Diabetes Care 2014; 37(5): 1360-6. [http://dx.doi.org/10.2337/dc13-1468] [PMID: 24574355]

[21] Shen X-J, Zhou J-D, Dong J-Y, Ding W-Q, Wu J-C. Dietary intake of n-3 fatty acids and colorectal cancer risk: A meta-analysis of data from 489 000 individuals. Br J Nutr 2012; 108(9): 1550-6. [http://dx.doi.org/10.1017/S0007114512003546] [PMID: 22906228]

[22] Gupta SC, Patchva S, Aggarwal BB. Therapeutic roles of curcumin: Lessons learned from clinical trials. AAPS J 2013; 15(1): 195-218. [http://dx.doi.org/10.1208/s12248-012-9432-8] [PMID: 23143785]

[23] Garcea G, Berry DP, Jones DJ, *et al.* Consumption of the putative chemopreventive agent curcumin by cancer patients: Assessment of curcumin levels in the colorectum and their pharmacodynamic

consequences. Cancer Epidemiol Biomarkers Prev 2005; 14(1): 120-5. [PMID: 15668484]

[24] Nahar PP, Slitt AL, Seeram NP. Anti-inflammatory effects of novel standardized solid lipid curcumin formulations. J Med Food 2015; 18(7): 786-92. [http://dx.doi.org/10.1089/jmf.2014.0053] [PMID: 25490740]

[25] Halder RC, Almasi A, Sagong B, Leung J, Jewett A, Fiala M. Curcuminoids and ω-3 fatty acids with anti-oxidants potentiate cytotoxicity of natural killer cells against pancreatic ductal adenocarcinoma cells and inhibit interferon γ production. Front Physiol 2015; 6: 129. [http://dx.doi.org/10.3389/fphys.2015.00129] [PMID: 26052286]

[26] Munoz G, Morse M. Pharmaceutical product, medical food or dietary supplement for preventing cancer and inflammatory diseases. WO2016046347, 2016.

[27] Diaz P, Munoz Fernandez G, Morse G. Pharmaceutical product, medical food or dietary supplement for preventing cancer and inflammatory diseases. WO2016046347, 2015.

[28] Diaz P, Carlos M, Munoz Fernandez G, Morse M. Pharmaceutical product, medical food or dietary supplement for preventing cancer and inflammatory diseases. US20160106696, 2016.

[29] Singh Ranger G. The role of aspirin in colorectal cancer chemoprevention. Crit Rev Oncol Hematol 2016; 104: 87-90. [http://dx.doi.org/10.1016/j.critrevonc.2016.05.011] [PMID: 27289249]

[30] Schiffmann S, Maier TJ, Wobst I, *et al.* The anti-proliferative potency of celecoxib is not a class effect of coxibs. Biochem Pharmacol 2008; 76(2): 179-87. [http://dx.doi.org/10.1016/j.bcp.2008.04.017] [PMID: 18547544]

[31] Guillem-Llobat P, Dovizio M, Bruno A, *et al.* Aspirin prevents colorectal cancer metastasis in mice by splitting the crosstalk between platelets and tumor cells. Oncotarget 2016; 7(22): 32462-77. [http://dx.doi.org/10.18632/oncotarget.8655] [PMID: 27074574]

[32] Grösch S, Maier TJ, Schiffmann S, Geisslinger G. Cyclooxygenase-2 (COX-2)-independent anticarcinogenic effects of selective COX-2 inhibitors. J Natl Cancer Inst 2006; 98(11): 736-47. [http://dx.doi.org/10.1093/jnci/djj206] [PMID: 16757698]

[33] Coulter I, McDonald BF, Aversa V. Celecoxib formulations useful for treating colorectal cancer. WO2015176780, 2015.

[34] Atari-Hajipirloo S, Nikanfar S, Heydari A, Noori F, Kheradmand F. The effect of celecoxib and its combination with imatinib on human HT-29 colorectal cancer cells: Involvement of COX-2, Caspase-3, VEGF and NF-κB genes expression. Cell Mol Biol 2016; 62(2): 68-74. [PMID: 26950454]

[35] Lu Y, Shi C, Qiu S, Fan Z. Identification and validation of COX-2 as a co-target for overcoming cetuximab resistance in colorectal cancer cells. Oncotarget 2016; 7(40): 64766-77. [PMID: 27074568]

[36] Tuncer S, Banerjee S. Eicosanoid pathway in colorectal cancer: Recent updates. World J Gastroenterol 2015; 21(41): 11748-66. [http://dx.doi.org/10.3748/wjg.v21.i41.11748] [PMID: 26557000]

[37] Sarveswaran S, Chakraborty D, Chitale D, Sears R, Ghosh J. Inhibition of 5-lipoxygenase selectively triggers disruption of c-Myc signaling in prostate cancer cells. J Biol Chem 2015; 290(8): 4994-5006. [http://dx.doi.org/10.1074/jbc.M114.599035] [PMID: 25540201]

[38] Zhou G-X, Ding X-L, Wu S-B, *et al.* Inhibition of 5-lipoxygenase triggers apoptosis in pancreatic cancer cells. Oncol Rep 2015; 33(2): 661-8. [http://dx.doi.org/10.3892/or.2014.3650] [PMID: 25483364]

[39] Meng Z, Cao R, Yang Z, Liu T, Wang Y, Wang X. Inhibitor of 5-lipoxygenase, zileuton, suppresses prostate cancer metastasis by upregulating E-cadherin and paxillin. Urology 2013; 82(6): 1452.e7-

1452.e14.
[http://dx.doi.org/10.1016/j.urology.2013.08.060] [PMID: 24295266]

[40] Collin P, Yang P, Newman R. Method to inhibit lipoxygenase and cancer cell proliferation. WO2001076588, 2001.

[41] Che X-H, Chen C-L, Ye X-L, *et al.* Dual inhibition of COX-2/5-LOX blocks colon cancer proliferation, migration and invasion *in vitro.* Oncol Rep 2016; 35(3): 1680-8.
[http://dx.doi.org/10.3892/or.2015.4506] [PMID: 26707712]

[42] Ghatak S, Vyas A, Misra S, *et al.* Novel di-tertiary-butyl phenylhydrazones as dual cyclooxygenase-2/5-lipoxygenase inhibitors: Synthesis, COX/LOX inhibition, molecular modeling, and insights into their cytotoxicities. Bioorg Med Chem Lett 2014; 24(1): 317-24.
[http://dx.doi.org/10.1016/j.bmcl.2013.11.015] [PMID: 24295787]

[43] Patsos HA, Hicks DJ, Dobson RR, *et al.* The endogenous cannabinoid, anandamide, induces cell death in colorectal carcinoma cells: A possible role for cyclooxygenase 2. Gut 2005; 54(12): 1741-50.
[http://dx.doi.org/10.1136/gut.2005.073403] [PMID: 16099783]

[44] Van Dross RT, Ladin DA, Burns CS, Danell AS. J-series prostaglandin-ethanolamides as novel therapeutics. US9328060, 2016.

[45] Kuo YH, Tang FY, Lin HY. Inhibition of cancer cell proliferation using oleoylethanolamide. US20130172407, 2013.

[46] Santos CR, Schulze A. Lipid metabolism in cancer. FEBS J 2012; 279(15): 2610-23.
[http://dx.doi.org/10.1111/j.1742-4658.2012.08644.x] [PMID: 22621751]

[47] Kuemmerle NB, Rysman E, Lombardo PS, *et al.* Lipoprotein lipase links dietary fat to solid tumor cell proliferation. Mol Cancer Ther 2011; 10(3): 427-36.
[http://dx.doi.org/10.1158/1535-7163.MCT-10-0802] [PMID: 21282354]

[48] Lupu R, Menendez JA. Pharmacological inhibitors of Fatty Acid Synthase (FASN)-catalyzed endogenous fatty acid biogenesis: A new family of anti-cancer agents? Curr Pharm Biotechnol 2006; 7(6): 483-93.
[http://dx.doi.org/10.2174/138920106779116928] [PMID: 17168663]

[49] Kothamasu SS, Sah A, Asapu US, Arumalla MR. Orlistat pharmaceutical formulations. WO2009039157, 2009.

[50] Pallasch CP, Schwamb J, Königs S, *et al.* Targeting lipid metabolism by the lipoprotein lipase inhibitor orlistat results in apoptosis of B-cell chronic lymphocytic leukemia cells. Leukemia 2008; 22(3): 585-92.
[http://dx.doi.org/10.1038/sj.leu.2405058] [PMID: 18079738]

[51] Smathers RL, Petersen DR. The human fatty acid-binding protein family: Evolutionary divergences and functions. Hum Genomics 2011; 5(3): 170-91.
[http://dx.doi.org/10.1186/1479-7364-5-3-170] [PMID: 21504868]

[52] Wang G, Bonkovsky HL, de Lemos A, Burczynski FJ. Recent insights into the biological functions of liver fatty acid binding protein 1. J Lipid Res 2015; 56(12): 2238-47.
[http://dx.doi.org/10.1194/jlr.R056705] [PMID: 26443794]

[53] Lawrie LC, Dundas SR, Curran S, Murray GI. Liver fatty acid binding protein expression in colorectal neoplasia. Br J Cancer 2004; 90(10): 1955-60.
[http://dx.doi.org/10.1038/sj.bjc.6601828] [PMID: 15138477]

[54] Dharmarajan S, Newberry EP, Montenegro G, *et al.* Liver fatty acid-binding protein (L-FABP) modifies intestinal fatty acid composition and adenoma formation in ApcMin/+ mice. Cancer Prev Res (Phila) 2013; 6(10): 1026-37.
[http://dx.doi.org/10.1158/1940-6207.CAPR-13-0120] [PMID: 23921281]

[55] Yamazaki T, Kanda T, Sakai Y, Hatakeyama K. Liver fatty acid-binding protein is a new prognostic

factor for hepatic resection of colorectal cancer metastases. J Surg Oncol 1999; 72(2): 83-7. [http://dx.doi.org/10.1002/(SICI)1096-9098(199910)72:2<83::AID-JSO8>3.0.CO;2-C] [PMID: 10518104]

[56] Shen X, Yue M, Meng F, Zhu J, Zhu X, Jiang Y. Microarray analysis of differentially-expressed genes and linker genes associated with the molecular mechanism of colorectal cancer. Oncol Lett 2016; 12(5): 3250-8. [PMID: 27899990]

[57] Ohmachi T, Inoue H, Mimori K, *et al.* Fatty acid binding protein 6 is overexpressed in colorectal cancer. Clin Cancer Res 2006; 12(17): 5090-5. [http://dx.doi.org/10.1158/1078-0432.CCR-05-2045] [PMID: 16951225]

[58] Kawaguchi K, Senga S, Kubota C, Kawamura Y, Ke Y, Fujii H. High expression of fatty acid-binding protein 5 promotes cell growth and metastatic potential of colorectal cancer cells. FEBS Open Bio 2016; 6(3): 190-9. [http://dx.doi.org/10.1002/2211-5463.12031] [PMID: 27047747]

[59] Lengyel E, Nieman K, Kenny H. Compositions and methods for treating and/or preventing cancer by inhibiting fatty acid binding proteins. US20120289570, 2012.

[60] Lengyel E, Nieman K, Kenny H. Compositions and methods for treating and/or preventing cancer by inhibiting fatty acid binding proteins. US20140363522, 2014.

[61] Madni A, Sarfraz M, Rehman M, *et al.* Liposomal drug delivery: A versatile platform for challenging clinical applications. J Pharm Pharm Sci 2014; 17(3): 401-26. [http://dx.doi.org/10.18433/J3CP55] [PMID: 25224351]

[62] Ichihara H, Nagami H, Yamamoto K, Matsumoto Y, Ueoka R. Chemotherapy with hybrid liposomes without any drug *in vivo.*. Yakugaku Zasshi 2003; 123(1): 25-34. [http://dx.doi.org/10.1248/yakushi.123.25] [PMID: 12607942]

[63] Ueoka R, Matsumoto Y, Goto K, Ichihara H, Komizu Y. Membrane targeted chemotherapy with hybrid liposomes for tumor cells leading to apoptosis. Curr Pharm Des 2011; 17(17): 1709-19. [http://dx.doi.org/10.2174/138161211796355128] [PMID: 21619525]

[64] Tanaka Y, Goto K, Matsumoto Y, Ueoka R. Remarkably high inhibitory effects of docosahexaenoic acid incorporated into hybrid liposomes on the growth of tumor cells along with apoptosis. Int J Pharm 2008; 359(1-2): 264-71. [http://dx.doi.org/10.1016/j.ijpharm.2008.03.045] [PMID: 18511224]

[65] Ichihara H, Hino M, Ueoka R, Matsumoto Y. Therapeutic effects of cationic hybrid liposomes on the hepatic metastasis of colon carcinoma along with apoptosis *in vivo.* Biol Pharm Bull 2014; 37(3): 498-503. [http://dx.doi.org/10.1248/bpb.b13-00764] [PMID: 24583871]

[66] Calle D, Negri V, Ballesteros P, Cerdán S. Magnetoliposomes loaded with poly-unsaturated fatty acids as novel theranostic anti-inflammatory formulations. Theranostics 2015; 5(5): 489-503. [http://dx.doi.org/10.7150/thno.10069] [PMID: 25767616]

[67] Moreno Egea F, Cerdan Garcia Esteller S, Calle Hernandez D. Compositions containing liposomes, long-chain omega-3 polyunsaturated fatty acids and superparamagnetic nanoparticles, and the use thereof in the treatment of malignant tumours. WO2015107244, 2015.

[68] Moreno Egea F, Cerdan Garcia Esteller S, Calle Hernandez D. Composiciones que contienen liposomas, ácidos grasos poliinsaturados omega-3 de cadena larga y nanopartículas superparamagnéticas y su uso en el tratamiento de tumores malignos. WO2015107244, 2015.

[69] Mathisen JS. Use of a composition comprising fish oil and juice for the treatment and/or post treatment of cancer. US20160067202, 2016.

[70] Mathisen JS. Use of a composition comprising fish oil and juice for the treatment and/or post treatment of cancer. WO2014175748, 2014.

[71] Schiffrin E. Nutritional support of the immune system during anti-cancer treatment. WO2010033424, 2010.

[72] De Carlo F, Witte TR, Hardman WE, Claudio PP. Omega-3 eicosapentaenoic acid decreases CD133 colon cancer stem-like cell marker expression while increasing sensitivity to chemotherapy. PLoS One 2013; 8(7): e69760.
[http://dx.doi.org/10.1371/journal.pone.0069760] [PMID: 23874993]

[73] Vasudevan A, Yu Y, Banerjee S, *et al.* Omega-3 fatty acid is a potential preventive agent for recurrent colon cancer. Cancer Prev Res (Phila) 2014; 7(11): 1138-48.
[http://dx.doi.org/10.1158/1940-6207.CAPR-14-0177] [PMID: 25193342]

[74] Cai F, Sorg O, Granci V, *et al.* Interaction of ω-3 polyunsaturated fatty acids with radiation therapy in two different colorectal cancer cell lines. Clin Nutr 2014; 33(1): 164-70.
[http://dx.doi.org/10.1016/j.clnu.2013.04.005] [PMID: 23672803]

[75] Daenen LG, Cirkel GA, Houthuijzen JM, *et al.* Increased plasma levels of chemoresistance-inducing fatty acid 16:4(n-3) after consumption of fish and fish oil. JAMA Oncol 2015; 1(3): 350-8.
[http://dx.doi.org/10.1001/jamaoncol.2015.0388] [PMID: 26181186]

[76] Schlotzer W, Krampitz B, Suchner U. Composition comprising a combination of DHA and EPA for administration prior to commencement of chemotherapy. US20150297549, 2015.

[77] Schlotzer W, Krampitz B, Suchner U. Application intraveineuse d'huile de poisson/DHA + EPA avant ou au début de la chimiothérapie. EP2425833, 2012.

[78] Burattin L. Mixture of fatty acids for use in the treatment of inflammatory pathologies. US20160015666, 2016.

[79] van der Meij BS, Langius JA, Smit EF, *et al.* Oral nutritional supplements containing (n-3) polyunsaturated fatty acids affect the nutritional status of patients with stage III non-small cell lung cancer during multimodality treatment. J Nutr 2010; 140(10): 1774-80.
[http://dx.doi.org/10.3945/jn.110.121202] [PMID: 20739445]

[80] Driscoll DF. Omega-3 enriched fish oil-in-water parenteral nutrition emulsions. US9034389, 2015.

[81] Courtney EDJ, Leicester R, Bennett A. Eicosapentaenoic acid for the treatment of cancer. WO2006067498, 2006.

[82] Liang SC, Orlandi RD. Eicosapentaenoic acid concentrate. US20130046020, 2013.

[83] Liang SC, Orlandi RD. An eicosapentaenoic acid concentrate. WO2012109539, 2015.

[84] Bandarra NM, Lopes PA, Martins SV, *et al.* Docosahexaenoic acid at the sn-2 position of structured triacylglycerols improved n-3 polyunsaturated fatty acid assimilation in tissues of hamsters. Nutr Res 2016; 36(5): 452-63.
[http://dx.doi.org/10.1016/j.nutres.2015.12.015] [PMID: 27101763]

[85] Cruz-Hernandez C, Destaillats F, Thakkar SK, *et al.* Monoacylglycerol-enriched oil increases EPA/DHA delivery to circulatory system in humans with induced lipid malabsorption conditions. J Lipid Res 2016; 57(12): 2208-16.
[http://dx.doi.org/10.1194/jlr.P070144] [PMID: 27707818]

[86] Lawson LD, Hughes BG. Human absorption of fish oil fatty acids as triacylglycerols, free acids, or ethyl esters. Biochem Biophys Res Commun 1988; 152(1): 328-35.
[http://dx.doi.org/10.1016/S0006-291X(88)80718-6] [PMID: 3358766]

[87] Davidson MH, Johnson J, Rooney MW, Kyle ML, Kling DF. A novel omega-3 free fatty acid formulation has dramatically improved bioavailability during a low-fat diet compared with omega-3-acid ethyl esters: The ECLIPSE (Epanova(®) compared to Lovaza(®) in a pharmacokinetic single-dose evaluation) study. J Clin Lipidol 2012; 6(6): 573-84.
[http://dx.doi.org/10.1016/j.jacl.2012.01.002] [PMID: 23312053]

CHAPTER 2

Microtubules as Anti-Cancer Drug Targets

Biswa P. Chatterji*, **Needa N. Bagban** and **Riddhi I. Bhavsar**

Department of Biotechnology, St. Xavier's College (Autonomous), Mumbai- 400001, India

Abstract: In developmental biology, all cellular events are suitably synchronized to ensure proper growth and development of any multicellular organism. A healthy adult tissue is often characterized by stem cells that can undergo orchestrated cell division and differentiation. Disruption of these events often leads to cancer resulting from the accretion or accumulation of the genetic and epigenetic changes that occur at the somatic as well as the germ line levels. In the recent years, significant progress has been made in the early detection, treatment and prevention of cancer. Targeted cancer therapies include the use of apoptosis inducing drugs and drugs that target microtubules among others. Over the past few years, drugs that inhibit microtubule dynamics have been successfully used as anticancer drugs. They can either be microtubule stabilizers (Vincristine, Vinblastine, Colchicine etc.) or microtubule destabilizers (Paclitaxel, Docetaxel, Epithilones, Taccalonolides etc.). Recently, new classes of compounds have been identified that interfere with cell growth and proliferation as a consequence of binding to tubulin αβ- dimers. Natural compounds like Curcumin have shown to inhibit tubulin activity. Whereas some antimitotic agents like Aurora A/B, Pentoxifylline, benzimidazole derivatives, combrestatin, polymeric nanoparticles etc. have been reported to show significant effect in the treating several types of cancer which were previously deemed untreatable. The following chapter acknowledges the presence of these anti-tumor compounds and how they target microtubules and further aid in the treatment of various cancers afflicting human beings.

Keywords: Antimitotic agents, Aurora A, Apoptosis, Cancer, Combretastatin analogs, Colchicine, Curcumin, Docetaxel, Epothilones, Microtubules, Microtubule polymerizers, Microtubule depolymerizers, Paclitaxel, Pentoxifylline, Taccalonolides, Taxanes, Tubulin, Vinca alkaloids, Vinblastine, Indexing words: Microtubules, Anti-cancer drug targets, Microtubule stabilizers, Taxanes, Epothilones, Taccalonolides, Microtubule destabilizers, Vinca alkaloids, Colchicine, Halichondrin B, Dolostatin 10, Aurora A, Curcumin, Pentoxifylline, Combretastatin, Benzimidazole derivatives, Casein K2 peptide inhibitor, Nanoparticles.

* **Corresponding author Biswa P. Chatterji**: Department of Biotechnology, St. Xavier's College (Autonomous), Mumbai- 400001, India; Tel: +91-9920010371; E-mail: biswaprasun@gmail.com

Atta-ur-Rahman and Khurshid Zaman (Eds.)

1. INTRODUCTION

1.1. Cancer

Cancer is the second leading cause of death in the world with the first position being conferred to cardiovascular diseases. The word cancer finds its origin from the Greek word *Karkinos* which was the term used by the Greek physician, Hippocrates (460-370 B.C) to describe carcinoma tumours. Within the developing embryo, events such as stem cell divisions, their fate determination, proliferation of cells and their migration followed by apoptosis need to be orchestrated. In an adult, the constant turnover of cells as well as their optimal functioning is ensured by the division and differentiation of the stem cells that are present in small numbers in the healthy tissues [1]. Cancer is thought to be the disruption of this critical organisation resulting from the accretion or accumulation of the genetic and epigenetic changes that occur at the somatic as well as the germ line levels [2]. This causes uncontrolled proliferation of normal cells and subsequently leads to the formation of cancerous cells which proceed to grow, proliferate and re-divide giving rise to abnormal cells instead of undergoing apoptosis. These cells have several features in common with stem cells. The observation of these similarities led to the advent of two alternative hypotheses, one stating that the stem cells might themselves be the targets of the mutations that transform them while the other suggesting that the dedifferentiation of those cells that are transformed and terminally differentiated gives rise to cancer stem cells (CSCs), thereby manifesting the disease [3] Cells of different types of cancer migrate via the blood circulation or lymph vessels to the other regions of the body and begin to grow in that target region. This phenomenon is termed as "metastasis". These cells are incapable of DNA repair and hence can be considered malignant (cancerous). However, some tumors do not possess the capacity to grow and migrate to the other parts of the body and are, therefore, categorized as benign (non-cancerous) [4].

Cancer is a multistage disease however; work carried out on cancer recognizes a link between chronic inflammation and cancer with Virchow (1863) hypothesising that cancer originates at the sites of chronic inflammation [4]. More advanced studies on cancer suggest that the inflammatory cells are actually involved in the promotion of cancer progression [5]. Most of the malignancies have been observed to be initiated by chronic inflammation or tissue injury, which can be associated to known parasitic, viral or bacterial infections [6].

Worldwide estimates about 15% of the malignancies (1.2 million/year) attributed to chronic infections instances of which include liver cancer caused due to Hepatitis B and C infection, cervical cancer caused due to human papilloma virus and gastric cancer resulting from *Helicobacter pylori (H. pylori)* infection. Individuals susceptible to an increased risk of cancer exhibit increased polymorphisms in the genes encoding pro-inflammatory cytokines. Population-based studies have established that when tissues are chronically inflamed, the susceptibility to cancer increases and also the risk of many cancers reduces significantly as a consequence of long- term use of NSAIDs, thereby demonstrating the vital role of inflammation in the pathogenesis of cancer [7].

1.2. Hallmarks of Cancer

Advances in cancer research has gained new insights and it is thought to be a disease that involves dynamic changes in the genome; the basis of which has been built on the discovery of mutations that lead to the production of oncogenes and tumour suppressor genes. ***Oncogenes*** are the genes which have gained dominance over the function. They drive the normal cells towards unrestrained growth and develop into cancer cells. Proto-oncogenes are the normal genes of the cell that regulate the frequency of cell division as well as the extent of its differentiation. Oncogenes arise when mutations occur in the proto-oncogenes. ***Tumor suppressor genes*** are the normal genes that are involved in regulating cell division, DNA repair and signalling of apoptosis. Tumor suppressor genes experience recessive loss of function. Any dysfunction in a tumor suppressor gene results in an uncontrollable growth of cells thereby causing cancer [8].

Cancer cells possess impaired regulatory circuits that are responsible for normal cell proliferation and maintenance of homeostasis. More than 100 distinct types of cancer exist with many subtypes of tumors being found within specific organs. The vast catalog of cancer genotypes is thought to be manifested due to six of the crucial alterations in the physiology of cells which eventually lead to a malignant growth. The six alterations seen are as follows:

1. Loss of sensitivity to growth-inhibitory signals: Tissue homeostasis is maintained when cells respond to anti-proliferative signals during G1 phase. However cancerous cells become insensitive to such signals due to the disruption of retinoblastoma proteins which helps in filtering anti proliferative signals.
2. Evasion from apoptosis: Cancerous cells grow in number not only because they become proliferative but also because they tend to evade cell death mechanisms.
3. Self- sufficiency in growth signals: Once a normal cell gets transformed into a cancerous cell, their dependency on exogenous stimulatory growth factor is scaled down. This is due to the fact that the oncogenes tend to mimic the growth signals in one form or the other.

4. Incessant replication: The above 3 characteristics allow cancerous cells to become insensitive to external cell to cell signalling. Maintaining telomere during replication is one of the reasons for extensive replication in cancerous cells.
5. Sustained angiogenesis: Tumor cells tend to alter gene transcription which eventually disrupts the balance between angiogenesis inducers and countervailing inhibitors.
6. Metastasis and tissue invasion: This is a state wherein the tumor cells tend to invade adjacent tissue or migrate over a new terrain in the body. This is achieved by cell adhesion molecules.

Each of the above mentioned physiologic alterations are the novel capabilities that a tumor acquires during their development and epitomizes the successful breaching of the anti- cancer defense mechanism that is in-built into the cells and tissues [8].

2. METHODS TO TREAT CANCER

Previous work on cancer has identified chemicals (carcinogens), viruses, inheritance of damaged DNA from ancestors and radiation as the causative agents of cancer. Therefore various treatments and therapies have been developed in the past few years to circumvent cancer. Following are the treatments currently used against cancer.

2.1. Chemotherapy

Over the last few years, novel methods for the treatment of cancer involving the combination of surgery with chemotherapy and radiation have been developed. Further studies identified nitrogen mustard as an effective agent against rapidly proliferating cancerous lymphoma cells. Many types of cancers have been successfully treated by the use of chemotherapeutic drugs. Currently, many novel approaches are being tested so as to reduce the side effects of chemotherapy. These approaches include:

(a) Use of novel combinations of drugs.

(b) Specific targeting of cancer cells by the use of monoclonal antibody and liposomal therapy.

(c) Use of chemo protective agents.

(d) Use of agents possessing the capacity to overcome multidrug resistance.

(e) Hematopoietic stem cell transplantation [9].

2.2. Hormonal Therapy

In 1878, Thomas Beatson observed that the ability of rabbits to produce milk was lost following the removal of the ovaries. Later, investigations identified that removal of the testes resulted in significant regression of metastatic prostate cancer. Currently, novel categories of drugs such as aromatase inhibitors are being considered for the treatment of breast and prostate cancers. Understanding the mechanism by which hormones impact cancer growth has greatly aided in reducing the risk of breast and prostate cancers [9].

2.3. Radiation Therapy

Initially, radiation was used to diagnose as well as treat cancer. Presently, a wide range of radiation therapies are being used for the treatment of cancer. These include:-

1. **Stereotactic surgery and stereotactic therapy-** This involves the use of a gamma knife to treat brain tumor.
2. **Conformal proton beam therapy-** This involves the use of a proton beam instead of X-rays for targeting tumor cells.
3. **Intra-operative radiation therapy-** This involves the surgical removal of the cancer followed by radiation therapy to the adjacent tissues [9].

2.4. Adjuvant Therapy

Adjuvant therapy involves the usage of chemotherapy following the surgical removal of cancer so as to destroy the few remnant cancer cells in the body. Adjuvant therapy has been employed for the treatment of testis and colon cancer [9].

2.5. Immunotherapy

Several biological agents possess the ability to mimic a few of the natural signals used by the body to regulate tumor growth. Use of such biological agent forms the basis of immunotherapy. These natural biological agents which include interleukins, endogenous angioinhibitors, antigens, cytokines and interferons have been successfully produced in the laboratory. In the 1990's, therapeutic monoclonal antibodies- trastuzumab and rituximab were produced so as to specifically target lymphoma and breast cancer cells. The present focus is on the development of vaccines that are capable of boosting the body's immune response against cancer cells [9].

2.6. Targeted Cancer Treatments

The hallmarks of cancer (mentioned earlier) can alternatively be used as drug targets to overcome cancer in the following manner:

2.6.1. Growth Signal Inhibitors

Growth factors are responsible for signalling the cells to grow and divide. Earlier, the role of growth factors was recognized in tissue repair and fetal growth. Later investigations showed that any abnormality in the levels of growth factors and their signalling contributed to the growth of cancer cells. Current targeted therapies used to block the signalling of growth factors involve the use of imatinib, cetuximab, gefitinib and trastuzumab [9].

2.6.2. Apoptosis Inducing Drugs

Apoptosis refers to the natural process of progammed cell death in which the cellular DNA gets damaged. Apoptosis inducing drugs, therefore, result in the death of cancer cells without allowing the damaged DNA to be repaired.

2.6.3. Endogenous Angioinhibitors

Angiogenesis refers to the process of the formation of new blood vessels from the existing ones. Generally, the process of angiogenesis aids the body in healing wounds and repairing the damaged tissues, however, during the event of cancer, angiogenesis aids in the growth of cancer by supporting the formation of new blood vessels that supply the tumor with blood and its own nutrients. Angioinhibition refers to a form of targeted therapy that makes use of drugs with the ability to inhibit the formation of new blood vessels by tumors. In the year 2004, bevacizumab became the first angioinhibitor to be approved for clinical use. Presently, for the treatment of cancer, there are about 25 endogenous angioinhibitors under clinical trials and a large number under preclinical studies. Angioinhibitors have been categorised into two classes namely:

a. Small molecules or antibodies that target VEGF, bFGF or PDGF, which are the pro-angiogenic factors of tumor cells.
b. Endogenous angioinhibitors, for example, angiostatin, arresten, tumstatin, endostatin, interferons and thrombopondin- 1 that target the vascular endothelial cells and inhibit angiogenesis [9].

3. MICROTUBULES AS DRUG TARGETS

Microtubules are dynamic structures that are essential for a wide range of cellular processes. The cytoskeleton of a cell is composed of microtubules in addition to actin microfilaments and intermediate filaments. Intracellular trafficking of vesicles and organelles, mitotic chromosome segregation and cellular motility; all require the microtubules in a highly organized arrangement [10].

The formation of microtubules takes place by the association of α and β-tubulin heterodimers that are folded and unfolded as a heterodimer complex by chaperones [10]. These heterodimers assemble in a head-to-tail fashion to form linear protofilament that undergoes further polymerisation to form the characteristic hollow cylindrical structure of the microtubule with an internal diameter of 12nm and an external diameter of 25nm (Fig. **1A-1C**) [11]. The 3D structure of alpha-beta tubulin is illustrated in Fig. (**1D**).

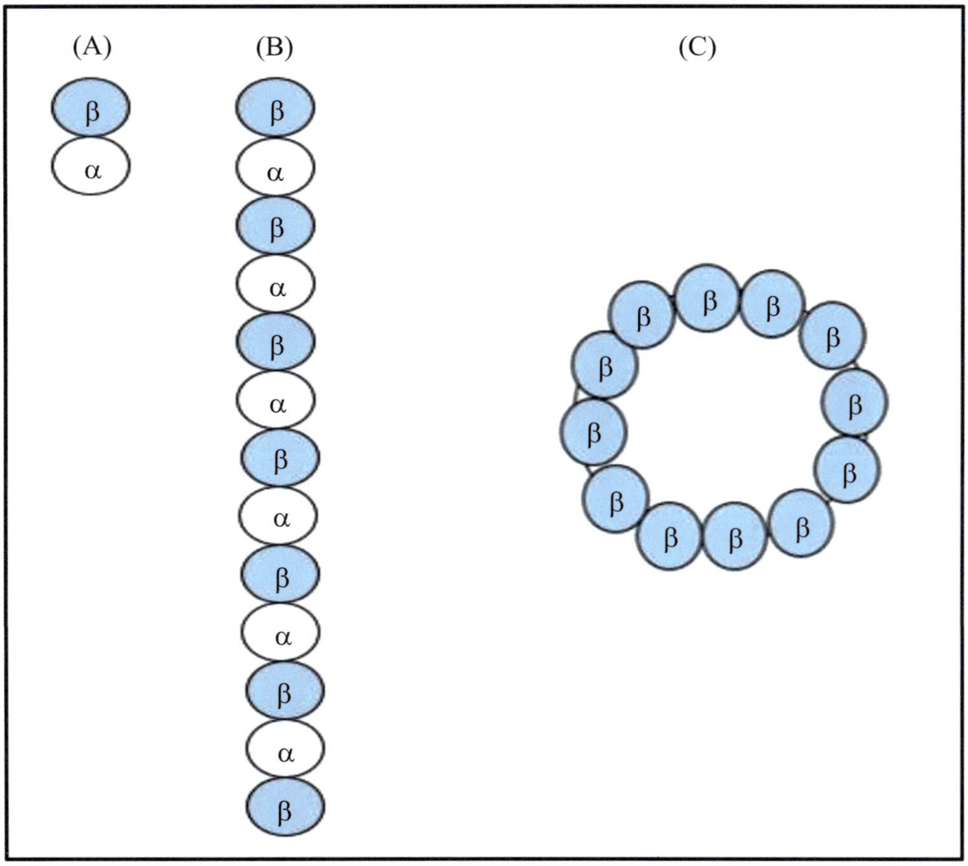

Fig. (1A-C). A). Tubulin protofilament is made up of α- and β- subunits that polymerize in a head- to tail fashion to form protofilaments. **(B & C)**. Thirteen such protofilaments come together to form the hollow cylindrical structure of the microtubule.

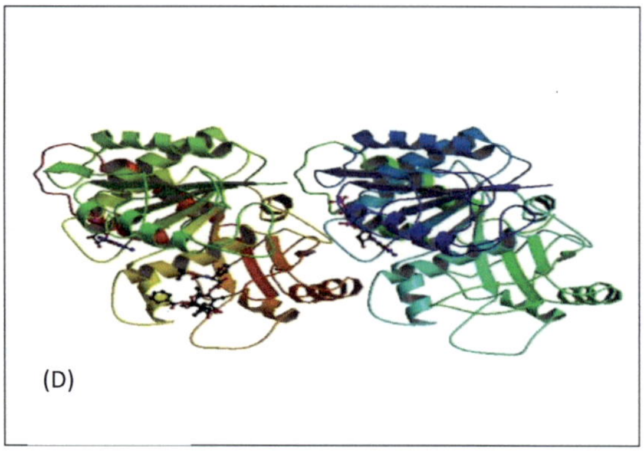

Fig. (1D). 3D structure of alpha-beta tubulin dimer obtained from PDB with DOI 10.2210/pdb1tub/pdb (http://www.rcsb.org/pdb/explore.do?structureId=1TUB last accessed on 07/07/2017).

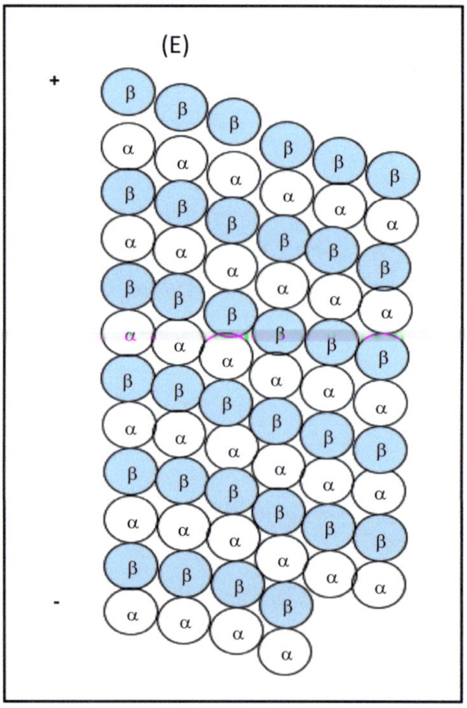

Fig. (1E). The structure of microtubule with α-tubulin exposed at the minus end (-) of microtubule and β-tubulin exposed at the plus (+) end of the microtubule.The α- tubulin subunit of the microtubule is exposed at one end (minus end) while the β-tubulin subunit is exposed at the other end (plus end), thus organising the final structure of the microtubule in a polar manner (**1E**). The microtubule polymer is highly stable at the dynamic plus end as dictated by the binding of GTP and hydrolysis on β-tubulin. Tubulin possesses two sites for the binding of GTP, a non-hydrolysable site on the α- subunit and a hydrolysable site on the β-subunit. For assembly into microtubules, the β-tubulin subunit should be bound to GTP at the hydrolysable site after which the GTP undergoes irreversible hydrolysis to form GDP. Consequently, the microtubule fiber has majority of the β-tubulin in the GDP-bound form and also "capped" with GTP-bound β-tubulin at the plus end.

When the GTP on a β-tubulin molecule undergoes hydrolysis into GDP prior to the addition of another GTP-bound β-tubulin, the exposed GDP- β-tubulin results in a change in conformation as a consequence of which, rapid depolymerisation of the microtubule takes place in an event referred to as microtubule catastrophe. The relatively rapid shortening and lengthening that occur at the plus end of the microtubule are known as dynamic instability. The gain of tubulin subunits at the plus end and loss of tubulin subunits at the minus end result in no net change in the microtubular mass (Fig. **1E**). This phenomenon is known as tread-milling. Microtubule- associated proteins (MAPs) and drugs that interact with microtubules have the ability to enhance or inhibit microtubule catastrophe in addition to affecting the rate of microtubule shortening and growth [12].

3.1. Microtubule Dynamics in Mitosis

Microtubule dynamics play a vital role in mitosis. Microtubules form an intracellular lattice-like structure during a major portion of the cell cycle, however, this microtubule network undergoes reorganization into the mitotic spindle once the cells enter mitosis. Highly coordinated microtubule dynamics is imperative for carrying out the depolymerisation of the interphase microtubules and formation of the mitotic spindle, as well as for the location, attachment and separation of chromosomes. Hence, the agents that are capable of interfering with microtubule dynamics limit the proliferation of cells by inhibiting their ability to successfully complete mitosis [13].

Over the past few years, drugs that inhibit microtubule dynamics have been successfully used as anticancer drugs. These drugs bind to tubulin, and cause an alteration in the interphase microtubule mass when present at high concentrations. These compounds are classified into two categories namely **microtubule stabilizers**, when they cause an increase in the interphase microtubule mass and **microtubule destabilizers** when they cause a decrease in the interphase microtubule mass. However, it has been observed that both these classes of drugs, when used at lower, clinically relevant concentrations, resulted in mitotic arrest and apoptosis by following a similar mechanism of slowing down microtubule dynamics [14, 15]. Although, microtubule- targeting agents have been successfully used as chemotherapeutics, innate and acquired drug resistance are the significant downfalls that still remain to their use. Consequently, novel agents that are capable of targeting microtubule dynamics are currently under investigation.

4. MICROTUBULE DESTABILIZING AGENTS

4.1. Vinca Site-Binding Agents

The vinca alkaloids were first identified for their myelosuppressive effects. They are potent microtubule destabilizing agents that are isolated from the periwinkle plant, *Catharanthus roseus* [16] Vincristine (Oncovin®) and Vinblastine (Velban®) were the original members of the vinca family that underwent clinical development and were introduced in the late 1950's (Fig. **2**) Moreover, vindesine (Eldisine®), vinflunine and vinorelbine (Navelbine®) are some of the second-generation semi-synthetic vinca analogs that have been developed and used in a variety of cancer treatments [17, 18].

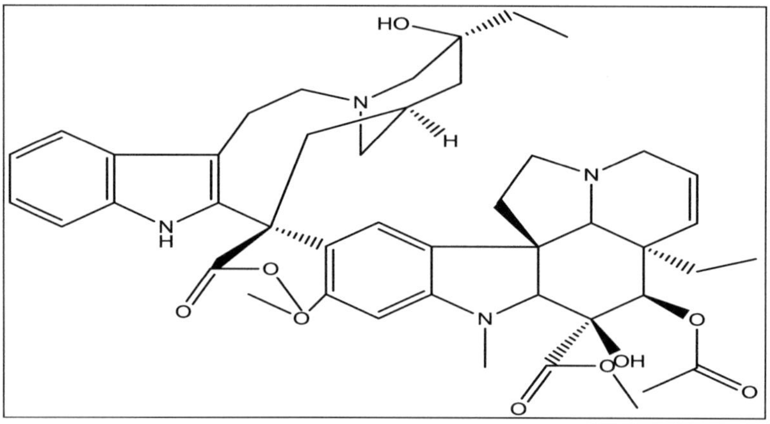

Fig. (2). Molecular structure of vinblastine.

The vinca alkaloids bind to β-tubulin close to the site of GTP-binding site [17, 18]. This binding takes place at the exposed plus end at low and clinically relevant concentrations which results in decreased dynamics and mitotic arrest (Fig. **3**) [19]. As a result, the vincas are also referred to as "end poisons". The vincas can give rise to tubulin paracrystals attributing to their affinity to free tubulin heterodimers at high concentrations [20]. Although, the antineoplastic properties of the vinca alkaloids are credited to tubulin binding and suppression of microtubule dynamics, many of these properties also result in the observed side effects of the vinca alkaloids [21].

Various vinca alkaloids differ slightly from each other in structure, however, they possess characteristic niches as chemotherapeutic agents. For instance, vincristine has been most promising in the curative treatment of sarcomas, leukemias and lumphomas. Moreover, a formulation of liposomal sphingosomal vincristine sulfate (Marqibo®; Tekmira) that may possess favourable pharmacokinetic properties and increased antitumor activity is presently in the stage of clinical trials and has already shown great promise in the treatment of acute lymphoblastic leukemia [22, 23]. Vincristine has a formyl group instead of methyl group found in vinblastine (Fig. **4**). It is effective in the treatment of lymphoma, Hodgkin's disease and advanced testicular cancer.

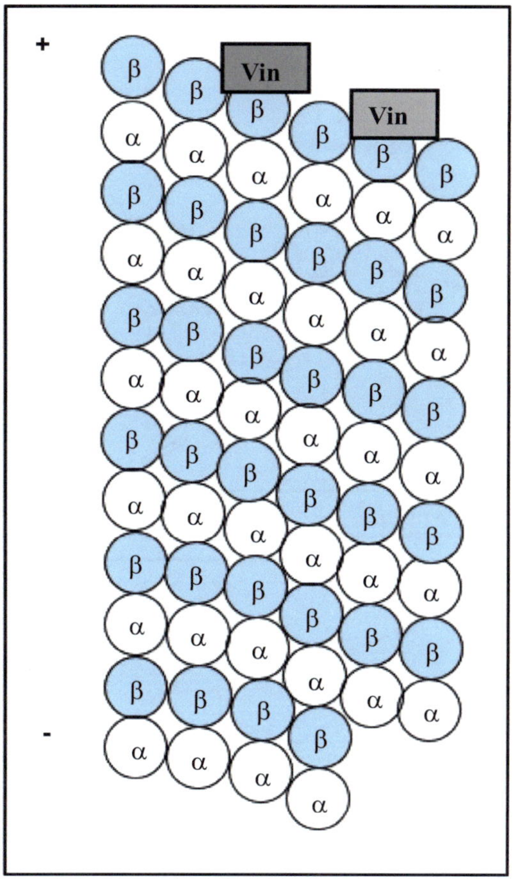

Fig. (3). Binding site of Vinblastine on tubulin: Vinblastine binds to β-tubulin close to the site of GTP-binding at the plus end of the microtubule.

Currently, vinorelbine is used as a single agent in the treatment of non-small cell lung cancer or in a combination with cisplatin. Moreover, the treatment of lymphoma, advanced ovarian carcinoma and metastatic breast cancer using vinorelbine is presently in the clinical trial stage. Vindesine (Fig. **5**) is currently under clinical investigation as a cure for acute lumphocytic leukemia [23]. Vinfluine is the newest member of the vinca alkaloid family that has proved to be more efficacious than vinblastine in several tumors and is presently under clinical investigation for its activity against solid tumors [24]. The dose-limiting toxicities of the vinca alkaloids differ with their structure; neutropenia being the most serious side effect of most of the vinca alkaloids and neurotoxicity being the most commonly associated dose-limiting toxicity of vincristine [21].

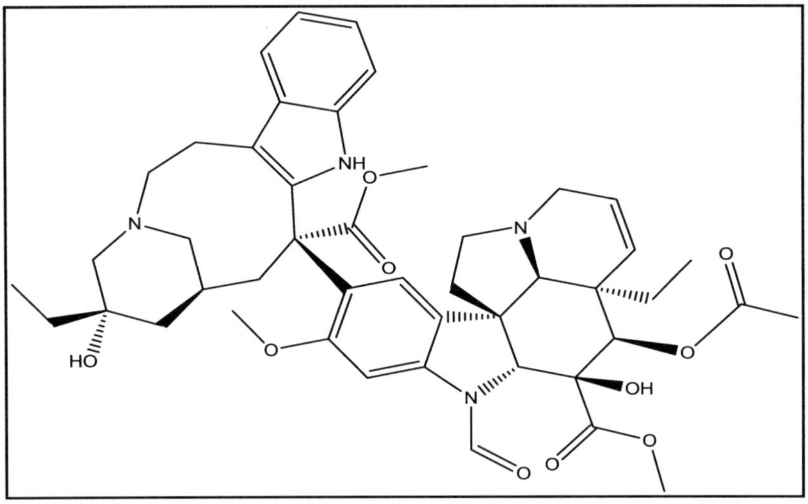

Fig. (4). Molecular structure of Vincristine.

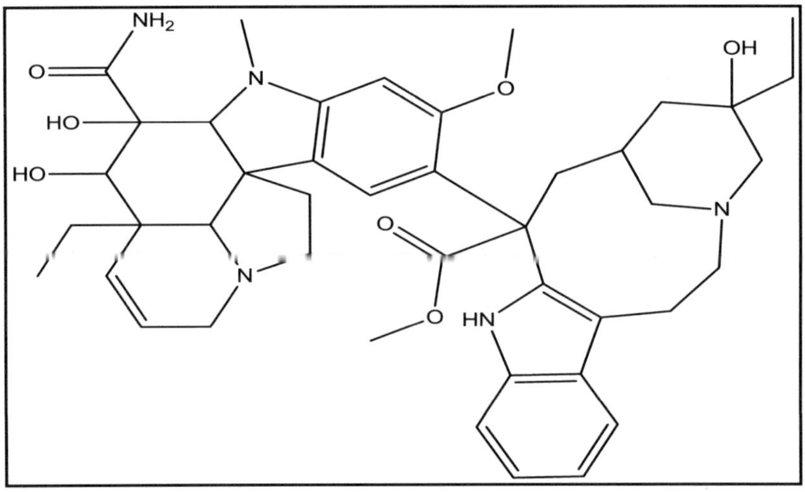

Fig. (5). Molecular structure of Vindesine.

Halichondrin B (Fig. **6**) is a macrolide lactone polyether that was isolated from various species of marine sponges attributing to its microtubule depolymerising property. Halichondrin B is unique in structure from the vinca alkaloids, however, it noncompetitively inhibits the binding of the vinca alkaloid to tubulin through an allosteric interaction [25]. Therefore, both the peptide-binding site and the vinca-binding site constitute the "vinca domain" [26].

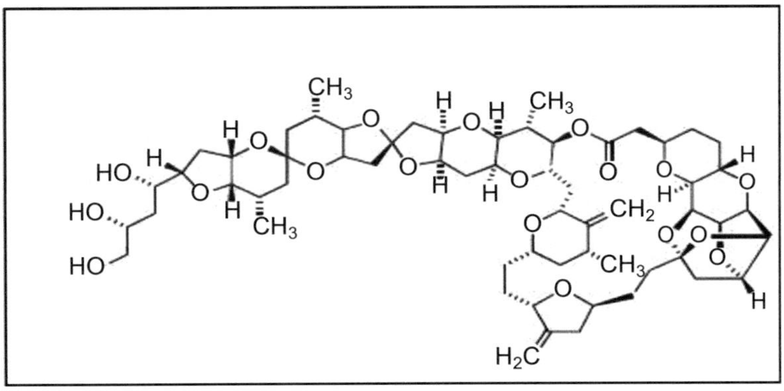

Fig. (6). Molecular structure of Halichondrin B [25].

Although, clinically useful quantities of Halichondrin B have been difficult to synthesize or isolate, several synthetic derivatives that are structurally simplified have been developed by Eisai. Currently, as a treatment option for solid tumors, a halichondrin derivative, E7389 (Eribulin®; Eisai) as a single agent or in combination with cisplatin, carboplatin or gemcitabine (Gemzar®; Lilly) is in Phase I of clinical trials [23]. For indications that include head and neck tumors, breast cancer, gynecological tumors, non-small cell lung cancer, prostate cancer and sarcomas, E7389 is under Phase II of clinical investigations. Also, a Phase III trial is underway to compare the effect of E7389 with capecitabine (Xeloda®) in breast cancer [23].

Several naturally occurring microtubule depolymerizing peptides exist that bind near or at the vinca-binding site present on tubulin and result in microtubule destabilization, for instance, hemiasterlin and dolastatins 10 and 15. **Dolastatin 10** failed to show any efficacy in multiple clinical trials when used as a single agent and hence was dropped out from clinical trials [27 - 30]. Cemadotin, a synthetic analog of dolastatin 15 could not advance through the clinical trials since it resulted in severe cardiac toxicity [31].

Tasidotin (TZT-1027; Genzyme), which is a water soluble and metabolically stable derivative of cemadotin, showed very little success in case of solid tumors when administered intravenously [32]. However, tasidotin is currently a candidate for advanced testing as an oral formulation owing to its desirable properties such as water solubility and low toxicity. Also, recent *in vitro* studies indicate that tasidotin may be effective in childhood sarcomas [33].

Cryptophycin is a depsipeptide of fresh water origin that may be considered as a very potent microtubule depolymerizer due to its properties such as competing for vinca binding and retention of efficacy in multidrug- resistant tumors [34, 35]. Cryptophycin 52 (LY355703), a synthetic derivative of cryptophycin, showed no success in clinical trials due to lack of measurable responses and severe toxicity [36].

5. AGENTS THAT BIND AT THE COLCHICINE SITE

Colchicine is a natural microtubule depolymerising agent that binds at the interface of the α/β-tubulin heterodimer, close to the GTP-binding site of α-tubulin (Fig. 7) [37]. Colchicine forms a stable complex by binding preferentially to the unpolymerized tubulin heterodimers in solution and results in the effective inhibition of microtubule dynamics when it binds to the microtubule ends [38].

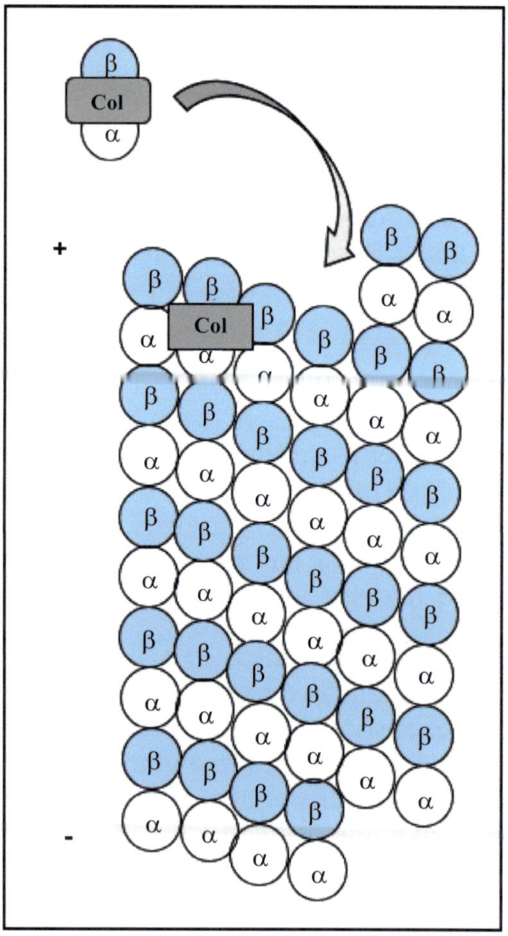

Fig. (7). Binding site of Colchicine on tubulin.

Colchicine (Col) binds to the umpolymerized tubulin at the interface of α/β-tubulin close to the GTP- binding site of α-tubulin. Binding of Colchicine to the plus end of microtubule results in a decrease in microtubule dynamicity.

Colchicine (Fig. **8**) inhibits the lateral contacts between the protofilaments, thereby causing microtubule depolymerisation [39]. Albeit antimitotic properties and potency as a microtubule deploymerizer of colchicine has not been therapeutically developed as an antitumor agent due to the elicitation of severe toxicity at the doses that result in antitumor effects. However, lower doses of colchicine have immunomodulating properties that are beneficial in the treatment of gout [40].

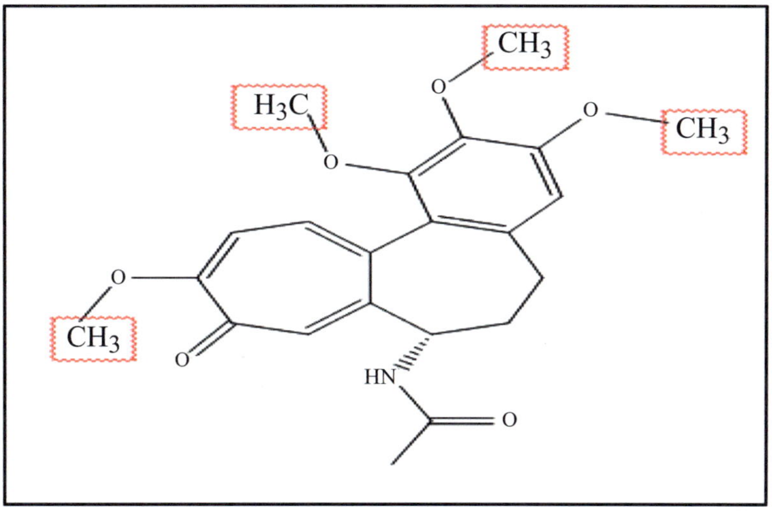

Fig. (8). Molecular structure of colchicine.

Another microtubule depolymerising agent that binds to the colchicine site is Methoxyestradiol (2ME2; Panzem®; Entremed). Although being an estrogen metabolite, 2ME2 does not bind effectively to the estrogen receptors and the antimitotic properties displayed by it are not dependent on the status of cellular estrogen receptor [41]. Evaluation of 2ME2 in clinical trials has been carried out for indications such as ovarian, prostate and breast cancers, glioblastoma and multiple myeloma. Existence of an oral formulation and inhibition of angiogenesis are the unique properties possessed by 2ME2 [42, 43]. However, the bioavailability of 2ME2 was observed to be low during the pharmacodynamics study in Phase I clinical trials, the probable reason being its metabolism to 2-methoxyestrone (2ME1), which is another estrogenic agent [44, 45].

Phase I studies in advanced solid tumors are underway for ENMD 1198 (Entremed) which is a 2ME2 analog with improved metabolic stability [46, 47].

LP-261, has the ability to competitively bind at the colchicine binding site is currently being developed as a drug candidate by Locus Pharmaceuticals [48]. LP-261 possesses anti-angiogenic and antimitotic properties and is orally bioavailable. Moreover, the development of LP-261 in Phase I studies of solid tumors has been advanced owing to its efficacy and low toxicity.

NPI-2358 (Nereus) and SSR97225 (Sanofi-Aventis) are two other drugs that bind at the colchicine- binding site and breakdown tumor vasculature. Good tolerability was observed in patients with lymphoma and solid tumors in Phase I study for NPI-2358. Also, blood supply to the tumor was inhibited, as suggested by mechanistic studies [49]. For the determination of the optimal dosing of NPI-2358 as a single agent as well as in combination with docetaxel, additional Phase I studies are underway. Also, early clinical development is being carried out for SSR97225 [23].

6. MICROTUBULE STABILIZERS

6.1. Agents that Bind at the Taxane Site

The taxane- binding site is the third of the well characterized drug- binding sites on microtubules. Taxanes are the agents that bind to the polymerized microtubules within the lumen of the polymer and target the microtubules (Figs. **9** & **10**). These agents straighten the GDP- bound β-tubulin protofilaments into a conformation that resembles the more stable GTP- bound structure and stabilizes them [50].

Paclitaxel binds to the interior lumen of microtubules and, at low concentrations, decreases microtubule dynamicity.

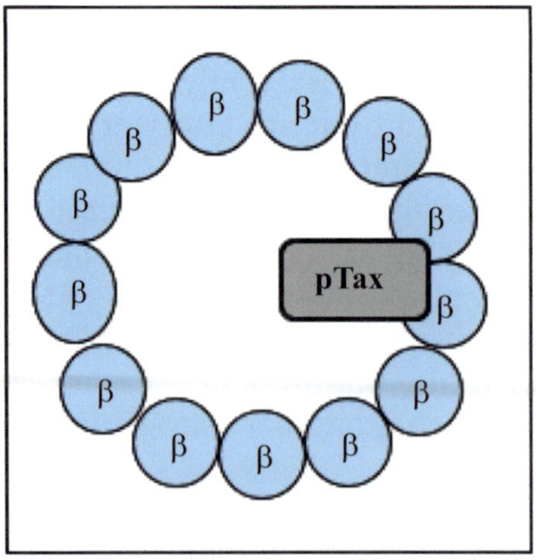

Fig. (9). Binding site of Paclitaxel (pTax) on microtubule.

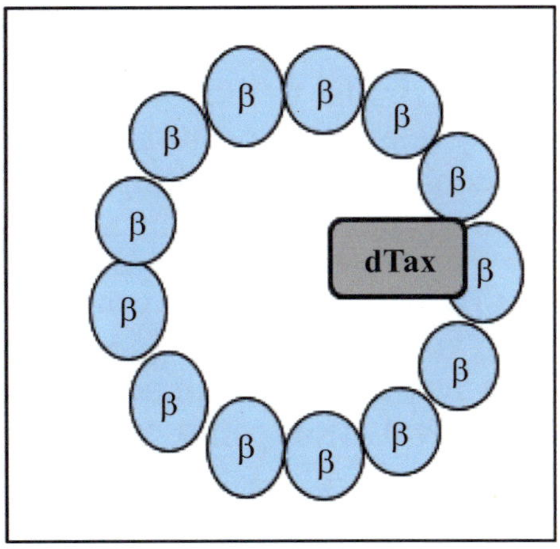

Fig. (10). Binding site of Docetaxel (dTax) on microtubule.

Docetaxel binds to the interior lumen of microtubules and results in a decrease in the dynamicity at low concentrations.

Paclitaxel (Taxol®, Bristol-Meyers Squibb) (Fig. **11**) which is a taxane, has been observed to possess the unique property of inducing the formation of microtubules that contain 12 protofilaments instead of the typical 13 protofilaments [51]. Binding of taxane results in the bundling of interphase microtubules by causing a shift in the equilibrium of the tubulin heterodimers from the soluble form to the polymerized form [52].

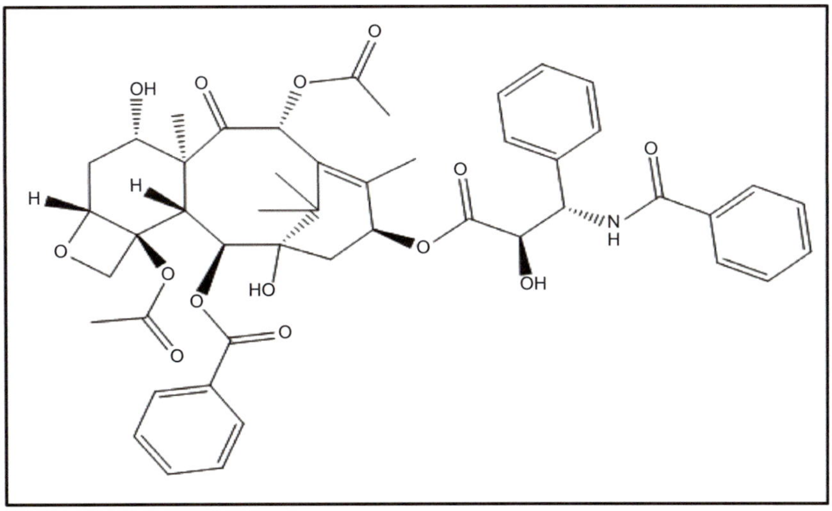

Fig. (11). Molecular structure of Paclitaxel (Taxol).

Taxanes follow a mechanism similar to that of agents that binds to the vinca and colchicines site at clinically relevant concentrations and cause a decrease in the microtubule dynamicity consequently resulting in irregular formation of the mitotic spindle, mitotic arrest and initiation of apoptosis [6, 53].

Paclitaxel and docetaxel (Taxotere®, Sanofi-Aventis) (Fig. **12**) are indispensable in the treatment of ovarian and breast cancer [54]. Taxanes have been clinically successful for many years however inherent,acquired drug resistance and dose limiting toxicities of peripheral neuropathy and immunosuppression are their serious limitations [55].

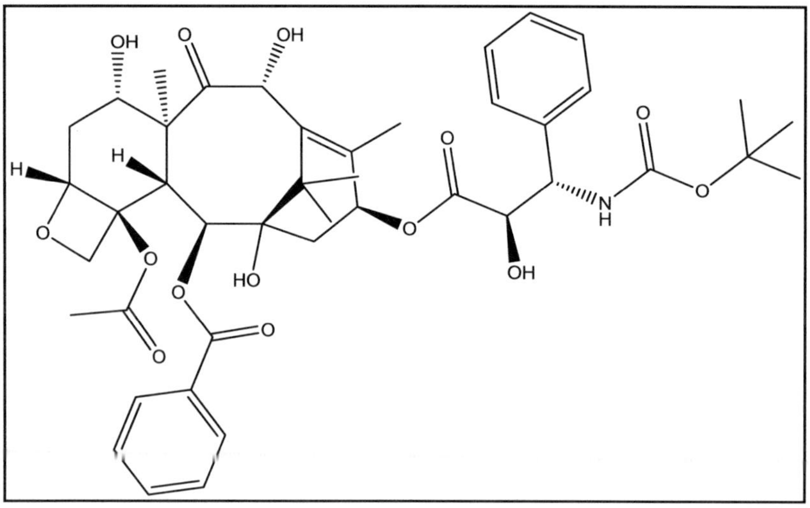

Fig. (12). Molecular structure of Docetaxel.

Overexpression of the βIII isotype of tubulin, which is specifically expressed in neuronal tissues is a mechanism of taxane resistance that is clinically relevant [56]. Although, taxane resistance has been correlated to mutations in the tubulin-binding site, unsuccessful reproduction of this original observation suggests that it may be clinically irrelevant [57]. Many novel agents that bind to taxane as well as taxane-based formulations that have enhanced tumor delivery or lowered toxicity are presently under clinical investigation.

One of the major problems hindering the development of taxanes is their poor solubility. Consequently, it became essential that the taxanes be formulated in cremaphor, an agent that requires patient pretreatment and results in hypersensitivity reactions. Abraxane® (Abraxis), a paclitaxel derivative, eliminates the need for cremaphor since the conjugation of albumin to paclitaxel confers it with an increased intrinsic solubility which dramatically reduces the drug administration time from 3h to 30 min [58]. Currently, Abraxane® is under clinical investigation against solid tumors and is approved for use in metastatic breast cancer [23].

XRP9881 (Larotaxel®; Sanofi-Aventis) is a semi-synthetic derivative of paclitaxel that is presently in Phase II trials as a single agent or in combination with trastuzumab (Herceptin®) for Her2+ breast cancer [23]. Also, trials are underway to test the efficacy of Larotaxel® with cisplatin when used as a combination therapy for non-small cell lung cancer. TPI287 (Tapestry) is another semi-synthetic paclitaxel derivative that is orally active and in the initial stages of Phase II trials as a single agent in pancreatic and prostate cancer [23].

6.2. Epothilones

The epothilones (Fig. **13**) are the agents of myxo-bacterial origin making them favourable for large- scale culture and isolation and possess microtubule stabilizing properties. The epothilones have a unique pharmacophore that has a binding site near or at the taxane- binding site and consequently results in a mechanism of action that is similar but slightly distinct to that of taxanes (paclitaxel) [59].

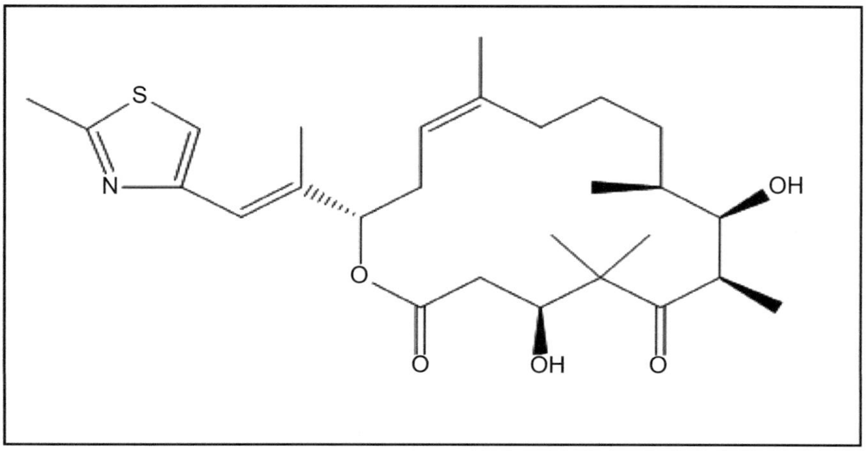

Fig. (13). Molecular structure of Epothilone.

Many epothilone derivatives, individually and in combination with other agents, are in clinical development for indications like lymphoma and solid tumors. Ixabepilone (Ixempra®; Bristol-Meyers Squibb) is a semi- synthetic epothilone derivative that was approved for metastatic or locally advanced taxane- resistant breast cancer in the year 2007 [60]. Phase II studies to examine the effect of ixabepilone on chemotherapy- resistant lymphoma are underway [23]. ZK-EPO (Sagopilone®; Bayer), Epothilone B (Patupilone®) and KOS-1584 (Kosan

Biosciences) are other epothilones that are undergoing clinical development [61, 62]. Despite the efficacy displayed by ixabepilone in tumors that were previously unresponsive, peripheral neuropathy in approximately 65% of the treated patients remains a major dose-limiting toxicity [60]. Dictyostatin, sarcodictyins, discodermolide (XAA296) and eleutherobin are other agents of marine origin that have microtubule- stabilizing properties [63, 64].

6.3. Taccalonolides

The taccalonolides are natural steroids derived from plants, possess microtubule stabilizing properties and do not bind to or enhance the polymerization of purified tubulin which suggests that they have a mechanism of action that is distinct from other microtubule- targeting agents [65]. Bundling of interphase microtubules and mitotic arrest with multiple abnormal spindles are some of the effects on cells that taccalonolides have in common with taxanes [66]. Moreover, taccalonolides are quite effective in the cell lines expressing βIII- tubulin unlike vinblastine, paclitaxel, docetaxel and epothilone B which are not effective [67]. Owing to the unique mechanistic and structural properties of taccalonolides as well as their capability of evading multiple modes of clinically relevant taxane- resistance, continued efforts of studying this group of agents have been encouraged.

7. PATENTS ON NOVEL AGENTS THAT TARGET MICROTUBULES

7.1. Aurora A

7.1.1. US Patent 9012475 by Hirai and Sootome (2015)

Anti-tumor agents like vinca alkaloids and taxanes fails to show satisfactory therapeutic effect due to the evolved resistance and refractoriness by the tumor cells.

The US Patent 9012475 by Hirai and Sootome (2015) described an enhanced method for treating tumor by combining a microtubule- targeting drug and an Aurora A selective inhibitor.

Aurora A is a serine/threonine kinase, reported to be involved in spindle kinetics, formation and maturation of centrosome, alignment of the chromosomes in the mitotic Phase of the cell cycle and regulation of mitotic division. Aurora A is expressed excessively in a wide range of carcinomas. Moreover, in a tumor cell, inhibition of Aurora A results in the induction of mitotic arrest and apoptosis. Aurora B, which is a subtype of Aurora A, acts on the mitotic Phase (M phase) of the cell cycle similar to Aurora A. Both of these molecules reduce the activity of spindle assembly checkpoints. It has been reported that an effect of paclitaxel or docetaxel is enhanced if Aurora A is inhibited. It is expected that if an agent selectively inhibiting Aurora A kinase when used in combination with a taxane antitumor agent, its antitumor effect can be enhanced to produce a higher therapeutic effect.

Under the above circumstance, MK5108, a piperidine compound, was reported as an Aurora A selective inhibitor. Enhancement of an antitumor effect was seen when MK5108 was administered orally along with docetaxel in nude rats. Although it's therapeutic effect was not sufficient. Furthermore, according to the administration schedule of the invention, a side effect of microtubule targeting drug was suppressed to a minimum. Also tumor cells, which have developed resistance and refractory to the microtubule targeting drug showed anti-tumor effect on administering piperidine in combination with MK5108 [68].

7.2. Synergistic Drug Combinations for Cancer Therapy

7.2.1. US Patent Application 20150140125 by Zaid et al. (2015)

The US Patent Application 20150140125 by Zaid *et al.* (2015) describes a synergistic drug combination for cancer. The therapeutic combination comprises of therapeutically amalgamated amounts of at least one chemotherapeutic agent and a fortified decoction dosage form. The fortified decoction dosage form comprises of plant extract of the genus *Arum*, fortified with effective amounts (about 10mg to about 6,000mg) of βsitosterol (phytosterol), isovanillin (phenolic aldehyde), and linolenic acid (fatty acid) not derived from the plant extract. These combinations have therapeutic effects on cancerous tissue which is greater than the sum of the individual therapeutic effects of the fortified decoction dosage form and the at least one chemotherapeutic agent on the cancerous tissue. The extracts, βsitosterol, isovanillin, and linolenic acid were optionally dispersed or dissolved in a solvent system (e.g., in suspension or solution) and administered in combination with a chemotherapeutic agent by subjects undergoing chemotherapy. In other words it can be said that the fortified decoction dosage acts as an adjunctive therapy along with a chemotherapeutic agent or vice versa. The fortified decoction dosage form in combination with the said chemotherapeutic agent advantageously achieved a therapeutic synergy in treating cancer in the subject. As such, the cancer of the subject was improved as compared to a subject treated with a chemotherapeutic agent without any decoction. The respective amounts of the fortified decoction and chemotherapy were coordinated with each other so as to obtain the desired therapeutic synergy, i.e., preselected amounts of each were employed to achieve the ends of the invention [69].

7.3. Pentoxifylline

7.3.1. US Patent Application 20150374702 by Kuh and Kim (2015)

In the US Patent Application 20150374702 by Kuh and Kim (2015), an anticancer adjuvant containing pentoxifylline was described. Pentoxifylline is a methylxanthine derivative and has a structure similar to caffeine (Fig. **14**). Pentoxifylline is a drug which improves the deformability of damaged erythrocytes and leukocytes, suppresses thrombocyte aggregation, and improves hemorheologic effects which lower blood viscosity and enhance erythrocyte flexibility. It is known to have activity as an inhibitor of phosphodiesterase as well as activity against other biological targets. Pentoxifylline has been widely used for treating circulatory disturbances (ischemia and cerebral arteriosclerosis such as apoplexy, vertigo, headaches, and amnesia) [70]. In addition to this, pentoxifylline is also believed to have anti-inflammatory and anti-fibrotic properties.

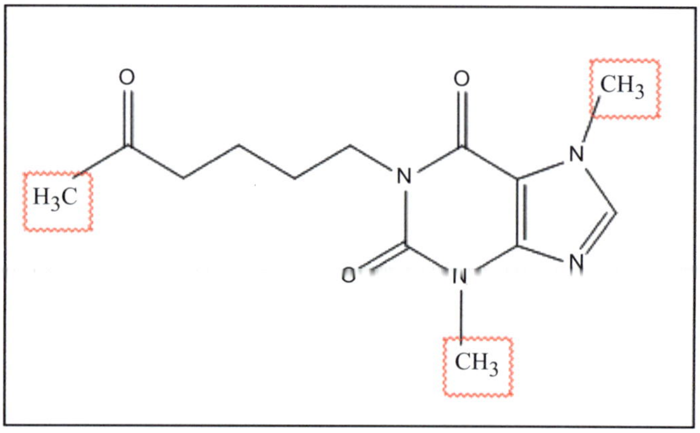

Fig. (14). Molecular structure of Pentoxifylline.

Meanwhile, the extracellular matrix of tumors is known to block the access of anticancer agents thereby reducing the therapeutic effects of anticancer agents. This extracellular matrix is composed mainly of collagen which is a connective tissue. Therefore, in order to increase the therapeutic effects of the anticancer agent, it is necessary to increase the penetration of the anticancer agent into tumor cells by suppressing the synthesis of collagen in the tumor. Therefore the present invention also states the use pentoxifylline along with an anticancer agent to inhibit the synthesis of collagen in the tumor and increase the distribution of an anticancer agent or the sensitivity of cancer cells, thereby enhancing the therapeutic effects of the anticancer agent [71].

In the given patent, the anticancer agent was one or more, selected from the group consisting of metabolic antagonists, alkylating agents, topoisomerase antagonists, microtubule antagonists, anticancer antibiotics, plant derived alkaloids, antibody anticancer agents, and molecular targeted anticancer agents. Also, the anticancer agent could be a nanoparticle preparation, for example, a liposome preparation. For the anticancer adjuvant, pentoxifylline was first administered followed by the anticancer agent. The invention claimed by the given patent was directed against pancreatic cancer, ovarian cancer, colorectal cancer, rectal cancer, liver cancer, breast cancer, lung cancer, stomach cancer, gallbladder cancer, bladder cancer, lymphoma, brain cancer, uterine cancer, prostate cancer, or malignant melanoma.

7.4. Benzimidazole Derivatives

7.4.1. US Patent Application 20160002214 by Ahmed et al. (2016)

The targeting of tubulin is an important mechanism for cancer chemotherapy and tubulin binding agents such as taxanes and vinca alkaloids have played a crucial role in the treatment of diverse human cancers [72] The tubulin binding agents like vinca alkaloids and taxanes have several limitations such as poor water solubility, development of drug resistance, toxic effects which has inspired to further search for novel effective antitumor agents that targets tubulin. Therefore, identification of new molecules with tubulin binding mechanism and with minimal toxicity to the normal tissues led to the discovery and development of novel anticancer agents.

The US Patent Application 20160002214 by Ahmed *et al.* (2016) is related to benzimidazole (Fig. **15**) derivatives as anticancer agents and the process of their preparation. Benzimidazole substituted derivatives are known as inhibitors of tubulin polymerisation and are useful for inhibiting cell proliferation for the treatment of cancer [73]. Among the anticancer benzimidazoles, an important position is held by 2aryl/ heteroarylbenzimidazole derivatives that are found to be more potent and hence the design and synthesis of 2 aryl benzimidazoles are the potential area of research [74]. For instance, Bisbenzimidazole derivatives such as Hoechst 33258 has undergone Phase II clinical evaluation as an anticancer agent and the inhibition of topoisomerase and DNA helicase has been proposed as its mechanism of action [75].

Similarly, there has been wide interest in compounds containing the 1,2,4 oxadiazole scaffold because of their broad range of biological activities such as antimicrobial, antiviral, anti-inflammatory, and antineoplastic properties [76]. Among the oxadiazoles, the 3,5 disubstituted 1,2,4 oxadiazoles derivatives are reported in literature for their anticancer potential. The inventors have found out that by incorporating 2 aryl benzimidazole with oxadiazole scaffold. Enhanced anticancer activity can be achieved that might work through inhibition of tubulin polymerization [77].

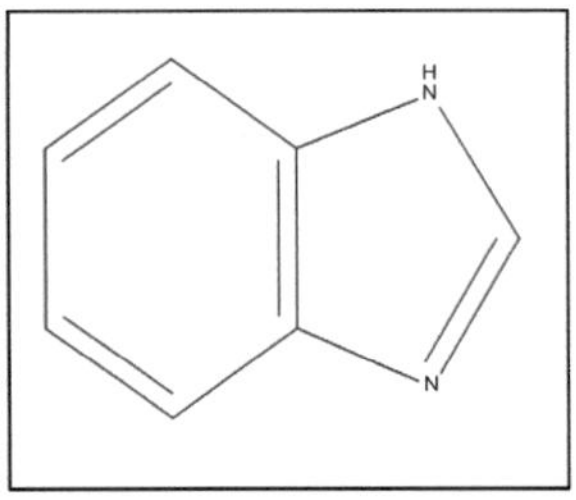

Fig. (15). Molecular structure of Benzimidazole.

In the said patent, it was claimed that by incorporating 2 aryl benzimidazole with oxadiazole scaffold, enhanced anticancer activity can be achieved that might work through inhibition of tubulin polymerization. In this invention, the synthesized compounds showed significant anticancer activity with less toxicity to normal cells. One of the compounds, (3(4(5Methoxy1Hbenzo[d]imidazol2yl)phenyl)5(3, 4,5trimethoxyphenyl)1,2,4oxadiazole) 5i showed potent cytotoxicity on SR (leukemia cell line) and BT549 (breast cancer cell line) with GI values of 0.71 and 0.52μM/ml respectively (Table **1**) [78].

Table 1. GI Values of (3¬(4¬(5¬Methoxy¬1H¬benzo[d]imidazol¬2¬yl)phenyl)¬5¬(3,4,5¬trimethoxy-phenyl)¬1,2,4-oxadiazole) 5i for Two Different Cell Lines.

Cell Line	GI_{50} Value (μM/ml)
Leukemia cell line (SR)	0.71
Breast cancer cell line (BT549)	0.52

7.5. Combination of Casein Kinase 2 (CK2) Peptide Inhibitor (Termed P15) with Standard Chemotherapeutic Agents

7.5.1. US Patent 9278118 by Rodriguez et al. (2016)

Drug resistance is recognized as the primary cause of chemo resistance. Apart from the suboptimal drug concentration on the tumor milieu that could influence the drug resistance, other factors like cellular origin, intracellular detoxification, changes on the cellular response, tolerance to stress and defects on the apoptosis signaling pathways [79]. The GlycoproteinP and the Gluthathione Stransferase are the major proteins that mediate the intracellular detoxification process linked to the drug resistance phenomenon in cancer [80, 81]. Other proteins like betatubulins have been reported to be involved on the drug resistance phenomenon and their levels directly correlate with the tumor resistance to

Paclitaxel [82]. Also, cisplatin resistance has been reported to be influenced by the over expression of different proteins like Tplastin [83], the Heat Shock Protein (HSP70) and (HSP90) [84] and the transcription factor YB1 [85].

Nucleophosmin is a protein which plays a central role in cell cycle promotion, inhibition of apoptosis and it has been regarded as a poor prognosis marker in cancer [86]. Likewise, the CK2 enzyme plays an important role in cell survival and the resistance of tumor cells toward apoptosis [87]. Previous findings have revealed the elevation of CK2 activity from 3 to 7 fold in epithelial solid tumors with respect to the normal tissues [87, 88].

Furthermore, the CK2 activity is an important cellular event for the malignant transformation and it constitutes a tumor progression marker [89]. The fact that the CK2 phosphorylation represents a strong signal to protect tumor cells from apoptosis, leads to the consideration of this enzyme as an antiapoptotic mediator on the physiology of the cell [90].

Different strategies can be used to inhibit the CK2 phosphorylation using independent approaches. Using these approaches, the US Patent 9278118 by Rodriguez *et al.* (2016) has demonstrated the proof of principle that the CK2 inhibition lead to apoptosis in tumor cells. These findings reinforce the experimental validation of CK2 as a suitable target to develop anticancer drugs. Inhibition of CK2 phosphorylation includes use of any chemical or peptidic compound that blocks either the substrate or the enzyme itself. The strategy is to bypass the tumor chemo-resistance toward the conventional cytostatic drugs. The invention claimed the use of pharmaceutical combination that contained two ingredients: a CK2 phosphorylation inhibitor (P15 peptide) and a cytostatic drug that is pharmaceutically acceptable. The cytostatic drug was pharmaceutically accepted for solid tumors and those from hematopoietic origin. The preferred cytostatics are cisplatin and carboplatin, paclitaxel and docetaxel, vincristin and vinblastin, 5fluorouracil, doxorubicin, cyclophosphamide, etoposide, mitomycin C, imatinib, iressa, and velcade (Bortezomib), cytarabine (Ara C), fludarabine, and mitoxantrone, mixed with appropriated vehicles. The administration of this pharmaceutical combination was performed by systemic, topic or oral routes. Thus, this pharmaceutical combination achieved 10 to 100 fold reduction of the effective dose for each cytostatic drug mentioned in this invention. An effective dose is that which achieves 50% antineoplastic effect which is also termed Inhibitory Concentration 50% (IC50) in proliferation assays *in vitro*. In this invention, “suboptimal doses” referred to those lower than the IC50. The sequential administration of the ingredients from this pharmaceutical combination demonstrated that P15 treatment bypasses the tumor chemoresistance both *in vitro* and *in vivo*. In this invention, it was understood that “bypassing of tumor chemoresistance or chemosensibilization" referred to the event of reducing the drug dose needed to produce the 50% of the antitumor effect after pretreatment with the P15 peptide. Thus tumor's chemosensibilization elicited after sequential administration of the ingredients from this pharmaceutical combination represented a great advantage [91].

7.6. Curcumin

7.6.1. WO Patent Application WO2015067282 by Fawzy (2015)

Another novel agent with anti cancer activity that was claimed in WO Patent Application WO2015067282 by Fawzy, I.M. (2015) was Curcumin (Fig. **16**). Curcumin [1,7bis(4hydroxy3methoxyphenyl)l, 6heptadien3,5dione] which is extracted from the rhizome of the plant *curcuma longa* was found to possess anti-proliferative activities against tumor cells *in vitro* and was found to have inhibition activity on tubulin. It also interferes with the microtubule formation, which is essential in cellular processes such as mitosis and cell replication [92].

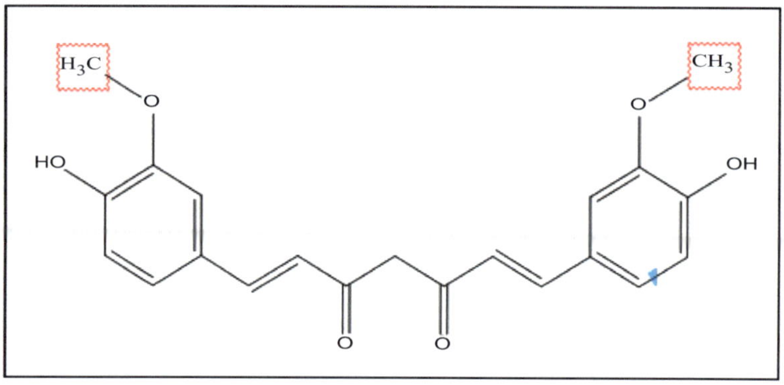

Fig. (16). Molecular structure of Curcumin.

Novel Curcumin analogs were designed and synthesized using 1, 5diaryl3oxo1,4 pentadienyl pharmacophore and evaluated for their antitumor activities in 5 different cell lines; ovarian cancer (A2780), renal adenocarcinoma (ACHN), prostate cancer (PC3), colorectal cancer (Hct116) and a leukemic monocyte lymphoma (U937GTB). Compounds VII and IV (Fig. **17**) of the invention exhibited highly potent cytotoxic activity with IC50 values in the range of 12.5μM and 11.423μM, respectively. Also, *in vitro* tubulin polymerization assay was performed for both analogs to test their effect on tubulin and the results showed that both analogs IV and VII stabilize microtubules with 79.8% and 60.6% respectively (Table **2**) causing cancer cell apoptosis with the same mechanism as Paclitaxel which it was compared to during the assay.

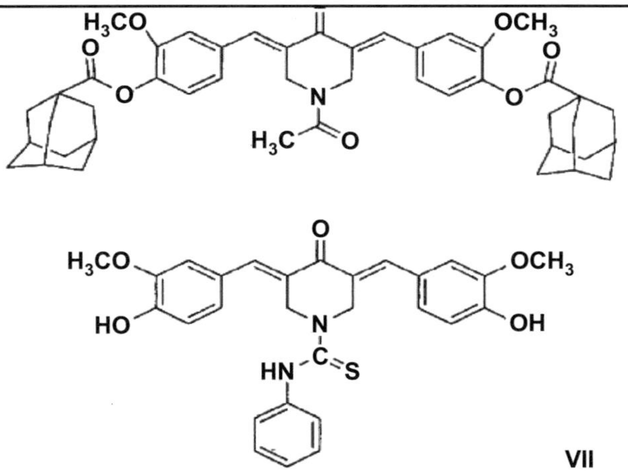

Fig. (17). Structure of newly designed curcumin analogs- Compounds 1V and VII [92].

Table 2. IC50 Values of Curcumin Analogs VII and IV against Cell Lines.

Compound (Curcumin Analog)	IC50 Value
VII	12.5μM
IV	11.423μM

Tubulin Polymerization assay was carried out using 10μM of the analogs VII and IV compared to positive control drug Vincristine and negative control drug Paclitaxel where, both control drugs affect tubulin and inhibit microtubule polymerization cycle but through two different mechanisms; Vincristine via inhibition of tubulin assembly while Paclitaxel via stabilization of microtubules. The results showed that both analogs acted on tubulin with the same mechanism as Paclitaxel by stabilizing microtubules and thus disrupting the tubulin assembly and polymerization cycle leading to cancer cell arrest and apoptosis.

7.7. Anticancer Drug and/ or Therapeutically Active Molecule

7.7.1. WO Patent Application WO2015193702 by Lavitrano et al. (2015)

Currently, the major limitation of anticancer treatments is the poor sensitivity of tumors cells to the cytotoxic action of various chemotherapeutic agents, and the subsequent resistance. For stage III colon carcinoma, since the early 90's the postsurgical treatment of choice is chemotherapy based on 5 fluorouracil (5FU), usually in combination with feucovorin or oxaliplatin (OxPt). Till date, the range of effective drugs is very limited although combination chemotherapy protocols have been developed (such as 5FU in combination with OxPt, capecitabine, tegafur or biologic agents such as bevacizumab and cetuximab) in order to overcome this drawback. However, Combination of 5FU with other chemotherapy drugs (such as oxaliplatin) leads to an increase in response up to 40-50%, a value not yet completely satisfactory for effective therapeutic action against cancer pathologies

Cells undergo several morphological changes in the course of apoptosis. Cells undergo fragmentation to form apoptotic bodies, which are phagocytosed by macrophages. The method described in the patent **WO2011123103** by Perrée and Hallquist (2011) makes use of the iCK (microculture kinetic) assay in order to assess whether cancer cells derived from known tumor cell lines undergo apoptosis in response to a particular drug which is known to be active against one or more types of cancer [93]. This allows identification of anticancer drugs or their combination that are sensitive, and identification of patients in whom chemotherapy is ineffective due to the development of drug resistance, the **WO Patent Application WO2015193702** by Lavitrano, M. *et al.* (2015) came into effect. The invention claimed by the patent application related to a method of assessing sensitivity or resistance of at least one cancer cell to at least one anticancer drug, at least one therapeutically active molecule capable of inhibiting growth (proliferation and/or metabolism) or of inducing death of the said tumor cell, and/or capable of restoring in resistant tumor cells the sensitivity at least one anticancer drug, and at least one combination of one anticancer drug and one therapeutically active molecule [94].

In the patent, neoplastic cells of any tumor stage or classification, derived from epithelial tumors, mesenchymal tumors, tumors of the nervous tissue, cells from colon carcinoma, breast cancer, ovarian cancer, stomach cancer, lung carcinoma, renal carcinoma, thyroid carcinoma or pancreatic carcinoma, but also circulating cancer cells, sarcomas and melanomas were tested. “Anticancer drug” comprised of classical chemotherapeutic drugs such as 5 fluorouracil (5FU), capecitabine, oxaliplatin and other platinum coordination compounds; And “therapeutically active molecule” referred to a molecule capable of inhibiting growth (proliferation and/or metabolism) or inducing death of said tumor cell and/or capable of restoring in resistant cancer cells the sensitivity to said at least one anticancer drug. Examples of such molecules are biological drugs such as monoclonal antibodies, preferably Cetuximab, Panitumumab, Bevacizumab and kinase inhibitors such as gefitinib, erlotinib, vermurafenib, sorafenib, ibrutinib and dasatinib [94].

7.8. Pharmaceutical Compositions Comprising Polymeric Nanoparticles of Anticancer Drugs

7.8.1. WO Patent Application WO2016020697 by Shrikhande et al. (2016)

According to the invention claimed by the WO Patent Application WO2016020697 by Shrikhande *et al.* (2016), a pharmaceutical composition comprising polymeric nanoparticles of one or more anticancer drugs that have been engineered to have an affinity for target tissues through passive or active targeting mechanisms, and optionally one or more pharmaceutically acceptable excipients has been provided. The composition was formulated to deliver the said anticancer drugs to the target site of action as well as to decrease or avoid side effects. Anticancer drugs according to the present invention included alkylating agents, antitumor antibiotics, antimicrotubule agents, DNA linking agents, bisphosphonates, topoisomerase inhibitors, antimetabolites, biological agents and nucleoside analogues, or any combinations thereof. Suitable alkylating agents included mechlorethamine, mustine, cyclophosphamide, nitrosoureas, tetrazine and the like or their combinations

The process of preparation comprised of dissolving one or more of the anticancer drugs in an aqueous solution of human serum albumin or gelatin; adding a desolvating agent for formation of nanoprecipitates; cross linking and neutralization of the formed nanoparticles with other pharmaceutically acceptable excipients; Optionally freeze drying the purified nanoparticles; and processing into a dosage form. The composition was directed towards the treatment of hepatocellular carcinoma [95].

Suitable DNA linking agents included cisplatin, carboplatin, nedaplatin, oxaliplatin, satraplatin and the like or their combinations. Suitable antitumor antibiotics and topoisomerase inhibitors according to the present invention included bleomycin, daunorubicin, epirubicin, doxorubicin, idarubicin, mitoxantrone, mitomycin, actinomycin, pirarubicin and the like or their combinations. Suitable antimetabolites included fluorouracil, capecitabine, asparaginase, and the like or their combinations. Suitable biological agents according to the present invention included bevacizumab, cetuximab, regorafenib, ibrutinib, axitinib, crizotinib, dabrafenib, ponatinib, afatinib, dasatinib, nilotinib ruxolitinib, trametinib, erlotinib, sorafenib, gefitinib, imatinib, interferon, trastuzumab and their combinations

The pharmaceutical composition according to the invention comprised of human serum albumin nanoparticles as well as gelatin nanoparticles of cisplatin. The term "cisplatin" used in the patent was used in a broad sense to include not only "cisplatin" but also its pharmaceutically acceptable derivatives. The pharmaceutical composition according to the invention comprised of polymeric nanoparticles of one or more anticancer drugs which can be administered by varying routes of administration such as oral, parenteral (subcutaneous, intravenous, intramuscular, intradermal, intraperitoneal) or topical or localized (directly at the site) etc. [95].

7.9. Tubulin inhibitors

7.9.1. US Patent 8883793 by Chen et al. (2014)

Cancer along with other autoimmune disorders such as lupus, multiple sclerosis or arthritis, infection, or immune rejection response of organ transplant results from abnormal proliferation of cells. Anti- mitotic agents that interfere with dynamic equilibrium of microtubules/ tubulin may lead to the appearance of typical hallmarks of cancer as a result of mitotic arrest at the level of nuclear membrane, chromosomes, G2/M cells and mitotic spindle. Anti- mitotic agents, for example, vinca alkaloids, such as vinblastine and vincristine have enjoyed considerable clinical success and have been used for the treatment of non- small- cell lung carcinoma and haematological malignancies. Also, taxanes such as docetaxel and paclitaxel have been successful in the treatment of non- small-cell lung carcinoma and breast cancer. Regardless of the success of most of the available anti- mitotic agents, there exist certain limitations to their use. For instance, the use of docetaxel or paclitaxel can lead to neuropathy. Moreover, use of both the taxanes and vinca alkaloids can induce tumor cells to become drug resistant. Therefore, it is imperative that novel drugs that can be used to treat abnormal cell proliferation be developed. Low cytotoxicity, ease of synthesis, good therapeutic index, high bioavailability and absence of drug resistance are the desirable properties of a powerful anti- mitotic agent.

With this intent, the US8883793 by Chen *et al.* (2014) made available the methods for the use and preparation of chemical compounds with anti- mitotic activity. The invention claimed by the patent related to compounds that had a structure described by the formula

R^2 YZ-Q-A-R^1 as inhibitors of tubulin polymerisation by means of binding at the colchicine site and which were effective in the treatment of gout, cancers and other disorders associated with abnormal cell proliferation.

A is a direct bond or one selected from the group consisting of alkyl, alkene, O, S, N-R and piperazine;

Q is selected from the group consisting of aryl and heteroaryl, wherein said aryl and heteroaryl are each optionally substituted with one or more substituents selected from R.

Z is a direct bond or one selected from the group consisting of aryl, heteroaryl, alkyl, alkene, piperazine, O, and S.

Y is a direct bond or one selected from the group consisting of alkyl, alkoxy, O-alkyl, S-alkyl.

R.sup.1 and R.sup.2 are independently selected from the group consisting of: halogen, aryl, heteroaryl, heterocycloalkyl, cycloalkyl, alkyl- aryl, alkyl-heteroaryl, cycloalkyl-aryl, cycloakyl-heteroaryl, alkyl-heterocycloalkyl [96].

7.10. Bicyclic and Tricyclic Pyrimidine Tyrosine Kinase Inhibitors with Antitubulin Activity

7.10.1. US Patent 9139590 by Gangjee (2015)

Anti-tubulin agents have had considerable clinical success as effective chemotherapeutic agents for cancer. Depending on their binding on tubulin, three distinct classes of anti-tubulin agents have been identified.

The first class of antitubulin agents are the taxanes, including docetaxel and paclitaxel, that are used as monotherapy as well as in combination with other agents for the treatment of lung, breast, head and neck and ovarian cancer among others.

The second class of antitubulin agents is the Vinca alkaloids, including vinblastine, vincristine, vindesine and vinorelbine. They are clinically significant in the treatment of small cell lung cancer, lymphomas and leukemias. Also, contrary to the taxanes, the Vincas are inhibitors of microtubule polymerization.

The colchicine site binding agents make up the third class of antitubulin agents and include colchicine in addition to other small molecules that bind to β-tubulin at the interface with α-tubulin. Compounds of this class are inhibitors of tubulin polymerization.

The compositions of the invention claimed by the US9139590 by Gangjee A. (2015) bind to the colchicine site and evade the resistance conferred by βIII-tubulin. Moreover, the recent approval of ixabepilone by the FDA indicates the need to overcome βIII- tubulin resistance. Clinical evidence suggests βIII- tubulin to be associated with failure of treatment with the taxanes and vincas. Thus, it is crucial that new drugs that have the ability to circumvent βIII- tubulin mediated tumor resistance be developed so as to aid the large number of patients that are either unresponsive or have develop resistance to the Vincas or taxanes. The compounds of the invention showed great promise in accomplishing this objective.

The clinical use of taxanes as well as ixabepilone has been plagued with poor water solubilty. Continuous efforts are being made to develop formulations of anti-mitotics that are soluble. The compositions of the invention exhibited high water solubility as their HCl salts and evaded the solubility issues associated with antimitotics [97].

The invention claimed by the patent related to bicyclic and tricyclic pyrimidine tyrosine kinase inhibitors possessing antitubulin activity. The compositions of the invention exhibited dual activity in a single agent owing to their exhibition of potency as inhibitors of vascular endothelial growth factor receptor in addition to being cytotoxic. The compositions mentioned in the invention could be made into water soluble salts with the intent of providing orally active antiangiogenic agents [97].

7.11. Combretastatin A-1 Phosphate and Combretastatin B-1 Phosphate Prodrugs.

7.11.1. US Patent 7078552 by Pettit et al. (2006)

An invention claimed by the US Patent 7078552 by Pettit *et al.* (2006) related to the synthesis of Combretastatin A1- Phosphate prodrugs and Combretastatin B1-phosphate prodrugs and their utilisation in the treatment of neoplastic diseases. The isolation and synthesis of combretastatin A-1 and B-1 from the South African willow tree *Combretum caffrum* (Combretaceae) was reported in 1987 (Pettit *et al.*, 1987). Both these natural products were shown to be effective inhibitors of cancer cell growth as well as antimitotic agents with an ED_{50} value of 0.99μg/ml and 1.7μg/ml respectively against the murine P388 lymphocytic leukemia *in vitro* system. Also, these compounds inhibited the assembly of microtubules *in vitro* with IC_{50} values of 2μM and 3μM (Table **3**) [98].

Table 3. ED50 and IC50 Values of Combretastatin A-1 and Combretastin B-1 against Murine P388 Lymphocytic Leukemia *In Vitro* System.

Compound	ED_{50} Value	IC_{50} Value
Combretastatin A-1	0.99μg/ml	2μM
Combretastatin B-1	1.7 μg/ml	3μM

With the intent of improving the solubility for drug delivery and also to increase the stability, the synthesis of combretastatin A-1 and B-1 phosphate prodrugs was undertaken. The biological activities of the metal cation prodrugs analysed in the invention resembled to the antimitotic properties of combretastatin A-1 which appeared to be among the most potent antagonists of colchicine binding to tubulin known and inhibit the polymerization of tubulin with about 99% inhibition of colchicine binding at equal concentrations. Several cations have been suggested to play an important role in the assembly and disassembly of microtubules. Divalent cations interact with tubulin in complex manners and bind to them in low as well as high- affinity sites. Magnesium has been demonstrated to be crucial for the assembly of microtubules and has been suggested to bind at the exchangeable GTP (guanosine 5′- triphosphate) site as a complex with a nucleotide. A substantial concentration of potassium cations is required to facilitate the formation of microtubules and could be replaced by sodium ions. Calcium ions inhibit the polymerization of tubulin and when added to preassembled microtubules result in their disassembly, while binding weakly to tubulin at the magnesium site. Zinc cations have been demonstrated to interfere with the lateral binding between the protofilaments of microtubules [98].

The invention claimed by the patent related to the syntheses of Combretastatin A1- Phosphate prodrugs and Combretastatin B1- phosphate prodrugs (Figs. **18** & **19**) and their utilisation in the treatment of neoplastic diseases. The prodrugs described in the invention had the following structure.

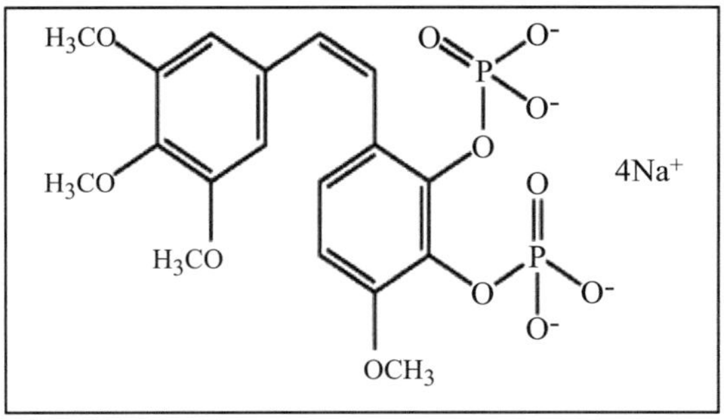

Fig. (18). Sodium phosphate prodrug of Combretastatin A-1 [98].

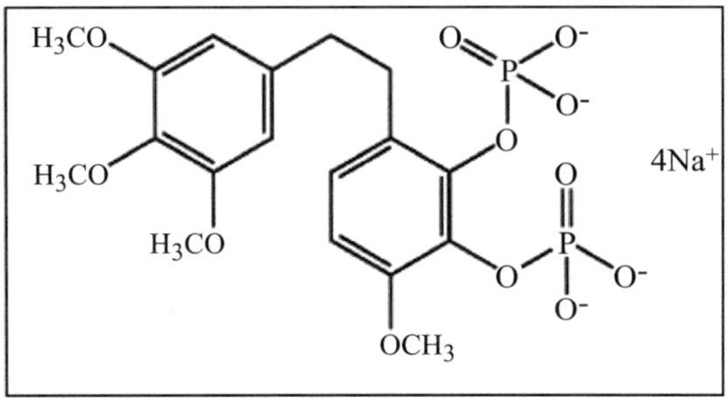

Fig. (19). Combretastatin prodrug B-1 [98].

7.12. Combretastatin Analogs

7.12.1. US Patent 7429681 by Pinney et al. (2008)

A separate class of antivascular chemotherapeutics that are of great significance are the Vascular Targeting Agents ("VTAs"), also known as vascular damaging agents or vascular disrupting agents. Contrary to the anti-angiogenic drugs which disrupt the formation of new microvessels of the developing tumor, VTAs selectively target the established tumor vasculature and lead to the extensive shutdown of blood flow to the tumor .It induces nutrient depletion and hypoxia, eventually leading to tumor necrosis. Combretastatin A4 phosphate prodrug (CA4P) is among the most potential new candidate compounds that possess vascular targeting activity. It is currently the lead drug under clinical development from among a group of tubulin- binding VTAs. It has been suggested that the VTAs result in the selective destabilisation of the microtubule cytoskeleton of the tumor endothelial cells, leading to a significant alteration in the cell shape which cause occlusion or blocking of the tumor blood vessel and the ultimate shutdown of blood flow to the tumor [99].

The invention claimed by the US Patent US7429681 by Pinney *et al.* (2008) addressed this need by making available a class of tubulin binding agent compositions that are structurally novel and possess potent tumor cell cytotoxicity and antiproliferative activity. The said invention related to the discovery of analogs of Combretastatin that act as tubulin binding agents and possess the ability of inhibiting tumor cell proliferation and tubulin assembly. The Combretastatin analogs resulted from combining a non- tubulin binding molecular template which was suitably modified with structural features such as arylalkoxy groups and hydroxyl moieties. Moreover, the given invention provided compounds that were vital for the prevention and treatment of the symptoms of neoplastic diseases and vascular proliferative disorders. Moreover, these compounds proved to be of great importance in decreasing the flow of blood to a portion of the neoplastic region and also inhibiting the polymerization of tubulin.

The IC_{50} values for tubulin polymerisation were determined for the compounds of the invention and were as follows (Table **4**):

Table 4. IC_{50} Values of Different Combretastin Analogs for Tubulin Polymerisation.

In Vitro Inhibition of Tubulin Polymerization	
Compound	**IC_{50} (μM)**
CA-4	0.73
1	~ 40

(Table 4) contd.....

In Vitro Inhibition of Tubulin Polymerization	
Compound	**IC_{50} (µM)**
2	1.4 ± 0.2
3	~ 40
23	~ 40
24	~ 40

The newly synthesised compounds were evaluated for their cytotoxic activity against different cell lines derived from human tumors. The cytotoxic activity of several compounds was evaluated against human P388 leukemia cell lines. The effective dose or ED_{50} value, which is defined as the effective dosage that is required to inhibit 50% of the cell growth, was measured. The compounds were evaluated in terms of their activity of growth inhibition against several other human cancer cell lines. These cell lines included that of non- small cell lung cancer ("lung- NSC", NCI-H460), pancreas (BXPC-3), prostate (DU-145), breast (MCF-7), ovarian (OVCAR-3), colon (KM20L2) and central nervous system ("CNS", SF- 268). The growth inhibition GI_{50}, which is defined as the dosage required to inhibit the 50% of the tumor cell growth was also measured. The results were as listed in Table **5**.

Table 5. ***In Vitro*** **Cytotoxicity against Human Cancer Cell Lines.**

ED50 (µM/ml) for Cell Line		**GI50 (µM/ml) for Cell Line**					
Compound	**P388**	**SF-268**	**BXP-3**	**NCI-H460**	**MCF-7**	**KM20L2**	**DU-145**
1	0.51	0.28	0.40	0.23	0.32	0.20	0.33
2	7.4	>10	>10	>10	>10	>10	>10
23	0.029	0.0090	0.017	0.023	0.0059	0.031	0.026

Thus, this invention made available several analogs of combetastatin which demonstrated remarkable ability to inhibit the polymerization of tubulin as well as impressive cytotoxicity. These compounds could prove to be significant clinical candidates for cancer treatment in humans. Moreover, most of the ligands, when used as pro-drugs, may prove to be effective chemotherapeutic agents that selectively target tumor vasculature and eventually result in the selective prevention and destruction of non-malignant vasculature with proliferative capabilities.

CONCLUSION

Cancer finds its place amongst the diseases that result in the highest number of fatalities worldwide. Several therapies and treatments like chemotherapy, hormonal therapy, immunotherapy, radiation therapy, adjuvant therapy, targeted therapy etc. have been developed in recent years to combat the disease. However available conventional methods for the treatment of cancer are accompanied by constant relapses and harmful side - effects. Therefore there is a need to develop a therapy which will eliminate cancer as a whole. In order to do so, several cancer targets are under the study. One such target is microtubules and their dynamics as they play a very crucial role in cellular events. There exist several natural compounds and their synthetic analogs that possess the capacity of binding to tubulin. These compounds are significant as drugs or drug candidates. They exhibit remarkable potency in altering the dynamics as well as the polymer mass of microtubules. Microtubule dynamics i.e. dynamic instability and treadmilling are vital for regulating several cellular functions such as cell signalling, cell shape, mitosis and migration among others. Various categories like microtubule stabilizers and destabilizers have been identified which have shown effect on tubulin activity. Microtubule stabilizer includes Taxanes, epothilones and taccalonolides whereas microtubule destabilizers include Vinca alkaloids, olchicine, Halichondrin B, dolostatin 10. The affinity with which these compounds binds to the soluble tubulin heterodimers is a biochemical characteristic of the tubulin-targeting drug that can be readily determined. Since, microtubules play a vital role in the growth and proliferation of cells, including cancerous cells, developing novel drugs that target them specifically would prove to be a remarkable step towards curbing the menace of cancer. Therefore, development of more novel microtubule- targeting agents that have high efficacy, low dose requirements, are easy to administer and demonstrate low toxicity to normal tissues are the need of the hour. Cancer therapy regimens should focus their attention in achieving effective drug combinations which greatly reduce toxicity and also reduce the possibility of chemoresistance. Thus, one of the major goals today in cancer therapy is to increase the therapeutic index of the current cytostatic drugs by reducing the effective dose and the intrinsic toxicity displayed by this kind of medicines.

FUTURE OF CANCER TREATMENT

In the recent years, early identification and treatment strategies have greatly aided in extending the life span of millions of people afflicted with cancer. Current and future advances on cancer research are being made on many fronts as mentioned below:

Anti-Angiogenic Chemotherapy

Many of the clinical trials make use of very low doses of the conventional chemotherapy in combination with angioinhibitors. Single angioinhibitors have been approved for the treatment of cancer, however, the efficacy of using a combination of angioinhibitors will be the major focus of future cancer treatments. For instance, the synergistic action of bisphosphonates with natural angioinhibitors like endostatin, arrresten, canstatin, angiostatin etc. needs to be investigated. Preventive angioinhibitory therapy could be considered as a viable option in the future attributing to its lower toxicity as well as lower predisposition to the induction of acquired drug resistance.

Other Targeted Treatments

Delving deeper into the molecular biology of cancer cells has greatly aided in the development of new classes of molecules for the treatment of cancer such as small interfering RNA (siRNA) and antisense oligodeoxynucleotides which hold great promise in the future.

Nanotechnology

Nanotechnology involves the use of extremely minute particles for the purpose of diagnostic imaging and for more accurate location of tumors so that drugs can be specifically and efficaciously delivered into the cancer cells.

RNA Expression Profiling

Profiling of RNA expression facilitates in determining the relative amounts of several RNA molecules at one time. Extensive knowledge of the different kinds of proteins and RNA molecules present in the cancer cell aids in understanding cell behaviour and in predicting the likely response of tumor cells to certain drugs.

Although, the development of a single "cure-all" drug for the treatment of cancer has not yet been accomplished, a wide range of treatment methods and drug targets have been discovered. Extensive research and advanced clinical trials directed towards finding a cure for cancer are the need of the hour [9].

LIST OF ABBREVIATIONS

CSCs	Cancer Stem Cells
DNA	Deoxyribonucleic Acid
NSAIDs	Nonsteroidal Anti-Inflammatory Drugs
VEGF	Vascular Endothelial Growth Factor
bFGF	Basic Fibroblast Growth Factor

PDGF	Platelet-Derived Growth Factor
RNA	Ribonucleic Acid
siRNA	small interfering Ribonucleic Acid
GTP	Guanosine Triphosphate
GDP	Guanosine Diphosphate
mg	Milligram
IC_{50}	Inhibitory Concentration 50%
ED_{50}	Effective Dose-50%
GI_{50}	Growth Inhibition 50%
CK2	Casein Kinase -2
HSP	Heat Shock Protein
μM	Micro Molar
OxPt	Oxaliplatin
iCK	Intestinal Cell Kinase
VTAs	Vascular Targeting Agents

CONFLICT OF INTEREST

The authors declare no conflict of interest, financial or otherwise.

ACKNOWLEDGEMENTS

The authors of this chapter would like to extend their heartfelt gratitude to Bentham Science Publishers for providing the opportunity to contribute this chapter to be published in their Patent e-book series.

REFERENCES

[1] Michor F, Iwasa Y, Nowak MA. Dynamics of cancer progression. Nat Rev Cancer 2004; 4(3): 197-205.
[http://dx.doi.org/10.1038/nrc1295] [PMID: 14993901]

[2] Clarke MF. Epigenetic regulation of normal and cancer stem cells. Ann NY Acad Sci 2005; 1044(1): 90-3.
[http://dx.doi.org/10.1196/annals.1349.012] [PMID: 15958701]

[3] Reya T, Morrison SJ, Clarke MF, Weissman IL. Stem cells, cancer, and cancer stem cells. Nature 2001; 414(6859): 105-11.
[http://dx.doi.org/10.1038/35102167] [PMID: 11689955]

[4] Balkwill F, Mantovani A. Inflammation and cancer: Back to Virchow? Lancet 2001; 357(9255): 539-45.
[http://dx.doi.org/10.1016/S0140-6736(00)04046-0] [PMID: 11229684]

[5] Plytycz B, Seljelid R. From inflammation to sickness: Historical perspective. Arch Immunol Ther Exp (Warsz) 2003; 51(2): 105-9.
[PMID: 12776909]

[6] Macarthur M, Hold GL, El-Omar EM. Inflammation and Cancer II. Role of chronic inflammation and cytokine gene polymorphisms in the pathogenesis of gastrointestinal malignancy. Am J Physiol Gastrointest Liver Physiol 2004; 286(4): G515-20.
[http://dx.doi.org/10.1152/ajpgi.00475.2003] [PMID: 15010360]

[7] Houghton J, Morozov A, Smirnova I, Wang TC. Stem cells and cancer. Semin Cancer Biol 2007; 17(3): 191-203.
[http://dx.doi.org/10.1016/j.semcancer.2006.04.003] [PMID: 16762563]

[8] Hanahan D, Weinberg RA. The hallmarks of cancer. Cell 2000; 100(1): 57-70.
[http://dx.doi.org/10.1016/S0092-8674(00)81683-9] [PMID: 10647931]

[9] Sudhakar A. History of cancer, ancient and modern treatment methods. J Cancer Sci Ther 2009; 1(2): 1-4.
[http://dx.doi.org/10.4172/1948-5956.100000e2] [PMID: 20740081]

[10] Lopez-Fanarraga M, Avila J, Guasch A, Coll M, Zabala JC. Review: Postchaperonin tubulin folding cofactors and their role in microtubule dynamics. J Struct Biol 2001; 135(2): 219-29.
[http://dx.doi.org/10.1006/jsbi.2001.4386] [PMID: 11580271]

[11] Nogales E, Wang HW. Structural mechanisms underlying nucleotide-dependent self-assembly of tubulin and its relatives. Curr Opin Struct Biol 2006; 16(2): 221-9.
[http://dx.doi.org/10.1016/j.sbi.2006.03.005] [PMID: 16549346]

[12] Jordan MA, Kamath K. How do microtubule-targeted drugs work? An overview. Curr Cancer Drug Targets 2007; 7(8): 730-42.
[http://dx.doi.org/10.2174/156800907783220417] [PMID: 18220533]

[13] Rusan NM, Fagerstrom CJ, Yvon AM, Wadsworth P. Cell cycle-dependent changes in microtubule dynamics in living cells expressing green fluorescent protein-α tubulin. Mol Biol Cell 2001; 12(4): 971-80.
[http://dx.doi.org/10.1091/mbc.12.4.971] [PMID: 11294900]

[14] Okouneva T, Hill BT, Wilson L, Jordan MA. The effects of vinflunine, vinorelbine, and vinblastine on centromere dynamics. Mol Cancer Ther 2003; 2(5): 427-36.
[PMID: 12748304]

[15] Kelling J, Sullivan K, Wilson L, Jordan MA. Suppression of centromere dynamics by taxol in living osteosarcoma cells. Cancer Res 2003; 63(11): 2794-801.
[PMID: 12782584]

[16] Cutts JH, Beer CT, Noble RL. Biological properties of Vincaleukoblastine, an alkaloid in *Vinca rosea* Linn, with reference to its antitumor action. Cancer Res 1960; 20(7): 1023-31.
[PMID: 13719013]

[17] Gigant B, Wang C, Ravelli RB, *et al.* Structural basis for the regulation of tubulin by vinblastine. Nature 2005; 435(7041): 519-22.
[http://dx.doi.org/10.1038/nature03566] [PMID: 15917812]

[18] Lin CM, Hamel E. Effects of inhibitors of tubulin polymerization on GTP hydrolysis. J Biol Chem 1981; 256(17): 9242-5.
[PMID: 6114958]

[19] Toso RJ, Jordan MA, Farrell KW, Matsumoto B, Wilson L. Kinetic stabilization of microtubule dynamic instability *in vitro* by vinblastine. Biochemistry 1993; 32(5): 1285-93.
[http://dx.doi.org/10.1021/bi00056a013] [PMID: 8448138]

[20] Takanari H, Yosida T, Morita J, Izutsu K, Ito T. Instability of pleomorphic tubulin paracrystals artificially induced by Vinca alkaloids in tissue-cultured cells. Biol Cell 1990; 70(1-2): 83-90.
[http://dx.doi.org/10.1016/0248-4900(90)90363-8] [PMID: 2085693]

[21] Risinger AL, Giles FJ, Mooberry SL. Microtubule dynamics as a target in oncology. Cancer Treat Rev

2009; 35(3): 255-61.
[http://dx.doi.org/10.1016/j.ctrv.2008.11.001] [PMID: 19117686]

[22] Thomas DA, Kantarjian HM, Stock W, *et al.* Safety and efficacy of marqibo (Vincristine sulfate liposomes injection, OPTISOME™) in for the treatment of adults with relapsed or refractory acute lymphoblastic leukemia (ALL). Blood 2007; 110(11): 858.

[23] ClinicialTrials.gov. http://clinicaltrials.gov (Accessed on August 31, 2016).

[24] Yun-San Yip A, Yuen-Yuen Ong E, Chow LW. Vinflunine: Clinical perspectives of an emerging anticancer agent. Expert Opin Investig Drugs 2008; 17(4): 583-91.
[http://dx.doi.org/10.1517/13543784.17.4.583] [PMID: 18363522]

[25] Dabydeen DA, Burnett JC, Bai R, *et al.* Comparison of the activities of the truncated halichondrin B analog NSC 707389 (E7389) with those of the parent compound and a proposed binding site on tubulin. Mol Pharmacol 2006; 70(6): 1866-75.
[http://dx.doi.org/10.1124/mol.106.026641] [PMID: 16940412]

[26] Bai RL, Pettit GR, Hamel E. Binding of dolastatin 10 to tubulin at a distinct site for peptide antimitotic agents near the exchangeable nucleotide and vinca alkaloid sites. J Biol Chem 1990; 265(28): 17141-9.
[PMID: 2211617]

[27] Margolin K, Longmate J, Synold TW, *et al.* Dolastatin-10 in metastatic melanoma: A Phase II and pharmokinetic trial of the California Cancer Consortium. Invest New Drugs 2001; 19(4): 335-40.
[http://dx.doi.org/10.1023/A:1010626230081] [PMID: 11561695]

[28] Vaishampayan U, Glode M, Du W, *et al.* Phase II study of dolastatin-10 in patients with hormone-refractory metastatic prostate adenocarcinoma. Clin Cancer Res 2000; 6(11): 4205-8.
[PMID: 11106233]

[29] Hoffman MA, Blessing JA, Lentz SS. Gynecologic Oncology Group Study. A Phase II trial of dolastatin-10 in recurrent platinum-sensitive ovarian carcinoma: A Gynecologic Oncology Group study. Gynecol Oncol 2003; 89(1): 95-8.
[http://dx.doi.org/10.1016/S0090-8258(03)00007-6] [PMID: 12694660]

[30] Vaishampayan U, Glode M, Du W, *et al.* Phase II study of dolastatin-10 in patients with hormone-refractory metastatic prostate adenocarcinoma. Clin Cancer Res 2000; 6(11): 4205-8.
[PMID: 11106233]

[31] Mross K, Berdel WE, Fiebig HH, Velagapudi R, von Broen IM, Unger C. Clinical and pharmacologic Phase I study of Cemadotin-HCl (LU103793), a novel antimitotic peptide, given as 24-hour infusion in patients with advanced cancer. A study of the Arbeitsgemeinschaft Internistische Onkologie (AIO) Phase I Group and Arbeitsgruppe Pharmakologie in der Onkologie und Haematologie (APOH) Group of the German Cancer Society. Ann Oncol 1998; 9(12): 1323-30.
[http://dx.doi.org/10.1023/A:1008430515881] [PMID: 9932163]

[32] Mita AC, Hammond LA, Bonate PL, *et al.* Phase I and pharmacokinetic study of tasidotin hydrochloride (ILX651), a third-generation dolastatin-15 analogue, administered weekly for 3 weeks every 28 days in patients with advanced solid tumors. Clin Cancer Res 2006; 12(17): 5207-15.
[http://dx.doi.org/10.1158/1078-0432.CCR-06-0179] [PMID: 16951240]

[33] Garg V, Zhang W, Gidwani P, Kim M, Kolb EA. Preclinical analysis of tasidotin HCl in Ewing's sarcoma, rhabdomyosarcoma, synovial sarcoma, and osteosarcoma. Clin Cancer Res 2007; 13(18 Pt 1): 5446-54.
[http://dx.doi.org/10.1158/1078-0432.CCR-06-2661] [PMID: 17875774]

[34] Smith CD, Zhang X, Mooberry SL, Patterson GM, Moore RE. Cryptophycin: A new antimicrotubule agent active against drug-resistant cells. Cancer Res 1994; 54(14): 3779-84.
[PMID: 7913408]

[35] Smith CD, Zhang X. Mechanism of action cryptophycin. Interaction with the Vinca alkaloid domain of tubulin. J Biol Chem 1996; 271(11): 6192-8.

[http://dx.doi.org/10.1074/jbc.271.11.6192] [PMID: 8626409]

[36] Edelman MJ, Gandara DR, Hausner P, *et al.* Phase 2 study of cryptophycin 52 (LY355703) in patients previously treated with platinum based chemotherapy for advanced non-small cell lung cancer. Lung Cancer 2003; 39(2): 197-9.
[http://dx.doi.org/10.1016/S0169-5002(02)00511-1] [PMID: 12581573]

[37] Ravelli RB, Gigant B, Curmi PA, *et al.* Insight into tubulin regulation from a complex with colchicine and a stathmin-like domain. Nature 2004; 428(6979): 198-202.
[http://dx.doi.org/10.1038/nature02393] [PMID: 15014504]

[38] Brossi A, Yeh HJ, Chrzanowska M, *et al.* Colchicine and its analogues: Recent findings. Med Res Rev 1988; 8(1): 77-94.
[http://dx.doi.org/10.1002/med.2610080105] [PMID: 3278182]

[39] Bhattacharyya B, Panda D, Gupta S, Banerjee M. Anti-mitotic activity of colchicine and the structural basis for its interaction with tubulin. Med Res Rev 2008; 28(1): 155-83.
[http://dx.doi.org/10.1002/med.20097] [PMID: 17464966]

[40] Ben-Chetrit E, Levy M. Colchicine: 1998 update. Semin Arthritis Rheum 1998; 28(1): 48-59.
[http://dx.doi.org/10.1016/S0049-0172(98)80028-0] [PMID: 9726336]

[41] LaVallee TM, Zhan XH, Herbstritt CJ, Kough EC, Green SJ, Pribluda VS. 2-Methoxyestradiol inhibits proliferation and induces apoptosis independently of estrogen receptors α and β. Cancer Res 2002; 62(13): 3691-7.
[PMID: 12097276]

[42] Mabjeesh NJ, Escuin D, LaVallee TM, *et al.* 2ME2 inhibits tumor growth and angiogenesis by disrupting microtubules and dysregulating HIF. Cancer Cell 2003; 3(4): 363-75.
[http://dx.doi.org/10.1016/S1535-6108(03)00077-1] [PMID: 12726862]

[43] Fotsis T, Zhang Y, Pepper MS, *et al.* The endogenous oestrogen metabolite 2-methoxyoestradiol inhibits angiogenesis and suppresses tumour growth. Nature 1994; 368(6468): 237-9.
[http://dx.doi.org/10.1038/368237a0] [PMID: 7511798]

[44] Dahut WL, Lakhani NJ, Gulley JL, *et al.* Phase I clinical trial of oral 2-methoxyestradiol, an antiangiogenic and apoptotic agent, in patients with solid tumors. Cancer Biol Ther 2006; 5(1): 22-7.
[http://dx.doi.org/10.4161/cbt.5.1.2349] [PMID: 16357512]

[45] James J, Murry DJ, Treston AM, *et al.* Phase I safety, pharmacokinetic and pharmacodynamic studies of 2-methoxyestradiol alone or in combination with docetaxel in patients with locally recurrent or metastatic breast cancer. Invest New Drugs 2007; 25(1): 41-8.
[http://dx.doi.org/10.1007/s10637-006-9008-5] [PMID: 16969706]

[46] ENMD-1198 CAS. 864668-87-1. www.entremed.com/science/enmd-1198 (Accessed on June 19, 2017).

[47] LaVallee TM, Burke PA, Swartz GM, *et al.* Significant antitumor activity *in vivo* following treatment with the microtubule agent ENMD-1198. Mol Cancer Ther 2008; 7(6): 1472-82.
[http://dx.doi.org/10.1158/1535-7163.MCT-08-0107] [PMID: 18566218]

[48] LP-251. Locus Pharmaceuticals http://www.locuspharmaceuticals.com/programs/lp-261 (Accessed on June 19, 2017).

[49] Mita M, Spear M, Yee L, *et al.* Phase 1 dose escalation trial of the novel vascular disrupting agent NPI-2358. AACR Annual Meeting. 2008. San Diego, CA, (2008).

[50] Elie-Caille C, Severin F, Helenius J, Howard J, Muller DJ, Hyman AA. Straight GDP-tubulin protofilaments form in the presence of taxol. Curr Biol 2007; 17(20): 1765-70.
[http://dx.doi.org/10.1016/j.cub.2007.08.063] [PMID: 17919908]

[51] Andreu JM, Bordas J, Diaz JF, *et al.* Low resolution structure of microtubules in solution. Synchrotron X-ray scattering and electron microscopy of taxol-induced microtubules assembled from purified

tubulin in comparison with glycerol and MAP-induced microtubules. J Mol Biol 1992; 226(1): 169-84. [http://dx.doi.org/10.1016/0022-2836(92)90132-4] [PMID: 1352357]

[52] Rao S, He L, Chakravarty S, Ojima I, Orr GA, Horwitz SB. Characterization of the Taxol binding site on the microtubule. Identification of Arg(282) in β-tubulin as the site of photoincorporation of a 7-benzophenone analogue of taxol. J Biol Chem 1999; 274(53): 37990-4. [http://dx.doi.org/10.1074/jbc.274.53.37990] [PMID: 10608867]

[53] Okouneva T, Hill BT, Wilson L, Jordan MA. The effects of vinflunine, vinorelbine, and vinblastine on centromere dynamics. Mol Cancer Ther 2003; 2(5): 427-36. [PMID: 12748304]

[54] Montero A, Fossella F, Hortobagyi G, Valero V. Docetaxel for treatment of solid tumours: A systematic review of clinical data. Lancet Oncol 2005; 6(4): 229-39. [http://dx.doi.org/10.1016/S1470-2045(05)70094-2] [PMID: 15811618]

[55] Leonard GD, Fojo T, Bates SE. The role of ABC transporters in clinical practice. Oncologist 2003; 8(5): 411-24. [http://dx.doi.org/10.1634/theoncologist.8-5-411] [PMID: 14530494]

[56] Sève P, Dumontet C. Is class III β-tubulin a predictive factor in patients receiving tubulin-binding agents? Lancet Oncol 2008; 9(2): 168-75. [http://dx.doi.org/10.1016/S1470-2045(08)70029-9] [PMID: 18237851]

[57] Orr GA, Verdier-Pinard P, McDaid H, Horwitz SB. Mechanisms of taxol resistance related to microtubules. Oncogene 2003; 22(47): 7280-95. [http://dx.doi.org/10.1038/sj.onc.1206934] [PMID: 14576838]

[58] Gradishar WJ, Tjulandin S, Davidson N, *et al.* Phase III trial of nanoparticle albumin-bound paclitaxel compared with polyethylated castor oil-based paclitaxel in women with breast cancer. J Clin Oncol 2005; 23(31): 7794-803. [http://dx.doi.org/10.1200/JCO.2005.04.937] [PMID: 16172456]

[59] Kowalski RJ, Giannakakou P, Hamel E. Activities of the microtubule-stabilizing agents epothilones A and B with purified tubulin and in cells resistant to paclitaxel (Taxol(R)). J Biol Chem 1997; 272(4): 2534-41. [http://dx.doi.org/10.1074/jbc.272.4.2534] [PMID: 8999970]

[60] Padzur R, Keegan P. FDA approval for Ixabepilone. Cancer topics 2007. Available at: http://www.cancer.gov.cancertopics/druginfo/fda-ixbepilone

[61] Fumoleau P, Coudert B, Isambert N, Ferrant E. Novel tubulin-targeting agents: anticancer activity and pharmacologic profile of epothilones and related analogues. Ann Oncol 2007; 18 (Suppl 5): v9-v15. [http://dx.doi.org/10.1093/annonc/mdm173] [PMID: 17656562]

[62] Trivedi M, Budihardjo I, Loureiro K, Reid TR, Ma JD. Epothilones: A novel class of microtubule-stabilizing drugs for the treatment of cancer. Future Oncol 2008; 4(4): 483-500. [http://dx.doi.org/10.2217/14796694.4.4.483] [PMID: 18684060]

[63] Martello LA, McDaid HM, Regl DL, *et al.* Taxol and discodermolide represent a synergistic drug combination in human carcinoma cell lines. Clin Cancer Res 2000; 6(5): 1978-87. [PMID: 10815923]

[64] Huang GS, Lopez-Barcons L, Freeze BS, *et al.* Potentiation of taxol efficacy and by discodermolide in ovarian carcinoma xenograft-bearing mice. Clin Cancer Res 2006; 12(1): 298-304. [http://dx.doi.org/10.1158/1078-0432.CCR-05-0229] [PMID: 16397055]

[65] Buey RM, Barasoain I, Jackson E, *et al.* Microtubule interactions with chemically diverse stabilizing agents: Thermodynamics of binding to the paclitaxel site predicts cytotoxicity. Chem Biol 2005; 12(12): 1269-79. [http://dx.doi.org/10.1016/j.chembiol.2005.09.010] [PMID: 16356844]

[66] Tinley TL, Randall-Hlubek DA, Leal RM, *et al.* Taccalonolides E and A: Plant-derived steroids with

microtubule-stabilizing activity. Cancer Res 2003; 63(12): 3211-20.
[PMID: 12810650]

[67] Risinger AL, Jackson EM, Polin LA, *et al.* The taccalonolides: Microtubule stabilizers that circumvent clinically relevant taxane resistance mechanisms. Cancer Res 2008; 68(21): 8881-8.
[http://dx.doi.org/10.1158/0008-5472.CAN-08-2037] [PMID: 18974132]

[68] Hirai H, Sootome H. Method for enhancing anti-tumor effect of a microtubule-targeting drug, and a method for treatment of tumor. US9012475, 2015.

[69] Zaid GH, Burgoyne TW, Lisa S-B, Mary Ann L-S. Synergistic cancer therapy drug inventions. US20150140125, 2015.

[70] U.S. FDA Registration. http://www.fda.gov/cder/foi/nda/99/74962 (Accessed on June 19 , 2017).

[71] Kuh HJ, Kim JH. Anticancer adjuvant containing pentoxifylline. US20150374702, 2015.

[72] Jordan MA, Wilson L. Microtubules as a target for anticancer drugs. Nat Rev Cancer 2004; 4(4): 253-65.
[http://dx.doi.org/10.1038/nrc1317] [PMID: 15057285]

[73] Vasquez RJ, Howell B, Yvon AM, Wadsworth P, Cassimeris L. Nanomolar concentrations of nocodazole alter microtubule dynamic instability *in vivo* and *in vitro.* Mol Biol Cell 1997; 8(6): 973-85.
[http://dx.doi.org/10.1091/mbc.8.6.973] [PMID: 9201709]

[74] White AW, Almassy R, Calvert AH, *et al.* Resistance-modifying agents. 9. Synthesis and biological properties of benzimidazole inhibitors of the DNA repair enzyme poly(ADP-ribose) polymerase. J Med Chem 2000; 43(22): 4084-97.
[http://dx.doi.org/10.1021/jm000950v] [PMID: 11063605]

[75] Singh MP, Joseph T, Kumar S, Bathini Y, Lown JW. Synthesis and sequence-specific DNA binding of a topoisomerase inhibitory analog of Hoechst 33258 designed for altered base and sequence recognition. Chem Res Toxicol 1992; 5(5): 597-607.
[http://dx.doi.org/10.1021/tx00029a003] [PMID: 1280170]

[76] Kumar D, Patel G, Chavers AK, Chang KH, Shah K. Synthesis of novel 1,2,4-oxadiazoles and analogues as potential anticancer agents. Eur J Med Chem 2011; 46(7): 3085-92.
[http://dx.doi.org/10.1016/j.ejmech.2011.03.031] [PMID: 21481985]

[77] Jessen KA, English NM, Yu Wang J, *et al.* The discovery and mechanism of action of novel tumor-selective and apoptosis-inducing 3,5-diaryl-1,2,4-oxadiazole series using a chemical genetics approach. Mol Cancer Ther 2005; 4(5): 761-71.
[http://dx.doi.org/10.1158/1535-7163.MCT-04-0333] [PMID: 15897240]

[78] Ahmed K, Telukutla SR, Vunnam S, Ayinampudi VS, Nagula S, Madugulla VPSVV. Anticancer agent and process for the preparation thereof. US20160002214 2016.

[79] Luqmani YA. Mechanisms of drug resistance in cancer chemotherapy. Med Princ Pract 2005; 14 (Suppl. 1): 35-48.
[http://dx.doi.org/10.1159/000086183] [PMID: 16103712]

[80] Saeki T, Tsuruo T, Sato W, Nishikawsa K. Drug resistance in chemotherapy for breast cancer. Cancer Chemother Pharmacol 2005; 56(1) (Suppl. 1): 84-9.
[http://dx.doi.org/10.1007/s00280-005-0106-4] [PMID: 16273361]

[81] Hara T, Ishii T, Fujishiro M, *et al.* Glutathione S-transferase P1 has protective effects on cell viability against camptothecin. Cancer Lett 2004; 203(2): 199-207.
[http://dx.doi.org/10.1016/j.canlet.2003.09.005] [PMID: 14732228]

[82] Orr GA, Verdier-Pinard P, McDaid H, Horwitz SB. Mechanisms of taxol resistance related to microtubules. Oncogene 2003; 22(47): 7280-95.
[http://dx.doi.org/10.1038/sj.onc.1206934] [PMID: 14576838]

[83] Hisano T, Ono M, Nakayama M, Naito S, Kuwano M, Wada M. Increased expression of T-plastin gene in cisplatin-resistant human cancer cells: Identification by mRNA differential display. FEBS Lett 1996; 397(1): 101-7.
[http://dx.doi.org/10.1016/S0014-5793(96)01150-7] [PMID: 8941723]

[84] Jäättelä M. Escaping cell death: survival proteins in cancer. Exp Cell Res 1999; 248(1): 30-43.
[http://dx.doi.org/10.1006/excr.1999.4455] [PMID: 10094811]

[85] Fujita T, Ito K, Izumi H, *et al.* Increased nuclear localization of transcription factor Y-box binding protein 1 accompanied by up-regulation of P-glycoprotein in breast cancer pretreated with paclitaxel. Clin Cancer Res 2005; 11(24 Pt 1): 8837-44.
[http://dx.doi.org/10.1158/1078-0432.CCR-05-0945] [PMID: 16361573]

[86] Ye K. Nucleophosmin/B23, a multifunctional protein that can regulate apoptosis. Cancer Biol Ther 2005; 4(9): 918-23.
[http://dx.doi.org/10.4161/cbt.4.9.2072] [PMID: 16103750]

[87] Tawfic S, Yu S, Wang H, Faust R, Davis A, Ahmed K. Protein kinase CK2 signal in neoplasia. Histol Histopathol 2001; 16(2): 573-82.
[PMID: 11332713]

[88] Faust RA, Gapany M, Tristani P, Davis A, Adams GL, Ahmed K. Elevated protein kinase CK2 activity in chromatin of head and neck tumors: Association with malignant transformation. Cancer Lett 1996; 101(1): 31-5.
[http://dx.doi.org/10.1016/0304-3835(96)04110-9] [PMID: 8625279]

[89] Seldin DC, Leder P. Casein kinase II alpha transgene-induced murine lymphoma: Relation to theileriosis in cattle. Science 1995; 267(5199): 894-7.
[http://dx.doi.org/10.1126/science.7846532] [PMID: 7846532]

[90] Ahmed K, Gerber DA, Cochet C. Joining the cell survival squad: An emerging role for protein kinase CK2. Trends Cell Biol 2002; 12(5): 226-30.
[http://dx.doi.org/10.1016/S0962-8924(02)02279-1] [PMID: 12062170]

[91] Rodriguez SE, Negrin YT, Ulloa AR, *et al.* Pharmaceutical combination for the treatment and/or chemosensibilization of refractory tumors to anticancer drugs. US8871725, 2014.

[92] Fawzy IM, Youssef KM, Abouzid KAM, Mohamed NS. Novel curcumin analogs with anticancer activity. WO2015067282, 2015.

[93] Perrée M, Hallquist AE. System and method for anti-cancer drug candidate evaluation. WO2011123103, 2011.

[94] Lavitrano M, Dalpra L, Conconi D, Grassilli E. Methods for determining the sensitivity or resistance of cancer cells to at least one anticancer drug and/or therapeutically active molecule. WO2015193702, 2015.

[95] Shrikhande S, Bajaj AN, Malhotra G, Raut P. Pharmaceutical compositions of polymeric nanoparticles. WO2016020697, 2016.

[96] Chen M-H, Chuang S-H, Chen Y-J, *et al.* Tubulin inhibitors and methods of using the same. US8883793, 2014.

[97] Gangjee A. Bicyclic and tricyclic pyrimidine tyrosine kinase inhibitors with antitubulin activity and methods of treating a patient. US9139590, 2015.

[98] Pettit GR, Lippert JW. Combretastatin A-1 phosphate and Combretastatin B-1 phosphate prodrugs. US7078552, 2006.

[99] Pinney KG, Madhavi S. Combretastatin analogs with tubulin binding activity. US7429681, 2008.

CHAPTER 3

Effects of Inflammation, Mitochondria and Energy Metabolism in the Heart due to Cancer

Thomas G. Ikonomidis[1], **Timothy C. Tan**[1,2] and **Patsie Polly**[1,*]

[1] *Mechanisms of Disease and Translational Research Group, Department of Pathology, School of Medical Sciences, University of New South Wales, Sydney 2052, Australia*

[2] *Western Clinical School and Westmead Hospital, Westmead, New South Wales, Australia*

Abstract: Cancer cachexia is a paraneoplastic syndrome characterised by significant skeletal muscle wasting and cardiac atrophy. It occurs in 50% of patients with cancer and approximately 20% of cancer deaths are attributed to cachexia. Heart failure due to cancer cachexia is suggested to contribute to the high mortality rate and currently there is limited therapeutic intervention. The relationship between inflammation and energy metabolism as well as mitochondrial dysfunction in the heart in the context of cancer cachexia will be discussed. This chapter provides an understanding of potential, novel molecular mechanisms that could be of interest when considering therapeutic interventions for heart failure due to cancer cachexia. In summary, several interrelated molecular effects should be considered in cancer-induced cachexia in cardiomyocytes. TNF-α induced mitochondrial dysfunction may be important for the generation of ROS. IL-6 may induce an autophagic/mitophagic response as a result of downregulation of mitochondrial STAT3 due to mTOR suppression. An imbalance in mitochondrial dynamics may contribute to insulin-resistance and atrophy. Decreased expression of ANT1 may contribute to MPTP dysfunction and an altered energetic profile from adult to fetal metabolism. The effects of ANT1 expression in cardiac muscle during cancer cachexia is worth investigating in mouse models as discussed with reference to an ANT1 patent in this chapter. Furthermore, patents that are relevant for therapeutic strategies to ameliorate heart failure in cancer cachexia have also been discussed. Patents addressing interventions that could be applied to cancer cachexia-induced cardiac atrophy include: sodium selenite treatment, inhibitory agents of NADPH oxidase such as phycobilin, an AMPK inhibitor, modulation of mitochondrial biogenesis and modulation of mTOR. Understanding the underlying molecular mechanisms of mitochondrial dysfunction in cardiomyocytes during cancer cachexia-induced cardiac atrophy may reveal novel molecular targets for therapeutic intervention.

Keywords: Cancer, cancer cachexia, cardiac atrophy, cardiomyocyte, energy metabolism, heart failure, inflammation, inflammatory cytokines, mitochondria,

[*] **Corresponding author Patsie Polly:** Mechanisms of Disease and Translational Research Group, Department of Pathology, School of Medical Sciences, University of New South Wales, Sydney, NSW 2052, Australia; Tel: +61 2 9385 2924; Fax: +61 2 9385 1389; E-mail: patsie.polly@unsw.edu.au

Atta-ur-Rahman and Khurshid Zaman (Eds.)

mitochondrial dynamics, mitochondrial dysfunction, mitophagy, muscle wasting.

1. INTRODUCTION

Cancer cachexia is a multifaceted paraneoplastic syndrome occurring in approximately 50% of patients with cancer [1, 2]. It is a significant contributor to cancer morbidity and mortality, with approximately 20% of cancer deaths due to this syndrome [1, 2]. The disease is defined as progressive skeletal muscle wasting with anorexia, increased catabolic drive and functional impairment that is not effectively reversed with nutritional supplementation [3]. Heart failure and cardiac atrophy have also been reported in cancer cachexia [4]. Recent investigations suggest that cardiac atrophy may contribute to the high mortality rates in patients with cancer induced cachexia [5, 6]. The pathogenic mechanisms of cancer cachexia-induced cardiac failure are not well established.

Current research on cancer cachexia in cardiac tissue has relied on the development of animal and cell culture models due to the reduced availability and accessibility of human clinical samples [4]. Given the significant metabolic derangement in patients with cancer-induced cachexia, mitochondrial dysfunction may play a role in the pathogenesis of cancer cachexia-induced heart failure [7 - 9]. This chapter will focus on how known pathological mechanisms and previously identified key molecules relate to mitochondrial dysfunction in the heart in the context of cancer cachexia.

2. INFLAMMATORY CYTOKINES AND MITOCHONDRIAL DYSFUNCTION IN CARDIAC TISSUE

2.1. Tumour Necrosis Factor-α

Elevated inflammatory cytokines may facilitate heart failure in cancer cachexia by affecting cardiomyocyte mitochondrial function. Tumour Necrosis Factor (TNF)-α induced mitochondrial dysfunction in cardiomyocytes involves the generation of increased reactive oxygen species (ROS) [10, 11]. ROS may either induce, or result from, mitochondrial dysfunction. Therefore, investigating the source of ROS in cardiomyocytes may determine if mitochondrial dysfunction is a primary or secondary process in the pathogenesis of cancer cachexia in the heart. The main mitochondrial source of ROS in the heart is the electron transport chain (ETC), whilst non-mitochondrial sources in the heart include NADPH oxidases (Nox) and uncoupled nitric oxide synthases (NOS) [12]. TNF-α administered to a rat cardiomyocyte cell culture model demonstrated that the ETC was the major source of ROS [10]. Furthermore, in a ventricular pacing-induced canine model of

Congestive Heart Failure (CHF), TNF-α inhibition partially and completely restored cardiomyocyte mitochondrial complex III and ATP synthase activities respectively and ameliorated oxidative stress (Table **1**) [13]. Thus, demonstrating that ETC is a source of ROS. In another ventricular pacing-induced canine model of CHF, blocking the function of complex I in the ETC in cardiomyocytes increased ROS production 2.8-fold. Interestingly, complex I enzymatic activity was decreased in the context of heart failure, possibly contributing to uncoupling and ROS production in mitochondria [14]. Further evidence of an ETC source has also been observed in a fibrosarcoma cell culture model, where TNF-α primarily produced ROS at the ubiquinone site [15]. These studies suggest a potential role for TNF-α- induced alterations in mitochondrial function in cardiomyocytes. Future therapeutic strategies, such as sodium selenite treatment, could target mitochondrial dysfunction to ameliorate cancer cachexia-induced cardiac atrophy [16].

Table 1. Summary of the Effects of Inflammatory Cytokines on Mitochondria in the Heart.

Cytokine	Model	Effect of the Cytokine Studied	Mechanism or Signalling Pathway	Reference
TNF-α	Canine model of pacing-induced CHF	Mitochondrial production of ROS	Complex III and ATP synthase dysfunction	Moe *et al.*, 2004 [13]
	Adult human cardiomyocyte cell culture	Activation of NF-kβ	NADPH oxidase production of ROS	Moe *et al.*, 2014 [17]
	Adult male Sprague-Dawley rats	Decreased ANT protein levels Altered membrane permeability transition pore opening in mitochondria	Increased ROS Unknown - hypothesised to be due to down regulation of ANT1	Mariappan *et al.*, 2007 [19]
	Neonatal Wilstar rat ventricular cell culture	ROS mediated mitochondrial DNA damage	Sphingomyelin-ceramide pathway	Suematsu *et al.*, 2003 [10]
IL-6	Simulated ischemia/reperfusion in neonatal Sprague-Dawley rat ventricular cell culture	Increase inner mitochondrial membrane polarisation and increase mitochondrial Ca^{2+} loading	PI3-kinase/Akt pathway	Smart *et al.*, 2006 [32]

In addition to the ETC, there are other non-mitochondrial sources of ROS in the heart including Nox and NOS [12]. There is emerging evidence for TNF-α-induced ROS generation from NADPH oxidase in cardiomyocytes [17] and TNF-α/IL-6/IL-2 mediated NOS dysfunction in papillary muscle cells [18]. Mariappan *et al.* [19], demonstrated in a healthy adult Sprague-Dawley rat model treated with TNF-α, that the mRNA and protein expression of NADPH oxidase enzyme subunits gp91phox and Nox1 were increased following TNF-α treatment. This evidence implies that Nox is also a source of ROS following TNF-α signalling in cardiomyocytes [19]. However, administration of the Nox inhibitor, apocynin, to TNF-α treated rats only partially reversed superoxide anion levels, suggesting only a partial role of NADPH oxidase, and the existence of other sources of intracellular ROS induced by TNF-α [19]. Investigations of the relative contributions of ETC, NADPH oxidase and NOS for the generation of ROS in cancer cachexia-induced cardiac failure have yet to be fully conducted and offer potential areas for exploration. Therapeutic treatment inhibiting NADPH oxidase activity using phycobilin may be useful in the treatment of cancer cachexia-induced heart failure [20].

Mariappan *et al.*, also demonstrated in a healthy rat model that TNF-α induced the opening of the membrane permeability transition pore (MPTP) [19]. When treated with a superoxide dismutase mimetic, Tempol, the opening of MPTP was comparable to levels in controls, indicating a role of TNF-α-mediated oxidative stress in causing MPTP opening function [19]. The proteins that consist of the MPTP and their roles are still not fully elucidated. However, recent evidence indicates that Adenine Nucleotide Translocator (ANT) may regulate MPTP activity [21]. Our laboratory recently found that *SLC25a4*, the gene encoding ANT1 isoform, was down regulated in skeletal muscle in cancer cachexia [22]. Mariappan *et al.*, showed that TNF-α treated rats had reduced ANT protein expression in their hearts as shown by Western blotting. When TNF-α treated rats were given Tempol, ANT protein levels were restored to control levels, indicating that TNF-α induced ROS mediates ANT levels in cardiomyocytes [19]. This study suggests that TNF-α activated MPTPs have a disorganised structure likely due to decreased ANT protein levels, which leads to increased mitochondrial permeability and swelling [19]. A mouse model of altered ANT1 [23] may inform research investigating cardiac specific ANT1 reduced expression in a mouse model of cancer cachexia such as the colon 26 (C26) carcinoma model. This approach may explain the role of ANT1 in the pathogenesis of cardiac wasting and further define how MPTPs may be involved in TNF-α-mediated mitochondrial dysfunction.

Interestingly, in a primary cardiomyocyte cell culture model prepared from healthy neonatal Wistar rat heart ventricles, TNF-α induced an increase in mtDNA damage mediated by ROS, with possible involvement of the sphingomyelin-ceramide pathway [10]. Plasma ceramide levels are also elevated in patients with chronic heart failure and correlate to disease severity [24]. In another primary cardiomyocyte culture prepared from the ventricles of healthy neonatal Sprague-Dawley rats, ceramide mediated changes in mitochondrial functioning by stimulating mitochondrial fragmentation and increasing mitochondrial fission [25]. Further research should investigate the role of ceramide in stimulating mitochondrial fragmentation in a cardiac cell culture model of cancer cachexia.

2.2. Interleukin-6 and STAT3 Effects

There is limited direct evidence involving interleukin (IL)-6 action on cardiac muscle in patients with cancer cachexia. In patients with heart failure, IL-6 is raised and has been proposed as a possible biomarker indicating a key role in its pathogenesis [4, 26]. Signal transducer and activator of transcription (STAT) 3 is a known key mediator of skeletal muscle wasting in cancer cachexia and is a downstream IL-6 target [27]. IL-6-mediated phosphorylation of STAT3 at serine 727 enables its capacity to function in mitochondria within the heart [28]. In mouse cardiomyocytes, mitochondrial STAT3 (mitoSTAT3) functions in a transcription-independent manner to maintain complexes I and II of the ETC [28, 29]. MitoSTAT3 binds to complex I of the ETC by attaching to GRIM-19 (also known as NDUFA13), a complex I subunit [29, 30]. During ischaemia-induced cardiomyocyte stress, mitoSTAT3 may function to reduce ROS production and retain cytochrome C to prevent apoptosis [31]. Furthermore, in ischaemia/ reperfusion injury, IL-6 signalling mediates a cardioprotective function through the PI3-kinase/Akt pathway to increase mitochondrial calcium loading and polarisation of the inner mitochondrial membrane (Table **1**) [32]. However, GRIM-19 has been shown to mediate retinoic acid, TNF-α, and IFN-β induced cytotoxicity, by increasing ROS generation [30, 33].

Therefore, mitoSTAT3 and GRIM-19 have been implicated in both cytotoxic and cytoprotective processes in a range of both pathological and physiological conditions. This has been supported by observations in animal models where inhibition of STAT3 has been reported to ameliorate muscle wasting [34] and cardiomyocyte-restricted STAT3 knockout mice have developed marked cardiac fibrosis and dysfunction [35]. However, there is limited direct evidence involving IL-6 action on cardiac muscle in patients with cancer cachexia. Future research is still needed to determine whether mitoSTAT3 has a cytoprotective or cytotoxic role in response to IL-6/TNF-α signalling in cancer cachexia-induced cardiac failure.

In a mouse fibrosarcoma cell culture model, mitoSTAT3 cytotoxic effects were linked to TNF-α induced receptor-interacting serine/threonine-protein kinase (RIPK)-1 activity [30]. RIPK-1 signalling is involved in apoptosis via caspase-8

[36], whereas caspase-3 and caspase-9 did not increase in cardiomyocytes in the C26 mouse model, indicating a non-apoptotic mechanism of cardiac atrophy [37]. Therefore, RIPK-1 activity is less likely to induce mitoSTAT3 in cardiomyocytes in cancer cachexia. Furthermore, mTOR may phosphorylate serine 727 on STAT3 which does not result in cytotoxicity [38, 39]. In the $Apc^{Min/+}$ mouse model of cancer cachexia, IL-6 overexpression led to suppressed mTOR phosphorylation of glucose and an induction of STAT3 in skeletal muscle [40]. This may suggest that IL-6 signalling decreases mitoSTAT3 production whilst enhancing phosphorylation of tyrosine 705 on STAT 3 (pY705-STAT3).

3. MITOCHONDRIAL DYSFUNCTION AND CANCER CACHEXIA

Mitochondria may play a role in muscle protein degradation in cancer cachexia, most likely through dysfunction and imbalance of mitochondrial dynamics. Mitochondrial dynamics are the dynamic processes of fission, fusion, transport and mitophagy, which would in turn affect energy stress, apoptosis and generation of ROS processes [7, 41]. These processes activate downstream AMPK signalling and the FoxO gene network to cause muscle proteolytic activation [41, 42]. Therapeutic administration of an AMPK inhibitor may be useful in the treatment of cancer cachexia [43]. The imbalance of mitochondrial dynamics is suggested to favour an increase in mitochondrial fission and decrease in mitochondrial fusion in the skeletal muscle of mice with cancer cachexia. This imbalance in mitochondrial dynamics occurs in both oxidative and glycolytic muscle such as soleus and gastrocnemius [44]. Inhibition of muscle mitochondrial fission in obese mice improved insulin signalling and systemic sensitivity [45], suggesting that altered mitochondrial dynamics in cancer cachexia may contribute to the associated insulin-resistance. Furthermore, induction of mitochondrial fission proteins triggered skeletal muscle atrophy in mice [46]. While observed mitochondrial dynamics in cardiomyocytes in cancer cachexia are limited, it is feasible that similar mechanisms may be occurring in hearts to what is known in skeletal muscle.

Regulation of muscle protein degradation in skeletal muscle in cancer cachexia is via both ATP-dependent and ATP-independent mechanisms [42]. An ATP-dependent process occurs early in the progression of cancer cachexia and is related to the ubiquitin-proteasome system (UPS), whilst an ATP-independent process occurs later and is related to autophagy [42]. In animal models, ATP-mediated UPS is the major proteolytic pathway involved in the breakdown of skeletal muscle in cancer cachexia [47, 48]. Skeletal muscle samples from patients with weight loss >10% also demonstrated increased mRNA levels of proteasome subunits C2 and C5 [49]. Increased expression of two ubiquitin-protein ligases, atrogin-1 and MuRF-1, have been used as well-established markers for protein breakdown in the C26 model, however the reliability of atrogin-1 as a marker for muscle proteolysis has recently come under scrutiny [50]. Increased expression of MuRF-1 by 11-fold was observed in the skeletal muscle of C26 mice. However, in the same mice, expression of MuRF-1 did not increase in the atrophied hearts [37]. Interestingly contradictory evidence has been observed in C26 models where MuRF-1 was increased in cardiac tissue providing evidence for ubiquitination [51]. The discrepancies may be explained as the baseline expression of UPS is greater in cardiac muscle than skeletal muscle in rodents [52]. Indeed, findings from gene array experiments from our laboratory indicate that protein breakdown signalling pathways are not as prominent in C26 hearts when compared to C26 skeletal muscle [22]. Therefore, the role of UPS activity in protein degradation in cardiomyocytes in rodents remains unclear and further research is needed.

In the *Apc*$^{Min/+}$ mouse model of cancer cachexia, a reduction in muscle mitochondrial content was observed in intermediate and severe cancer cachexia. Furthermore, a parallel reduction in expression of mitochondrial proteins cytochrome C and Cox IV was observed [7]. The expression of mitochondrial fusion proteins mitofusin 1 (Mfn1) and Mfn2 were reduced while mitochondrial fission protein (FIS1) was increased [7]. IL-6 over expression also increased autophagy related protein levels and mRNA expression of ubiquitin related proteins [7]. IL-6 inhibition and exercise attenuated all of these findings, indicating that IL-6 is a key mediator of the observed mitochondrial dysfunction in the *Apc*$^{Min/+}$ mouse model. In this study, it was proposed that muscle mitochondrial loss does not occur early on in cachexia, rather mitochondrial loss progresses as cachexia progresses and coincides with apoptosis and induction of autophagy [7, 53]. A proposed mechanism suggests that suppression of mitochondrial biogenesis at onset of cachexia causes mitochondrial loss and dysfunction observed at later stages of cancer cachexia. Interestingly, it is suggested that suppression of mTORC1 complex and down-regulation of peroxisome proliferator-activated receptor-gamma co-activator 1 alpha (PGC-1α) causes a reduction of muscle mitochondrial content and may be involved with apoptosis [54, 55]. Future therapeutic treatments involving modulation of mitochondrial biogenesis may ameliorate skeletal muscle wasting in cancer cachexia [56].

Under normal physiological conditions in the heart, 60-90% of metabolism is via fatty acid oxidation whilst the remaining 10-40% is derived equally from glycolysis and lactate oxidation [57]. PGC-1α is a master regulator of metabolism, inducing mitochondrial biogenesis and fatty acid utilisation in the heart [58, 59]. Studies indicate that PGC-1α is involved in ROS regulation, and may be suppressed in skeletal muscle in cancer cachexia [44]. In a rat model of congestive heart failure, down regulation of PGC-1α was observed in the heart (Table **2**) [60].

Fatty acid oxidation is decreased in advanced heart failure, whereas glucose utilisation is increased as the failing heart changes to a fetal metabolic gene profile [61 - 63]. However, it has been reported that glucose utilisation decreases in advanced heart failure, and this may be due to increased insulin-resistance [64]. Reduction in PGC-1α also leads to impairment of oxidative phosphorylation and loss of contractile reserve in cardiomyocytes [65] suggesting its role as a modulator of muscle oxidative capacity in cardiac and skeletal muscles [60]. Furthermore, in skeletal muscle, overexpression of PGC-1α has a protective role in cardiac cachexia as it inhibits FoxO3 transcription and increases antioxidant gene expression [66]. Investigation on the level of PGC-1α in cardiomyocytes in cancer cachexia is required to identify the link to mitochondrial dysfunction.

Interestingly, there is also a change in the fetal gene expression pattern, demonstrating a predominance of carbohydrate metabolism in heart failure, possibly as an adaptive cardioprotective mechanism [63, 67]. This switch has also been observed in the hearts of C26 cachectic mice [51]. Peroxisome proliferator-activated receptor (PPAR)α is a regulator involved in the switch from fatty acids to glucose substrate utilisation in cardiomyocytes, where a decrease in PPARα in cardiac hypertrophy depresses fatty acid utilisation, and thus promotes glucose utilisation [64]. PPARα is shown to decrease in the cardiomyocytes of C26 mice, therefore the switch to glucose utilisation may be via a similar mechanism, indicating that the heart is attempting to protect itself as it is a vital organ [51].

Recently, the role of adenosine partial agonists as potential therapeutic agents has been described in heart failure [68]. In a microembolisation-induced canine model of heart failure, the administration of capadenoson (CAP), a partial adenosine receptor 1 (AR1) agonist, showed improvement in left ventricular systolic function and prevention of remodelling [69]. Further, treatment with CAP demonstrated an increase in muscle carnitine palmitoyl transferase (mCPT-1), an enzyme in the outer mitochondrial membrane involved in fatty acid metabolism. This may indicate that maintaining high levels of adenosine will prevent transition from adult to fetal metabolic gene expression in cardiomyocytes in heart failure. Further, in a Sprague-Dawley neonatal rat cardiomyocyte cell culture exposed to hypoxic conditions, addition of an adenosine agonist showed a reduction in MPTP opening and decreased ROS formation with involvement of downstream protein kinase C (PKC) activity [70]. Therefore, adenosine may have a role in maintaining mitochondrial function in cardiomyocytes, however the mechanism is unknown. Interestingly, in a C57BL/6J mouse macrophage cell culture model, treatment with adenosine increased IL-10 induced STAT3 phosphorylation, whilst inhibiting IL-6 induced STAT3 phosphorylation [71]. The STAT3 residue that was phosphorylated in the study was not mentioned; however, the differential regulation of adenosine on STAT3 via IL-10 and IL-6 signalling may indicate a mechanism in MPTP and ROS regulation in cardiomyocytes in cancer cachexia.

Recently, ketone oxidation has been shown to be increased in heart failure [72]. It is currently unknown whether the shift to ketone bodies is adaptive or maladaptive and future investigation into this mechanism is needed. Interestingly, in a female athymic nude mouse model with pancreatic injections of S2-013 cells to induce pancreatic cancer, the mice fed a ketogenic diet for 3 weeks had reduced tumour weight, tumour volume and a 45% increase in muscle weight [73]. The reductions in tumour cell proliferation were explained to be due to the lack of ketone oxidative capacity of the tumour leading to increased tumour apoptosis. In the same study, a cell culture model derived from differentiating mouse C2C12 premyocytes into myotubes was treated with Capan1 or S2-013 cancer cell-conditioned medium (CCCM) to mimic the effects of cancer cachexia on myotubes. Addition of ketone bodies to these C2C12 myotubes was protective against the effects of the CCCM [73]. Further, the ketone bodies caused a reduction in *MuRF1* and *Atrogin* mRNA levels which may have contributed to the reversal of myotube degradation [73]. Whilst this suggests a possible mechanism for the role of ketone bodies in the treatment of cancer cachexia there is a need for further supporting evidence. Also, given the mitochondrial dysfunction evident in cancer cachexia-induced heart failure, the role of ketone oxidative capacity in the heart of cancer patients is not certain. Therefore, further investigation into the ketone oxidative capacity in the hearts of cancer patients is required to determine if a ketogenic diet could propose as a therapeutic approach to cancer cachexia-induced heart failure.

Table 2. Summary of Mitochondrial Markers in Cancer Cachexia and Heart Failure.

Marker	**Process**	**Model**	**Increased, Decreased or Same**	**Reference**
Mfn1/Mfn2	Mitochondrial fusion	$Apc^{Min/+}$ mouse model; skeletal muscle of cancer cachexia	Decreased	White *et al.*, 2012 [7]
Fis1	Mitochondrial fission	$Apc^{Min/+}$ mouse model; skeletal muscle of cancer cachexia	Increased	White *et al.*, 2012 [7]
PGC-1α	Mitochondrial biogenesis Mitochondrial biogenesis	Rat model of congestive heart failure $Apc^{Min/+}$ mouse model; skeletal muscle of cancer cachexia	Suppressed Suppressed in severely cachectic mice	White *et al.*, 2011 [44] Garnier *et al.*, 2003 [60]

4. CANCER CACHEXIA-INDUCED CARDIOMYOCYTE AUTOPHAGY AND MITOPHAGY

Autophagy has been proposed as a major mechanism of protein degradation in cardiomyocytes in cancer cachexia [37]. Elevated LC3-II protein levels, which are a marker of autophagy detection, were significantly increased in cardiomyocytes of atrophied hearts in C26 bearing mice [37, 74]. Furthermore, autophagy was directly observed using electron microscopy of cardiomyocytes in C26 mice. Autophagy was evident as autophagosomes contained cytoplasm, myelin-like structures and mitochondria [37]. The mechanism of autophagy in cardiac pathology is unclear. Recent studies suggest that it is an adaptive response involved in prevention of protein aggregation due to increased protein turnover, and maintenance of myocyte size [75, 76]. Key regulators of cancer cachexia such as STAT3, FoxO3 and mTOR are mechanistically linked upstream of autophagy and thus may explain the observed autophagy in cardiomyocytes due to cancer [77 - 79]. Autophagy is an ATP-independent process in cancer cachexia models and occurs late in the course of disease progression [42].

Autophagy in cancer cachexia may be due to a reduced cardioprotective function of mitoSTAT3. A study on chronic alcohol induced myocardial autophagy and decreased cardiac contractility, showed that increased mTOR-STAT3 interaction may have cardioprotective effects [80]. Recent evidence suggests that inhibition of STAT3 and mTOR may also stimulate autophagy [39].

In C26 mouse skeletal muscle, there were increased levels of pY705-STAT3 in the myonuclei of the cells [81]. The levels of mitoSTAT3 in cancer cachexia have not been measured, however theoretically they may possibly be low due to suppressed mTOR phosphorylation activity in cancer cachexia. Indeed, evidence exists which implies a complex role for mTOR in autophagy induction, where its mechanism of action is not completely understood [82, 83]. Furthermore, since mitoSTAT3 negatively modulates nuclear STAT3 transcriptional activity, an increase in pY705-STAT3 indicates a decrease in mitoSTAT3 [84]. pY705-STAT3 and unphosphorylated STAT3 mediate a BNIP3 and FoxO3 pathway to autophagy respectively [77]. Future research may focus on the effects of mTOR suppression and activation on autophagy/mitophagy in cardiomyocytes in cancer cachexia. mTOR modulation could be used as a future therapeutic strategy in treating cancer cachexia-induced heart failure [85].

Unphosphorylated STAT3 may mediate a FoxO3 pathway for autophagy induction, which appears to be induced by IL-6 [77]. In skeletal muscle, FoxO3 mediates autophagy via Bnip3 and AKT signalling prevents autophagy by inhibiting FoxO3 activity [86]. Furthermore, FoxO3 independently controls both autophagy and UPS in skeletal muscle cells [86]. Research findings suggest that autophagy may be independent of mTOR activity in muscle cells *in vivo*, supporting a role for the AKT-FoxO pathway for autophagy induction (Fig. **1**) [86].

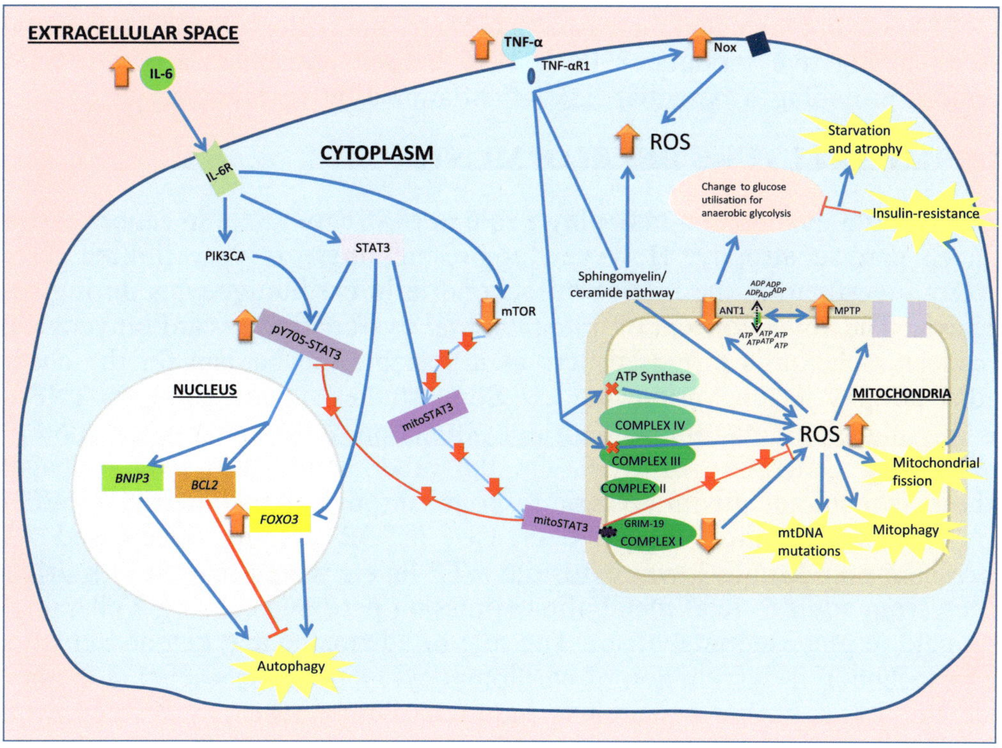

Fig. (1). A proposed mechanism of pro-inflammatory cytokine mediated mitochondrial dysfunction, autophagy and altered energy metabolism in cardiomyocytes in cancer cachexia. Upregulated IL-6 signalling increases PIK3CA levels and tyrosine phosphorylation of STAT3, resulting in pY705-STAT3. PY705-STAT3 translocates to the nucleus regulating BNIP3 and BCL2 expression to induce autophagy. Upregulated IL-6 signalling increases unphosphorylated STAT3 levels which translocate to the nucleus to increase FoxO3 which induces autophagy. Upregulated IL-6 signalling decreases mTOR serine phosphorylation of STAT3 leading to decreased levels of mitoSTAT3. Decreased mitoSTAT3 leads to decreased inhibition of pY705-STAT3 and decreased regulation of mitochondrial ROS. Upregulated TNF-α signalling causes dysfunction of complex III and ATP synthase which increases mitochondrial ROS. Upregulated TNF-α signalling causes up regulation of Nox enzymes, which increases intracellular ROS. Upregulation of TNF-α signalling activates the sphingomyelin/ceramide pathway to increase ROS which further drives mitochondrial fission. Downregulation of complex I by an unknown mechanism also contributes to increased mitochondrial ROS. Increased mitochondrial ROS leads to decreased ANT1 expression in the inner mitochondrial membrane. Increased mitochondrial ROS causes increased membrane permeability transport pores (MPTP) which interact with low levels of ANT1 to cause MPTP dysfunction and subsequent mitochondrial swelling. Increased mitochondrial ROS may also promote autophagy and mtDNA mutations leading to further mitochondrial dysfunction. Decreased ANT1 expression may mediate a reduction in cytosolic ATP levels leading to a change in energy metabolism to glucose for anaerobic glycolysis. Mitochondrial fission contributes to insulin-resistance which prevents anaerobic glycolysis, leading to cellular starvation and atrophy.

Recently, STAT1 was shown to localise to the mitochondria following simulated ischaemia-reperfusion injury and binds to LC3b, in a cardiomyocyte cell culture from the heart ventricle of healthy neonatal Sprague-Dawley rats [87]. Also, STAT1 knockout mice had increased mitophagy in cardiomyocytes, suggesting its role as a negative modulator [87]. IL-6 causes phosphorylation of STAT1, therefore providing a potential link of inflammation to mitophagy.

CURRENT & FUTURE DEVELOPMENTS

Mitochondrial dysfunction may play a role in cardiomyocytes in cancer cachexia-induced cardiac atrophy. However, at present, there is very limited research directly investigating the role of mitochondria in cardiomyocytes during cancer cachexia. The novel concept of mitochondrial dysfunction in cardiomyocytes due to cancer cachexia is proposed here as a possible mechanism for the observed cardiac atrophy seen in various models. Some studies suggest a role for TNF-α for possibly inducing direct mitochondrial dysfunction of the electron transport chain and causing generation of ROS. On the other hand, IL-6 may propagate a pathological autophagic/mitophagic response through mitochondrial STAT3 and STAT1 downregulation due to decreased mTOR activity. Decreased ANT1 expression may lead to lower cytosolic ATP levels which may in turn drive the switch from adult to fetal metabolic expression patterns, causing a change from fatty acid to glucose metabolism. The role of adenosine and ketone oxidation in the mitochondrial dysfunction of cardiomyocytes in cancer cachexia is not well understood and further research is required. Future research developments in mitochondrial dynamics in models of cancer cachexia may determine better mechanistic insights into heart failure due to cancer cachexia. Identification of key molecular mechanisms and molecular targets may provide potential avenues for therapeutic strategies to attenuate heart failure due to cancer.

CONFLICT OF INTEREST

The authors declare no conflict of interest, financial or otherwise.

ACKNOWLEDGEMENTS

Patsie Polly was the recipient of UNSW Sydney Faculty of Medicine Research Grant Funding.

REFERENCES

[1] Evans WJ, Morley JE, Argilés J, *et al.* Cachexia: A new definition. Clin Nutr 2008; 27(6): 793-9. [http://dx.doi.org/10.1016/j.clnu.2008.06.013] [PMID: 18718696]

[2] Inagaki J, Rodriguez V, Bodey GP. Proceedings: Causes of death in cancer patients. Cancer 1974; 33(2): 568-73. [http://dx.doi.org/10.1002/1097-0142(197402)33:2<568::AID-CNCR2820330236>3.0.CO;2-2]

[PMID: 4591273]

[3] Fearon K, Strasser F, Anker SD, *et al.* Definition and classification of cancer cachexia: An international consensus. Lancet Oncol 2011; 12(5): 489-95. [http://dx.doi.org/10.1016/S1470-2045(10)70218-7] [PMID: 21296615]

[4] Kazemi-Bajestani SM, Becher H, Fassbender K, Chu Q, Baracos VE. Concurrent evolution of cancer cachexia and heart failure: Bilateral effects exist. J Cachexia Sarcopenia Muscle 2014; 5(2): 95-104. [http://dx.doi.org/10.1007/s13539-014-0137-y] [PMID: 24627226]

[5] Springer J, Tschirner A, Haghikia A, *et al.* Prevention of liver cancer cachexia-induced cardiac wasting and heart failure. Eur Heart J 2014; 35(14): 932-41. [http://dx.doi.org/10.1093/eurheartj/eht302] [PMID: 23990596]

[6] Murphy KT. The pathogenesis and treatment of cardiac atrophy in cancer cachexia. Am J Physiol Heart Circ Physiol 2016; 310(4): H466-77. [http://dx.doi.org/10.1152/ajpheart.00720.2015] [PMID: 26718971]

[7] White JP, Puppa MJ, Sato S, *et al.* IL-6 regulation on skeletal muscle mitochondrial remodeling during cancer cachexia in the ApcMin/+ mouse. Skelet Muscle 2012; 2(1): 14. [http://dx.doi.org/10.1186/2044-5040-2-14] [PMID: 22769563]

[8] Fermoselle C, García-Arumí E, Puig-Vilanova E, *et al.* Mitochondrial dysfunction and therapeutic approaches in respiratory and limb muscles of cancer cachectic mice. Exp Physiol 2013; 98(9): 1349-65. [http://dx.doi.org/10.1113/expphysiol.2013.072496] [PMID: 23625954]

[9] McLean JB, Moylan JS, Andrade FH. Mitochondria dysfunction in lung cancer-induced muscle wasting in C2C12 myotubes. Front Physiol 2014; 5: 503. [http://dx.doi.org/10.3389/fphys.2014.00503] [PMID: 25566096]

[10] Suematsu N, Tsutsui H, Wen J, *et al.* Oxidative stress mediates tumor necrosis factor-α-induced mitochondrial DNA damage and dysfunction in cardiac myocytes. Circulation 2003; 107(10): 1418-23. [http://dx.doi.org/10.1161/01.CIR.0000055318.09997.1F] [PMID: 12642364]

[11] Nakamura K, Fushimi K, Kouchi H, *et al.* Inhibitory effects of antioxidants on neonatal rat cardiac myocyte hypertrophy induced by tumor necrosis factor-α and angiotensin II. Circulation 1998; 98(8): 794-9. [http://dx.doi.org/10.1161/01.CIR.98.8.794] [PMID: 9727550]

[12] Burgoyne JR, Mongue-Din H, Eaton P, Shah AM. Redox signaling in cardiac physiology and pathology. Circ Res 2012; 111(8): 1091-106. [http://dx.doi.org/10.1161/CIRCRESAHA.111.255216] [PMID: 23023511]

[13] Moe GW, Marin-Garcia J, Konig A, Goldenthal M, Lu X, Feng Q. *In vivo* TNF-alpha inhibition ameliorates cardiac mitochondrial dysfunction, oxidative stress, and apoptosis in experimental heart failure. Am J Physiol Heart Circ Physiol 2004; 287(4): H1813-20. [http://dx.doi.org/10.1152/ajpheart.00036.2004] [PMID: 15205165]

[14] Ide T, Tsutsui H, Kinugawa S, *et al.* Mitochondrial electron transport complex I is a potential source of oxygen free radicals in the failing myocardium. Circ Res 1999; 85(4): 357-63. [http://dx.doi.org/10.1161/01.RES.85.4.357] [PMID: 10455064]

[15] Schulze-Osthoff K, Bakker AC, Vanhaesebroeck B, Beyaert R, Jacob WA, Fiers W. Cytotoxic activity of tumor necrosis factor is mediated by early damage of mitochondrial functions. Evidence for the involvement of mitochondrial radical generation. J Biol Chem 1992; 267(8): 5317-23. [PMID: 1312087]

[16] Power R, Egan C, Yiannikouris A, *et al.* Compositions comprising selenium and use of same for the treatment and prevention of disease or conditions associated with mitochondrial dysfunction. US20160113977, 2016.

[17] Moe KT, Khairunnisa K, Yin NO, Chin-Dusting J, Wong P, Wong MC. Tumor necrosis factor---induced nuclear factor-kappaB activation in human cardiomyocytes is mediated by NADPH oxidase. J Physiol Biochem 2014; 70(3): 769-79. [http://dx.doi.org/10.1007/s13105-014-0345-0] [PMID: 25059721]

[18] Finkel MS, Oddis CV, Jacob TD, Watkins SC, Hattler BG, Simmons RL. Negative inotropic effects of cytokines on the heart mediated by nitric oxide. Science 1992; 257(5068): 387-9. [http://dx.doi.org/10.1126/science.1631560] [PMID: 1631560]

[19] Mariappan N, Soorappan RN, Haque M, Sriramula S, Francis J. TNF-α-induced mitochondrial oxidative stress and cardiac dysfunction: Restoration by superoxide dismutase mimetic Tempol. Am J Physiol Heart Circ Physiol 2007; 293(5): H2726-37. [http://dx.doi.org/10.1152/ajpheart.00376.2007] [PMID: 17675574]

[20] McCarty MF, Hendler SS, Rorvik DM, Inoguchi T. Compositions for inhibiting NADPH oxidase activity. US8709434, 2014.

[21] Kwong JQ, Molkentin JD. Physiological and pathological roles of the mitochondrial permeability transition pore in the heart. Cell Metab 2015; 21(2): 206-14. [http://dx.doi.org/10.1016/j.cmet.2014.12.001] [PMID: 25651175]

[22] Shum AM, Fung DC, Corley SM, *et al.* Cardiac and skeletal muscles show molecularly distinct responses to cancer cachexia. Physiol Genomics 2015; 47(12): 588-99. [PMID: 26395599]

[23] Wallace DC, Graham BH, MacGregor GR. Mouse lacking heart-muscle adenine nucleotide translocator protein and methods. US6013858, 2000.

[24] Yu J, Pan W, Shi R, *et al.* Ceramide is upregulated and associated with mortality in patients with chronic heart failure. Can J Cardiol 2015; 31(3): 357-63. [http://dx.doi.org/10.1016/j.cjca.2014.12.007] [PMID: 25746025]

[25] Parra V, Eisner V, Chiong M, *et al.* Changes in mitochondrial dynamics during ceramide-induced cardiomyocyte early apoptosis. Cardiovasc Res 2008; 77(2): 387-97. [http://dx.doi.org/10.1093/cvr/cvm029] [PMID: 18006463]

[26] Fülster S, Tacke M, Sandek A, *et al.* Muscle wasting in patients with chronic heart failure: Results from the studies investigating co-morbidities aggravating heart failure (SICA-HF). Eur Heart J 2013; 34(7): 512-9. [http://dx.doi.org/10.1093/eurheartj/ehs381] [PMID: 23178647]

[27] Zimmers TA, Fishel ML, Bonetto A. STAT3 in the systemic inflammation of cancer cachexia. Semin Cell Dev Biol 2016; 54: 28-41. [http://dx.doi.org/10.1016/j.semcdb.2016.02.009] [PMID: 26860754]

[28] Wegrzyn J, Potla R, Chwae Y-J, *et al.* Function of mitochondrial Stat3 in cellular respiration. Science 2009; 323(5915): 793-7. [http://dx.doi.org/10.1126/science.1164551] [PMID: 19131594]

[29] Tammineni P, Anugula C, Mohammed F, Anjaneyulu M, Larner AC, Sepuri NB. The import of the transcription factor STAT3 into mitochondria depends on GRIM-19, a component of the electron transport chain. J Biol Chem 2013; 288(7): 4723-32. [http://dx.doi.org/10.1074/jbc.M112.378984] [PMID: 23271731]

[30] Shulga N, Pastorino JG. GRIM-19-mediated translocation of STAT3 to mitochondria is necessary for TNF-induced necroptosis. J Cell Sci 2012; 125(Pt 12): 2995-3003. [http://dx.doi.org/10.1242/jcs.103093] [PMID: 22393233]

[31] Szczepanek K, Chen Q, Larner AC, Lesnefsky EJ. Cytoprotection by the modulation of mitochondrial electron transport chain: The emerging role of mitochondrial STAT3. Mitochondrion 2012; 12(2): 180-9. [http://dx.doi.org/10.1016/j.mito.2011.08.011] [PMID: 21930250]

[32] Smart N, Mojet MH, Latchman DS, Marber MS, Duchen MR, Heads RJ. IL-6 induces PI 3-kinase and nitric oxide-dependent protection and preserves mitochondrial function in cardiomyocytes. Cardiovasc Res 2006; 69(1): 164-77.
[http://dx.doi.org/10.1016/j.cardiores.2005.08.017] [PMID: 16219301]

[33] Huang G, Chen Y, Lu H, Cao X. Coupling mitochondrial respiratory chain to cell death: An essential role of mitochondrial complex I in the interferon-β and retinoic acid-induced cancer cell death. Cell Death Differ 2007; 14(2): 327-37.
[http://dx.doi.org/10.1038/sj.cdd.4402004] [PMID: 16826196]

[34] Bonetto A, Aydogdu T, Jin X, *et al.* JAK/STAT3 pathway inhibition blocks skeletal muscle wasting downstream of IL-6 and in experimental cancer cachexia. Am J Physiol Endocrinol Metab 2012; 303(3): E410-21.
[http://dx.doi.org/10.1152/ajpendo.00039.2012] [PMID: 22669242]

[35] Jacoby JJ, Kalinowski A, Liu M-G, *et al.* Cardiomyocyte-restricted knockout of STAT3 results in higher sensitivity to inflammation, cardiac fibrosis, and heart failure with advanced age. Proc Natl Acad Sci USA 2003; 100(22): 12929-34.
[http://dx.doi.org/10.1073/pnas.2134694100] [PMID: 14566054]

[36] Wang L, Du F, Wang X. TNF-α induces two distinct caspase-8 activation pathways. Cell 2008; 133(4): 693-703.
[http://dx.doi.org/10.1016/j.cell.2008.03.036] [PMID: 18485876]

[37] Cosper PF, Leinwand LA. Cancer causes cardiac atrophy and autophagy in a sexually dimorphic manner. Cancer Res 2011; 71(5): 1710-20.
[http://dx.doi.org/10.1158/0008-5472.CAN-10-3145] [PMID: 21163868]

[38] Yokogami K, Wakisaka S, Avruch J, Reeves SA. Serine phosphorylation and maximal activation of STAT3 during CNTF signaling is mediated by the rapamycin target mTOR. Curr Biol 2000; 10(1): 47-50.
[http://dx.doi.org/10.1016/S0960-9822(99)00268-7] [PMID: 10660304]

[39] Yokoyama T, Kondo Y, Kondo S. Roles of mTOR and STAT3 in autophagy induced by telomere 3′ overhang-specific DNA oligonucleotides. Autophagy 2007; 3(5): 496-8.
[http://dx.doi.org/10.4161/auto.4602] [PMID: 17617738]

[40] White JP, Puppa MJ, Gao S, Sato S, Welle SL, Carson JA. Muscle mTORC1 suppression by IL-6 during cancer cachexia: A role for AMPK. Am J Physiol Endocrinol Metab 2013; 304(10): E1042-52.
[http://dx.doi.org/10.1152/ajpendo.00410.2012] [PMID: 23531613]

[41] Romanello V, Sandri M. Mitochondrial biogenesis and fragmentation as regulators of muscle protein degradation. Curr Hypertens Rep 2010; 12(6): 433-9.
[http://dx.doi.org/10.1007/s11906-010-0157-8] [PMID: 20967516]

[42] White JP, Baynes JW, Welle SL, *et al.* The regulation of skeletal muscle protein turnover during the progression of cancer cachexia in the Apc(Min/+) mouse. PLoS One 2011; 6(9): e24650.
[http://dx.doi.org/10.1371/journal.pone.0024650] [PMID: 21949739]

[43] Algire C, Herzig S. Acip/peptide-based inhibition of cancer cachexia. WO2014180908, 2014.

[44] White JP, Baltgalvis KA, Puppa MJ, Sato S, Baynes JW, Carson JA. Muscle oxidative capacity during IL-6-dependent cancer cachexia. Am J Physiol Regul Integr Comp Physiol 2011; 300(2): R201-11.
[http://dx.doi.org/10.1152/ajpregu.00300.2010] [PMID: 21148472]

[45] Jheng H-F, Tsai P-J, Guo S-M, *et al.* Mitochondrial fission contributes to mitochondrial dysfunction and insulin resistance in skeletal muscle. Mol Cell Biol 2012; 32(2): 309-19.
[http://dx.doi.org/10.1128/MCB.05603-11] [PMID: 22083962]

[46] Romanello V, Guadagnin E, Gomes L, *et al.* Mitochondrial fission and remodelling contributes to muscle atrophy. EMBO J 2010; 29(10): 1774-85.
[http://dx.doi.org/10.1038/emboj.2010.60] [PMID: 20400940]

[47] Temparis S, Asensi M, Taillandier D, *et al.* Increased ATP-ubiquitin-dependent proteolysis in skeletal muscles of tumor-bearing rats. Cancer Res 1994; 54(21): 5568-73. [PMID: 7923198]

[48] Baracos VE, DeVivo C, Hoyle DH, Goldberg AL. Activation of the ATP-ubiquitin-proteasome pathway in skeletal muscle of cachectic rats bearing a hepatoma. Am J Physiol 1995; 268(5 Pt 1): E996-E1006. [PMID: 7539218]

[49] Khal J, Hine AV, Fearon KC, Dejong CH, Tisdale MJ. Increased expression of proteasome subunits in skeletal muscle of cancer patients with weight loss. Int J Biochem Cell Biol 2005; 37(10): 2196-206. [http://dx.doi.org/10.1016/j.biocel.2004.10.017] [PMID: 16125116]

[50] Attaix D, Baracos VE. MAFbx/Atrogin-1 expression is a poor index of muscle proteolysis. Curr Opin Clin Nutr Metab Care 2010; 13(3): 223-4. [http://dx.doi.org/10.1097/MCO.0b013e328338b9a6] [PMID: 20393275]

[51] Tian M, Asp ML, Nishijima Y, Belury MA. Evidence for cardiac atrophic remodeling in cancer-induced cachexia in mice. Int J Oncol 2011; 39(5): 1321-6. [PMID: 21822537]

[52] Liu Z, Miers WR, Wei L, Barrett EJ. The ubiquitin-proteasome proteolytic pathway in heart vs. skeletal muscle: Effects of acute diabetes. Biochem Biophys Res Commun 2000; 276(3): 1255-60. [http://dx.doi.org/10.1006/bbrc.2000.3609] [PMID: 11027619]

[53] Baltgalvis KA, Berger FG, Peña MM, Mark Davis J, White JP, Carson JA. Activity level, apoptosis, and development of cachexia in Apc(Min/+) mice. J Appl Physiol 2010; 109(4): 1155-61. [http://dx.doi.org/10.1152/japplphysiol.00442.2010] [PMID: 20651218]

[54] Romanino K, Mazelin L, Albert V, *et al.* Myopathy caused by mammalian target of rapamycin complex 1 (mTORC1) inactivation is not reversed by restoring mitochondrial function. Proc Natl Acad Sci USA 2011; 108(51): 20808-13. [http://dx.doi.org/10.1073/pnas.1111448109] [PMID: 22143799]

[55] Adhihetty PJ, Uguccioni G, Leick L, Hidalgo J, Pilegaard H, Hood DA. The role of PGC-1α on mitochondrial function and apoptotic susceptibility in muscle. Am J Physiol Cell Physiol 2009; 297(1): C217-25. [http://dx.doi.org/10.1152/ajpcell.00070.2009] [PMID: 19439529]

[56] Mootha VK, Altshuler D. Methods of regulating metabolism and mitochondrial function. WO2005003766, 2005.

[57] Stanley WC, Recchia FA, Lopaschuk GD. Myocardial substrate metabolism in the normal and failing heart. Physiol Rev 2005; 85(3): 1093-129. [http://dx.doi.org/10.1152/physrev.00006.2004] [PMID: 15987803]

[58] Lin J, Handschin C, Spiegelman BM. Metabolic control through the PGC-1 family of transcription coactivators. Cell Metab 2005; 1(6): 361-70. [http://dx.doi.org/10.1016/j.cmet.2005.05.004] [PMID: 16054085]

[59] Lehman JJ, Barger PM, Kovacs A, Saffitz JE, Medeiros DM, Kelly DP. Peroxisome proliferator-activated receptor γ coactivator-1 promotes cardiac mitochondrial biogenesis. J Clin Invest 2000; 106(7): 847-56. [http://dx.doi.org/10.1172/JCI10268] [PMID: 11018072]

[60] Garnier A, Fortin D, Deloménie C, Momken I, Veksler V, Ventura-Clapier R. Depressed mitochondrial transcription factors and oxidative capacity in rat failing cardiac and skeletal muscles. J Physiol 2003; 551(Pt 2): 491-501. [http://dx.doi.org/10.1113/jphysiol.2003.045104] [PMID: 12824444]

[61] Osorio JC, Stanley WC, Linke A, *et al.* Impaired myocardial fatty acid oxidation and reduced protein expression of retinoid X receptor-α in pacing-induced heart failure. Circulation 2002; 106(5): 606-12.

[http://dx.doi.org/10.1161/01.CIR.0000023531.22727.C1] [PMID: 12147544]

[62] Nascimben L, Ingwall JS, Lorell BH, *et al.* Mechanisms for increased glycolysis in the hypertrophied rat heart. Hypertension 2004; 44(5): 662-7.
[http://dx.doi.org/10.1161/01.HYP.0000144292.69599.0c] [PMID: 15466668]

[63] Razeghi P, Young ME, Alcorn JL, Moravec CS, Frazier OH, Taegtmeyer H. Metabolic gene expression in fetal and failing human heart. Circulation 2001; 104(24): 2923-31.
[http://dx.doi.org/10.1161/hc4901.100526] [PMID: 11739307]

[64] Neubauer S. The failing heart--an engine out of fuel. N Engl J Med 2007; 356(11): 1140-51.
[http://dx.doi.org/10.1056/NEJMra063052] [PMID: 17360992]

[65] Arany Z, He H, Lin J, *et al.* Transcriptional coactivator PGC-1 α controls the energy state and contractile function of cardiac muscle. Cell Metab 2005; 1(4): 259-71.
[http://dx.doi.org/10.1016/j.cmet.2005.03.002] [PMID: 16054070]

[66] Geng T, Li P, Yin X, Yan Z. PGC-1α promotes nitric oxide antioxidant defenses and inhibits FOXO signaling against cardiac cachexia in mice. Am J Pathol 2011; 178(4): 1738-48.
[http://dx.doi.org/10.1016/j.ajpath.2011.01.005] [PMID: 21435455]

[67] Rajabi M, Kassiotis C, Razeghi P, Taegtmeyer H. Return to the fetal gene program protects the stressed heart: A strong hypothesis. Heart Fail Rev 2007; 12(3-4): 331-43.
[http://dx.doi.org/10.1007/s10741-007-9034-1] [PMID: 17516164]

[68] Greene SJ, Sabbah HN, Butler J, *et al.* Partial adenosine A1 receptor agonism: A potential new therapeutic strategy for heart failure. Heart Fail Rev 2016; 21(1): 95-102.
[http://dx.doi.org/10.1007/s10741-015-9522-7] [PMID: 26701329]

[69] Sabbah HN, Gupta RC, Kohli S, *et al.* Chronic therapy with a partial adenosine A1-receptor agonist improves left ventricular function and remodeling in dogs with advanced heart failure. Circ Heart Fail 2013; 6(3): 563-71.
[http://dx.doi.org/10.1161/CIRCHEARTFAILURE.112.000208] [PMID: 23564604]

[70] Xiang F, Huang YS, Zhang DX, Chu ZG, Zhang JP, Zhang Q. Adenosine A1 receptor activation reduces opening of mitochondrial permeability transition pores in hypoxic cardiomyocytes. Clin Exp Pharmacol Physiol 2010; 37(3): 343-9.
[http://dx.doi.org/10.1111/j.1440-1681.2009.05300.x] [PMID: 19793110]

[71] Koscsó B, Csóka B, Kókai E, *et al.* Adenosine augments IL-10-induced STAT3 signaling in M2c macrophages. J Leukoc Biol 2013; 94(6): 1309-15.
[http://dx.doi.org/10.1189/jlb.0113043] [PMID: 23922379]

[72] Aubert G, Martin OJ, Horton JL, *et al.* The failing heart relies on ketone bodies as a fuel. Circulation 2016; 133(8): 698-705.
[PMID: 26819376]

[73] Shukla SK, Gebregiworgis T, Purohit V, *et al.* Metabolic reprogramming induced by ketone bodies diminishes pancreatic cancer cachexia. Cancer Metab 2014; 2(1): 18.
[http://dx.doi.org/10.1186/2049-3002-2-18] [PMID: 25228990]

[74] Barth S, Glick D, Macleod KF. Autophagy: Assays and artifacts. J Pathol 2010; 221(2): 117-24.
[http://dx.doi.org/10.1002/path.2694] [PMID: 20225337]

[75] Tannous P, Zhu H, Nemchenko A, *et al.* Intracellular protein aggregation is a proximal trigger of cardiomyocyte autophagy. Circulation 2008; 117(24): 3070-8.
[http://dx.doi.org/10.1161/CIRCULATIONAHA.107.763870] [PMID: 18541737]

[76] Nakai A, Yamaguchi O, Takeda T, *et al.* The role of autophagy in cardiomyocytes in the basal state and in response to hemodynamic stress. Nat Med 2007; 13(5): 619-24.
[http://dx.doi.org/10.1038/nm1574] [PMID: 17450150]

[77] You L, Wang Z, Li H, *et al.* The role of STAT3 in autophagy. Autophagy 2015; 11(5): 729-39.

[http://dx.doi.org/10.1080/15548627.2015.1017192] [PMID: 25951043]

[78] Sengupta A, Molkentin JD, Yutzey KE. FoxO transcription factors promote autophagy in cardiomyocytes. J Biol Chem 2009; 284(41): 28319-31.
[http://dx.doi.org/10.1074/jbc.M109.024406] [PMID: 19696026]

[79] Jung CH, Ro S-H, Cao J, Otto NM, Kim D-H. mTOR regulation of autophagy. FEBS Lett 2010; 584(7): 1287-95.
[http://dx.doi.org/10.1016/j.febslet.2010.01.017] [PMID: 20083114]

[80] Ge W, Ren J. mTOR-STAT3-notch signalling contributes to ALDH2-induced protection against cardiac contractile dysfunction and autophagy under alcoholism. J Cell Mol Med 2012; 16(3): 616-26.
[http://dx.doi.org/10.1111/j.1582-4934.2011.01347.x] [PMID: 21609394]

[81] Bonetto A, Aydogdu T, Kunzevitzky N, *et al.* STAT3 activation in skeletal muscle links muscle wasting and the acute phase response in cancer cachexia. PLoS One 2011; 6(7): e22538.
[http://dx.doi.org/10.1371/journal.pone.0022538] [PMID: 21799891]

[82] Nobukuni T, Kozma SC, Thomas G. HVPS34, an ancient player, enters a growing game: mTOR Complex1/S6K1 signaling. Curr Opin Cell Biol 2007; 19(2): 135-41.
[http://dx.doi.org/10.1016/j.ceb.2007.02.019] [PMID: 17321123]

[83] Lum JJ, DeBerardinis RJ, Thompson CB. Autophagy in metazoans: Cell survival in the land of plenty. Nat Rev Mol Cell Biol 2005; 6(6): 439-48.
[http://dx.doi.org/10.1038/nrm1660] [PMID: 15928708]

[84] Chung J, Uchida E, Grammer TC, Blenis J. STAT3 serine phosphorylation by ERK-dependent and -independent pathways negatively modulates its tyrosine phosphorylation. Mol Cell Biol 1997; 17(11): 6508-16.
[http://dx.doi.org/10.1128/MCB.17.11.6508] [PMID: 9343414]

[85] Finan P, Keigan JM, Murphy L, Nicklin PL, Triantafellow E. Compositions and Methods for Modulating mTOR Signaling. US20090258929, 2009.

[86] Mammucari C, Milan G, Romanello V, *et al.* FoxO3 controls autophagy in skeletal muscle *in vivo.* Cell Metab 2007; 6(6): 458-71.
[http://dx.doi.org/10.1016/j.cmet.2007.11.001] [PMID: 18054315]

[87] Bourke LT, Knight RA, Latchman DS, Stephanou A, McCormick J. Signal transducer and activator of transcription-1 localizes to the mitochondria and modulates mitophagy. JAK-STAT 2013; 2(4): e25666.
[http://dx.doi.org/10.4161/jkst.25666] [PMID: 24470977]

CHAPTER 4

Chalcone and Their Derivatives as Anticancer Agents

Zahoor A. Wani and **Suaib Luqman***

Molecular Bioprospection Department, CSIR-Central institute of Medicinal and Aromatic Plants, Lucknow-226015, Uttar Pradesh, India

Abstract: Cancer has eventually stepped into the molecular insights focussing on the development of new generation of anticancer drugs especially of natural origin and its analogues with less or no toxicity issues and targeting specific molecular signalling pathways. In various therapeutic areas, numerous natural products and their derivatives have been effectively used to treat many human diseases or disorders. Chalcones, as metabolic precursors of some flavonoids and isoflavonoids have a structure of open chain flavonoids (1,3-diaryl-2-propen-1-ones) present in fruits and vegetables, possessing a broad range of biological activities including cancer chemotherapeutic and chemopreventive property. The anticancer properties of chalcones have been improved by substituting aryl rings (e.g. methoxy substitution on both aryl rings A and B) and introducing heterocyclic moieties. Hybridization with other pharmacologically important moieties (benzodiazepines, benzothiazoles, imidazolones etc.) by taking the help of SAR (structure-activity relationship) studies with much ease in preparation and oral administration ultimately has made chalcone a safe therapeutic agent. Some clinical trials revealed that these compounds did not cause toxicity and are present in plasma at optimum concentrations. Nowaday's several chalcones are also used in cosmetic formulations and in food additives which could further be utilized for its chemopreventive potential. This book chapter briefly summarizes the demanding efforts made in the development of novel anticancer chalcones recorded in recent literatures with focussed cancer targets as well as presents an outline of the patents published in recent decades.

Keywords: Angiogenesis, antiproliferative, apoptosis, cancer, cell cycle arrest, cell line, chalcone, chalcone derivatives, chemoprevention, cytotoxicity, heterocyclic chalcone derivatives, IC_{50}, metastasis, NFκB, p53, p21, p23, TRIAL, tumor.

* **Corresponding author Suaib Luqman**: CSIR-Central Institute of Medicinal and Aromatic Plants, Lucknow-226015, Uttar Pradesh, India; Tel: +91-522-2718635; Fax: +91-522-2716141; E-mail: s.luqman@cimap.res.in

Atta-ur-Rahman and Khurshid Zaman (Eds.)

1. INTRODUCTION

Chalcones are phytomolecules belonging to the largest group of secondary metabolites of plant system with chemical structure of 1, 3-diphenyl-2-propen-e-1-ones, in which the two aromatic rings are linked by three carbon α, β-unsaturated carbonyl system (Fig. **1**). The name was derived from "*chalcos*" meaning bronze due to its variant colour and it was given by Kostanecki and Tambor [1]. These compounds have a conjugated system where *p*-electron systems are delocalized with conjugated double bonds on both the benzene rings [2]. Chalcones due to their Michael acceptor features and small structure, easily bind with different cellular metabolites resulting in profound molecular and cellular effect ultimately exhibiting a broad range of biological activities [3]. Chalcones in general have lower redox potential due to enone (alkene-ketone) system and therefore, it prefers more electron transfer reactions. They are assumed to be intermediate metabolites in the synthesis of flavonoids and isoflavonoids that serve mainly for the defense system in the plants and thus protecting them from ROS (Reactive Oxygen Species) and consequently minimizing molecular and environmental injury. Functionally, it serves to regulate cholesterol levels, maintaining blood glucose levels, decrease the blood pressure, remove joint and muscle pain, help in sleep, improves immune system, liver and kidney functions, and enhance vision, skin beauty, hair growth and memory [4].

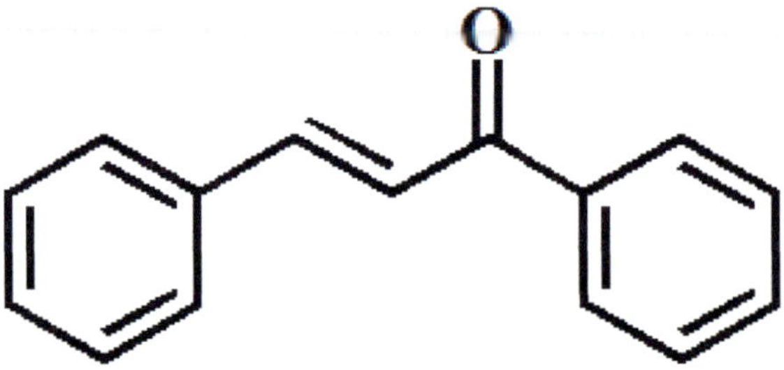

Fig. (1). Basic chalcone structure.

2. CONJUGATES AND DERIVATIVES OF CHALCONES

Chalcone has been widely used in organic synthesis to establish highly enantio-selective Michael adducts. The asymmetric catalytic conjugate adding a stabilized carbanion nucleophile to α, β-unsaturated carbonyl compounds shows one of the most essential carbon-carbon bond forming reactions in organic chemistry because the adducts are interesting intermediates for further optimization, such as amino-carbonyls, pyrrolidines and amino-alkanes. Many chalcone derivatives have also been prepared due to their convenient synthesis [3].

Madhavi *et al.* (2017) studied the synthesis of chalcones incorporating quinazoline derivatives as anticancer agents [5].

Bhale *et al.*, (2017) worked on the synthesis of protracted conjugated indolyl chalcones as the strong antioxidant, anti-inflammatory and anti-breast cancer agents [6]. Cai *et al.* (2017) studied the analogues of xanthones-chalcones and bis-chalcones as α-glucosidase inhibitors and anti-diabetes candidates [7]. Hawash and collaborators worked on the synthesis and bioactivity of novel pyrazolic chalcone derivatives as novel hepatocellular carcinoma therapeutics [8]. Ramaiah *et al.*, (2011) studied Chalcone-imidazolone conjugates and they found that these synthesized conjugates trigger DNA damage in the cells and show apoptosis [9]. Kamal *et al.*, (2015) studied about phenstatin/isocombretastatin-chalcone conjugates as effective tubulin polymerization inhibitors and mitochondrial apoptotic inducers [10]. Similarly, Khan (2009) published a patent on certain novel chalcones derivatives (in particular boronic chalcone derivatives) wherein he claimed that they possess anti-proliferative activity against cancer cells at micro molar concentrations. The invention provides the design and synthesis of novel boronic chalcone derivatives, and pharmaceutical compositions of chalcones derivatives. The invention also reveals the high activity and less toxicity of numerous compounds against breast cancer cell lines compared to normal MCF12A cells [11].

In glioblastoma cell lines, Indole chalcone has been recognized as a possible anticancer agent as it decreases the multiplication of cells under *in vitro* conditions. It was revealed that the indole chalcone battle for the binding site with colchicine and induces the inhibition of tubulin polymerization. Moreover, it distorted microtubule formation and triggered G2/M phase arrest and apoptosis. The molecule also worked as the dual inhibitor of Pgp and BCRP in glioblastoma cell line [12]. Chalcones are reported for both cancer chemotherapeutic action as well as for its chemopreventive mechanism as it possesses ability to inhibit carcinogenesis due to various modes like by increasing reduced glutathione levels and maintaining the optimum redox level [13].

TRAIL (Tumor necrosis factor related apoptosis inducing ligand) indicates programmed cell death specific to cancers and without any toxic effect to normal cells. TRAIL in association with the death receptor DR4 and/or DR5 mediates programmed cell death [14, 15]. However, decrease in the expression of pro-apoptotic proteins, TRAIL-R1 and TRAIL-R2 (death receptors) with concurrent upsurge in the level of anti-apoptotic proteins in tumor cells mediates TRAIL-resistance [16]. Szliszka *et al.* (2010) reported that the TRAIL-induced programmed cell death and cytotoxicity enhanced in prostate cancer cells by chalcones and dihydrochalcones such as phloretin. Their results show the remarkable role played by chalcones and dihydrochalcones in chemoprevention of prostate cancer by triggering the tumor cells to TRAIL-mediated programmed cell death [17].

Kamal *et al.* (2010) studied some of the chalcone derivatives against MCF-7 cell line and found that they trigger G0/G1-phase cell-cycle arrest, with decreased level of cyclins D1 and E1 and augmented expression of CDK4. Further, these molecules elicited distinctive features of programmed cell death by increasing the expression of p21, p27 and p53, thereby decreasing the NF-κB level and increasing caspase-9 expression [18]. Llango *et al.* (2010) synthesized various chalcones and evaluated them for anticancer activity by Microculture Tetrazolium Test Assay method against MCF-7 and T47D breast cancer cell lines. There was significant cytotoxicity observed against both the cell lines with IC_{50} ranging between 52-89μM [19]. Gloria *et al.* (2013) published a patent in which they claim that some novel chalcone like compounds (47a-e) significantly increased ($p < 0.01$) the cell death of two breast cancer cell lines namely MCF-7 (ER-positive) and MDA-MB435 (ER-negative). These compounds were safe on MCF-10 (normal breast epithelial cell line) [20].

Lin *et al.* (2011) synthesized 2′,5′dimethoxychalcone derivatives and asserted that these derivatives act as microtubule targeted tubulin polymerizing agents [21]. However, Rose and Hartman (2010) published a patent on modified chalcone compounds and stated that they are designed to interfere with the cell division processes in cancer cells, thereby reducing the unrestrained proliferation of cancer cells and/or decreasing tumor size [22].

Liu and Go (2007) synthesized mono as well as dibasic chalcones and interpreted that chalcones having one basic group were better anticarcinogenic agents compared to those possessing more than one basic group. Piperazinyl chalcone and piperidinyl chalcone possessing basic groups on Ring A were found to be potent cytostatic agents by interfering with cell cycle progression [23]. Bombardelli *et al.* (2003) claimed chalcone derivatives and chalcone analogues, particularly the compounds, in which the phenyl ring in 1-position is substituted by rings having one or more heteroatoms, possessing greater antiproliferative potential both on sensitive cancerous cells and on cells which are resistant to paclitaxel and docetaxel [24]. *In vitro* anticancer activity (MTT assay) of thiazolyl-chalcones has been demonstrated by Shi *et al.* (2010) against liver cancer cell line (BEL-7402), lung cancer (NCI-H460) and prostate cancer (PC-3). One of the compounds was further evaluated at 50mg/kg dose for *in vivo* anticancer activity against Sarcoma-180 tumor bearing mice, wherein it showed therapeutic efficacy of 23% [25].

4-Hydroxyderricin (a chalcone), isolated from *Angelica keiskei* by Kimura *et al.* (2004) was administered through the oral route at 50mg/kg x 2/day to Lewis lung carcinoma bearing mice. The compound inhibited lung metastasis of the tumor and enhanced the survival time of animals after surgical removal of subcutaneous tumors [26].

Nishimura *et al.* (2007) reported isobavachalcone and xanthoangelol H (both chalcones) to exhibit cytotoxic activity against IMR-32 and NB-39 cell lines without affecting the normal cells even at (10^{-4}M) concentration. The external morphologic features of apoptosis which include shrinkage of cells, chromatin condensation, fragmentation of nucleus and apoptotic body formation, were seen in isobavachalcone-treated cells. This molecule also significantly decreased pro-caspase-9 and 3, and subsequently enhanced the expressions of activated caspase-9 and 3 in NB-39 and IMR-32 cells, showing mitochondrial mediated apoptosis [27].

In view of the potent bioactivity of chalcones and imidazothiazoles, Kamal *et al.* (2013) synthesized imidazothiazole-chalcone derivatives and evaluated their anti-tumor activity. All the synthesized compounds exhibited significant anticancer activity against cell viability and NCI's cell panel assay with log GI_{50} values ranging from -7.51 to -4.00. It was observed that the levels of G1/S check point-related tumor suppressor proteins p53, p27, p21 and chk2 were upregulated that resulted in cell cycle arrest at G1 Phase. Their study also demonstrated upregulation of p53 and concurrent down-regulation of NF-kB by these compounds which finally lead to programmed cell death [28]. Kamal *et al.* (2011) published an application for the synthesis of imidazothiazolechalcone hybrids and claimed that the synthesized molecules exhibited significant cytotoxic activity against sixty human tumour cell lines [29]. Konieczny *et al.* (2011) synthesised some novel chalcone derivatives and published the patent in which they claimed that these novel derivatives are cytotoxic to various cancers and could be valuable as chemotherapeutic agents for the cure of neoplastic diseases [30].

Quinoxaline-chalcone derivatives were synthesized by Mielcke *et al.* (2012) against human glioma cell lines. Some of the analogs were synthesized as per the PI3K inhibitor AS605240. These derivatives were evaluated for their anticancer potential at different doses against U-138 MG and C6 glioma cell lines. The chalcone derivatives inhibited cell division with more efficacy than AS605240 that had methoxy groups on the A ring of chalcone. FACS analysis showed that the treatment on C6 cells triggered G1 phase cell cycle arrest, there by eliciting apoptosis with an efficacy greater than that of the positive control (AS605240) [31]. Florescence activated cell sorting examination revealed that the treatment of C6 cells arrested them in the G1 phase, showing an interference with programmed cell death [31].

A series of amidobenzothiazole-chalcone derivatives was synthesised and studied for their anti-tumor potential by Kamal *et al.* (2010). These molecules showed significant anticancer activity. In this series of synthesized molecules, two showed potent anticancer potential against different cancer cell lines with IC_{50} values between 0.85-3.3μM. Cell cycle analysis was done through flow cytometry, which revealed G2/M phase cell cycle arrest in lung cancer. Further these derivatives inhibit microtubule assembly in lung cancer cell lines. Conclusively, amidobenzothiazole-chalcone derivatives were observed to act as strong anticancer agents [32].

Xanthohumol, which is a natural chalconoid, induces programmed cell death in cancer cells by rising intracellular ROS level, that triggers the loss of mitochondrial membrane potential, activates caspase-3 and 7 and also shows the expression of cleaved PARP and discharge of cytochrome C [33]. Xanthohumol was also evaluated against Bcr-Abl (+) myeloid leukemia cells and K562 where it showed significant cytotoxicity by efficiently decreasing Bcr-Abl expression at mRNA and protein level. Cell death of leukemia by xanthohumol was associated with apoptotic induction, augmentation in p21 and p53 levels and decrease in survivin level [34]. Erker *et al.* (2013) published a patent related to vinylogous chalcone derivatives and they claimed that these derivatives can be used for treatment or prevention of cancer and malignant haematological disorders [35]. Chaudhuri *et al.* (2016) published a patent in which they synthesised various chalcone derivatives by making substitutions on both the rings of chalcone and they claim that these compounds are particularly useful for the prevention and treatment of cancer of the lungs, colon, pancreas, liver and kidney [36]. Vanura *et al.* (2016) claimed in one of their patent publications that hetero aromatic chalcone derivatives can be used in the prevention or treatment of cancer and especially in the hematologic malignancies [37]. Sashidhara *et al.* (2014) published a patent on coumarin chalcone derivatives and claimed that one of the molecules can be used for the treatment or prevention of cervical carcinoma, oral squamous cell carcinoma or lung or prostate carcinoma or brain tumour [38]. There are various patents filed from time to time on chalcones and their derivatives for their cancer chemotherapeutic and cancer chemopreventive properties (see Table **1**). Majority of them are thiazoline substituted chalcones, quinolone chalcones, O-phenyl chalcones, deoxydihydroxanthoangelol H chalcone, heteroaromatic chalcones, methoxy chalcone derivative, isoxazolyl aryl chalcone derivative, coumarin-chalcones, imidazolone-chalcones, boronic chalcones derivative etc. Figure (**2**) explains the diagrammatic synopsis of anticancer mechanism of various heterocyclic chalcone analogues.

3. CHALCONE AND CHALCONE DERIVATIVES AS TARGETED ANTICANCER AGENTS

Cancer cells over proliferate and possess extraordinary escape mechanisms driven by genetic and epigenetic alterations controlling their survival, migration and death. Most of these drastic changes map to intracellular signalling pathways. Some of these pathways and targets which are deregulated in cancer and are targeted by chalcones and its derivatives have been documented.

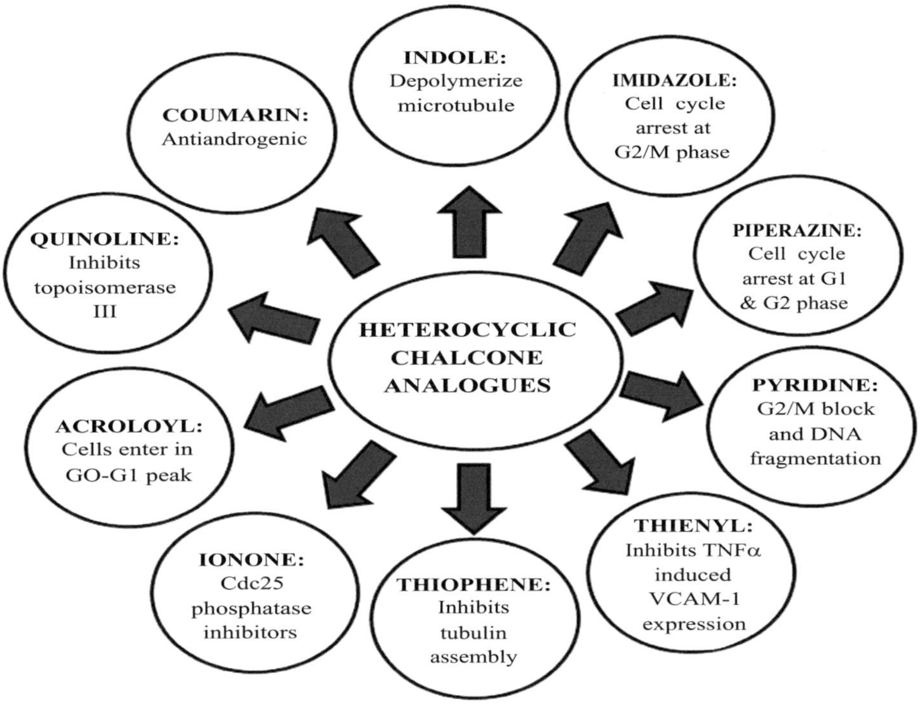

Fig. (2). Mechanisms involved in antitumor effect of heterocyclic chalcone analogues.

3.1. Chalcones as Inhibitors of Nuclear Factor κB (NFκB) Signalling Pathway

The NFκB transcription factor is a ubiquitous protein heterodimer (p65/p50) present in inactive forms with the inhibitor of κB protein (IκB) in the cytosol. Phosphorylation of IκB results in its degradation by proteasome which releases NFκB and then translocates to the nucleus where it trans-activates more than 500 target genes, of which some are involved in tumor promotion and progression especially angiogenesis and metastasis [39]. Mi *et al.* (2016) studied about Cardamonin which inhibited the viability of cells and tumor formation partly by obstruction of testes-specific protease 50-induced NFκB signaling pathway activation [40]. Moon *et al.* (2010) studied about Butein which downregulates the nuclear factor-kappa B-mediated MMP-9 and VEGF in prostate cancer cells [41].

Srinivasan *et al.* (2009) studied about SAR studies of chalcone leading to 3-hydroxy-4,3',4',5'-tetramethoxychalcone and its derivatives as strong NFκB inhibitors which showed effective antiproliferative potential [42]. Shen *et al.* (2007) studied about chalcone which arrests cell cycle and triggers programmed cell death by mitochondrial mediated pathway and inhibition of NFκB signalling in human bladder cancer cells [43].

3.2. Chalcones as Inhibitors of Histone Deacetylases (HDAC)

Histone acetylation is associated with commencement of cellular transcription machinery. It occurs after transcription on NH3 group of lysine residue which is implanted in N-terminal tails of core, leading to the development of more transcriptionally active chromatin (less compact). However, HDACs elminate acetyl group of lysine residue, thus terminating the transcription process. Hyperacetylation of histones takes place due to activation of histone deacetylases that have an effect on the expression of genes [44, 45]. Orlikova *et al.* (2012) worked on histone deacetylase enzymes' (HDAC) inhibitory potential of various natural chalcones. Since HDACs manage the expression of NFκB, these molecules were also tested for inhibition of NFκB activation. This study demonstrated that isoliquiritigenin, butein, homobutein and the glycoside marein showed HDAC inhibitory activity with IC_{50} ranging from 60-190μM, besides some compounds stalled the commencement of TNFα-induced NFκB expression with an IC_{50} ranging from 8-41μM. Furthermore, three chalcones, isoliquiritigenin, butein and homobutein, controlled total HDAC activity and TNFα-induced NFκB activity. Their study furthermore confirmed that chalcones can work as the dual inhibitors of inflammation and cancer [46].

Table 1. Patents Published on Chalcone (s) and/or their Derivatives [12, 20, 21, 30, 35 - 38, 47 - 65].

Patent Number	Filing Date	Publication Date	Activity and/or Title	Inventor	Ref.
CN106831376	1/24/2017	6/13/2017	Chalcone compound and its preparation method and application of the formulation having anticancer activity	Li, J.F., Ba, D., Zhou, S.Y., Yang, Zhao, X.	[47]
CN106674149	12/1/2016	5/17/2017	Thiazoline substituted chalcones, preparation methods and application for preparing the antineoplastic	Shi, H.B., Hu, W.X.	[48]

(Table 1) contd.....

Patent Number	Filing Date	Publication Date	Activity and/or Title	Inventor	Ref.
WO2017083979	11/18/2016	5/26/2017	Quinolone chalcone compounds and uses thereof	Lee, H., Trivedi, P., Karthikeyan, C., Lindamulage, I.K.	[49]
US20170044141	10/18/2016	2/16/2017	Alkyne-, azide- and triazole-containing flavonoids as modulators for multidrug resistance in cancers	Chow, L.M.C., Chan, T.H., Chan, K.F., Wong, I.L.K., Law, M.C.	[50]
CN106543155	9/26/2016	3/29/2017	Chalcone and flavone derivatives adopted as aurora kinase inhibitor	Zhao, Q.C., Fan, Y.H., Xu, Y.N., Zhou, Z.P.	[51]
CN105669630	1/12/2016	6/15/2016	Extraction method of deoxydihydroxanthoangelol H chalcone suitable to serve as liver cancer targeted drug	Li, Z.C., Zhong, J.Y., Guo, P.Z., Li, Q., Li, X.-W., Liu, F.F., Wang, L.P., Liu, Q.Q., Niu, C.F., Ma, M., Li, J.	[52]
CN106478560	9/1/2015	3/8/2017	Dihydrochalcone compound based on C-glycoside synthesis and synthetic method thereof	Fang, Z.J., Zhang, T.	[53]
CN104592132	2/26/2015	4/12/2017	Novel method for preparing chalcone derivatives and quinazoline application containing sulfide	Hu, D.Y., Wan, Z.H., Song, B.A., Xue, W., Jin, L.H., Li, X.Y., Xie, D.D., Zhang, W.Y.	[54]
CN104292140	8/25/2014	6/29/2016	Comprising the chalcone skeleton, and farnesyl thiosalicylic acid analogs preparation and use	Ling, Y., Wang, X.Y., Wang, Z.Q., Wang, X.M., Li, X.H., Xu, C.J., Chen, J., Chen, Y., Xia, C.	[55]

(Table 1) contd.....

Patent Number	Filing Date	Publication Date	Activity and/or Title	Inventor	Ref.
US20160333033	7/25/2016	11/17/2016	*O*-Phenyl Chalcone Compounds And Preparation Method And Use Thereof	Bu, X.Z., Zhu, C.G., Yue, X., Zuo, Y.L., Chen, Y., Wen, G.	[56]
CN103896932	4/18/2014	7/2/2014	Isoxazolyl aryl chalcone derivative as well as preparation method and application thereof	Wan, M.S., Li, L., Li, A.L., Zhang, L.M., Li, S.Q.	[57]
CN104292139	8/25/2014	4/13/2016	Farnesyl thioether substituted chalcone derivatives and preparation method and application	Ling, Y., Wang, Z.Q., Wu, C.X., Xu, C.J., Wang, X.M., Li, X.H., Zhao, Y., Tao, O.Y., Wu, T.A	[58]
CN104803927	3/31/2015	7/29/2015	Chalcone analogue containing 2-methyl-4-oxo-quinazoline-6-base, and preparation method and application thereof	Cao, S.L., Xu, X.Z., Liao, S.T., Pan, P.P., Ma, L., Zhang, J.J., Tang, X.	[59]
CN103755541	2/19/2014	9/2/2015	A class of chalcone derivatives and their preparation and use	Wu, Z., Fang, M.J., Zhou, Q., Xue, Y.H., Ao, M.T., Wu, J.J., He, Z., Ji, Y.F.	[60]
CN103102331	1/17/2013	5/27/2015	Pharmaceutical application of chalcone compound containing piperazine ring	Zhang, C., Cui, D.-M., Xia, Y.-P., Zhang, S.-Q.	[61]
CN103102332	1/17/2013	5/27/2015	Chalcone compound containing piperazine ring and preparation and application thereof	Zhang, C., Cui, D.M., Xia, Y.P., Qi, J.F., Zhang, S.Q.	[62]
CN103768042	10/19/2012	5/7/2014	Application of licochalcone A to prepare anticancer medicines or health-care products	Zhang, D.D.	[63]
WO 2016030510	8/28/2015	7/5/2017	Heteroaromatic chalcone derivatives and their medical use	Katrina, V.	[37]
US7514579	3/12/2009	9/10/2009	Boronic chalcone derivatives and uses thereof	Khan, S.R.	[12]

(Table 1) contd.....

Patent Number	Filing Date	Publication Date	Activity and/or Title	Inventor	Ref.
US20130123367	07/27/2011	05/16/2013	Vinylogous chalcone derivatives and their medical use	Erker, T., Brunhofer, G., Jäger, U., Vanura, K., Dirsch, V., Heiss, E.	[35]
WO2007133588	5/10/2010	10/8/2013	Modified chalcone compounds as antimitotic agents	Hartman, R.F., Rose, S.D.	[64]
US8450377	07/02/2011	05/28/2013	1-Adamantyl chalcones for the treatment of proliferative disorders	Anderson, G.L.	[20]
US20110306775	10/01/2010	12/15/2011	Synthesis and biological evaluation of 2',5'dimethoxychalcone derivatives as microtubule targeted anticancer agents	Lin, C.N.	[21]
WO 2011009826	07/16/2010	01/27/2011	Novel chalcone derivatives with cytotoxic activity	Konieczny, M.	[30]
WO 2012013725	8/28/2015	7/5/2017	Vinylogous chalcone derivatives and their medical use	Brunhofer, G.	[65]
WO 2015166040	05/01/2014	04/30/2015	Chalcone derivatives and their use in treating cancer	Chaudhuri, B.	[36]
US8815940	08/05/2011	08/26/2014	Coumarin chalcones as anticancer agents	Shashidhara, K.V.	[38]

3.3. Chalcones as Angiogenesis Inhibitors

Angiogenesis is the physiological phenomenon by which newer blood vessels are created from the older blood vessels. Angiogenesis directs the expression of angiogenin, VEGF, fibroblast growth factor, TGF-β, etc. which results in the enhancement of vascularisation of tumor. New blood vessels are formed from the older ones by the help of these factors. Inhibition of angiogenesis triggers inhibition of "angiogenic switching" that retains the activation of pro-angiogenic factors and consequently the cancer development discontinues [66, 67]. Bowen *et al.* (2002) published a patent about chalcone and its analogs in which they synthesised various chalcone derivatives and claimed that they show surprisingly good activity as angiogenic inhibitors. They also claimed that these analogs act as anticancer agents and can be used to treat various disease states where angiogenesis is a factor [68]. Sun *et al.* (2003) published a patent and described 2,4-dihydroxy-6-methoxy-3,5-dimethylchalcone that exhibit strong inhibitory activity against VEGF receptor tyrosine kinase that is a vital factor for angiogenesis. Receptor tyrosine kinase inhibition can be established as a valuable target for cancer prevention [69].

3.4. Chalcones as Inhibitors of Proteasome

The proteasomal enzyme complex functions for the degradation of proteins mainly short-lived regulatory proteins and the misfolded ones. Intracellular proteins are directed to degradation by proteasome through ubiquitin-conjugated machinery. The ubiquitin-proteasome machinery is crucial for various cellular activities. There has been great interest in targeting the ubiquitin-proteasome machinery for dealing cancer. Achanta *et al.* (2006) demonstrated the tumour growth inhibitory potential of a library of boronic chalcones in HCT116 cells that have wild-type p53 and their isogenic ones, which are without p53. Two molecules from the synthesised library exhibited significant anticancer potential. Their IC_{50} values were 1.5 and 3.9μM, respectively. Proteasome inhibition led to cytotoxicity in cancerous cells with increase in the expression of p53 and other ubiquitinated proteins [70].

3.5. Chalcones as Inhibitors of p53 Degradation

Tumor suppressor protein p53 protein functions as a guardian regulating cell cycle and other processes like apoptosis, genomic stability, mediating DNA repair and inhibiting angiogenesis and ultimately preventing the intracellular system from getting disbalanced and thus is crucial for preventing cancer and gene activation. Degradation of p53 protein occurs by MDM2, Sirtuin-1, etc. Inhibiting them is one of the ways for preventing the degradation of p53 protein which is an important strategical approach for anticancer therapy [71, 72]. Modzelewska *et al.* (2006) performed synthesis and screening on some chalcones and bis- chalcones having boronic acid. They also tested them for their anticancer potential especially in breast cancer cell lines both in ER-ve (MDA-MB-231) and ER+ve (MCF-7) cell lines and compared with their corresponding normal cell lines (MCF-10A and MCF-12A). Piperazine bis-chalcone was the most potent cancer cytotoxic agent, furthermore, it was also tested against two isogenic HCT 116 cancer cell lines having different expressions of p53. Their studies showed that the growth inhibition was p53-dependent [73].

4. STRUCTURE ACTIVITY RELATIONSHIP (SAR) OF CHALCONES

Structure-activity relationship (SAR) associates and relates the overall pattern of chemical structure (no of bonds, cis/trans, chirality, functional groups types and positions etc.) and its biological activity, property and effect linked with that chemical through both the ways i.e. qualitative as well as quantitative considerations eventually ranging from primary screening to lead optimization. Whether SAR really helps can only be predicted in a series of molecules through their bioactivities which can further provide clue to make structural modifications for optimum property and less toxicity. In case of chalcones, there are many evidences that proved that SAR helps in the development of novel targets with improved bioactivities with more safety profile. Easy synthesis and simple structure of chalcone derivatives make it an important object of study in drug discovery program [74]. The specific structural characteristics of chalcone derivatives had been shown to interact with the metabolites, proteins, lipids etc. which are important in different phases of carcinogenesis. There are some specific general conclusions drawn highlighting the importance of structural features of chalcones; for example, the presence of unsaturated ketone group and meta-dimethoxy motif on ring A in chalcones and its derivatives was postulated and accounted for different medicinal properties [75, 76]. There was no change in relative orientation of the two aryl rings (Fig. **3**) in which a substitution of double bond with a thiophene was done which resulted in anti-proliferative activity [77]. However the addition of different groups into aryl rings of chalcones made it more potent and active biologically [78]. Regarding the cis/trans orientation, it was verified that s-cis orientation of chalcones is crucial for the pharmacological activity [79]. Chalcone piperidine derivatives have a slight chance to form reactive metabolites, thus are better anticancer agents when compared to primary amino group of various heterocyclic molecules [80 - 82]. Similarly, SAR studies pointed out that for more target protein affinity and interactions with biological membranes, those chalcones derivatives which have isoprenoid chains were more potent than their non-prenylated analogs [27, 83]. Overall, as compared to other cytotoxic drugs, the chalcone derivatives exhibit less interaction affinity with deoxy ribonucleic acid that diminishes the harmful outcome of mutagenicity and carcinogenicity [84].

Some major biologically imperative compounds contain chalcone as a fundamental core exhibiting two absorption maxima at 280 and 340nm and possessing anti-malarial, anti-parasitic, anti-fungal, anti-bacterial, anti-platelet, anti-angiogenic, anti-arrhythmic, anti-diabetic, anti-filarial, anti-gout, anti-histaminic, anti-hypertensive, anti-inflammatory, anti-neoplastic, anti-nociceptive, anti-obesity and anti-oxidant, hypolipidemic, hypnotic, immunosuppressant, anti-protozoal, anti-retroviral, anti-spasmodic, anti-steroidal, anti-tubercular, anxiolytic and cardioprotective activities [85 - 87].

The existing evidences of chalcones and their derivatives or conjugates are still in the pre-clinical or clinical then in the first phase stage with an advantage of less toxicity [88]. The strenuous efforts among the scientists are focussed on the mechanistic study of chalcones and its derivatives taking the help of SAR. Chalcones which exhibit anti-inflammatory property, generally possess an α-β unsaturated bond which helps it to behave as a Michael acceptor for a nucleophilic moiety for example, GSH or proteins like IKK-β having cysteine residues [89]. The presence of electron-donating groups on the A ring decreases the acidity of the α-H and thus stabilizes the GSH adduct [23, 46]. Some major studies revealed that the anticancer activities are linked with the presence of one or more hydroxyl substituent on the chalcone scaffold which increases its potency against cancer cells [46]. Furthermore, as inflammation and carcinogenesis are interlinked with each other, the presence of 20-hydroxy group in the chalcones was considered to be crucial for augmentation of its anti-inflammatory properties which can be explained on the basis of electrophilic properties of α-β unsaturated ketone by hydrogen bonding between the carbonyl group and 20-hydroxy group. The creation of energetically favoured intramolecular hydrogen bonds becomes a major platform and reason for its RO(N)S radical scavenging ability; for example, chalcones with conformations in which the carbonyl group and the A ring are orthogonal, are more potent ROS radical scavengers [90] while, NO scavenging ability has been pinpointed to the presence of α-β double bond as compared to the single bond. Similar reflection has also been observed for inhibiting the activation of NF-κB transcription factor [42]. Different glycosidic substitutions on the aromatic rings decreases antiproliferative action as compared to aglycones, may be due to complexity caused by sugar moieties resulted in lower lipophilicity and less cellular uptake through passive diffusion by cell membrane [91]. Prenylation is an important protein post-translational modification, helps in increasing lipophilicity of protein and its targeting to membrane, thus prenylated chalcones had more chances for cellular uptake and subcellular localization [92].

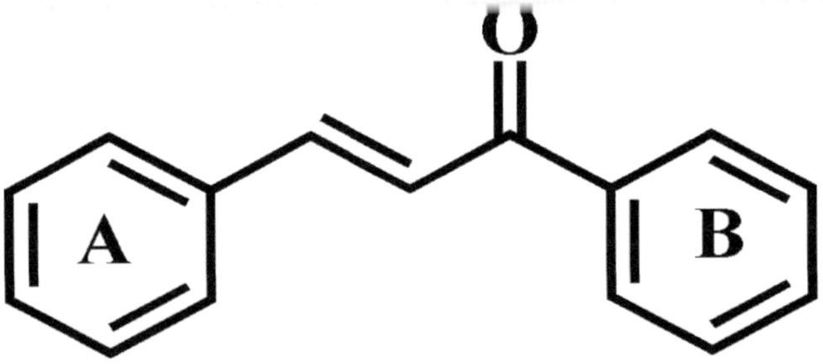

Fig. (3). Structure activity relationship of chalcone moeity.

CURRENT & FUTURE DEVELOPMENTS

Chalcones and their derivatives as well as conjugates are preferred structures, strategically effective in the discovery of drugs due to many reasons like already established synthetic methods are present which can provide a basic platform for different novel types, both by introducing different functional groups and chiral forms and also by modifying the main core structure. The conjugated system of chalcones with nucleophilic and electrophilic functional moieties helps them in obtaining varieties of different analogues/conjugates which are not only important for their bioactivity, less toxicity, more solubility but they are also helpful in obtaining fluorescent chemical probes for diagnosis, imaging and mechanistic studies. Although the chalcones obtained from natural sources with bioactivities are presumed to be safe, but they still need validation while the synthetic chalcones derivatives and conjugates need to be further studied for their safety and potency through SAR studies. Regarding the use of chalcones and their derivatives for clinical use, further studies are needed for analysing their solubility as well as the *in vivo* efficacy. Co-crystallization studies in which chalcone is co-crystallized with its target protein like tubulin, helps in its study for understanding its interaction as it is directly linked with the target protein. Some of these issues have been highlighted and further simplicity in the coming years is expected in synthesis and bioactivity testing as well as in validation so much that all these become clinically safe and effective. Clinical trials have shown that some specific chalcones and their derivatives are more bio available and less toxic and are thus, used for various ailments and treatments like stomach cancer etc, and in food additives and cosmetic formulations [93]. Nature offers chalcones, which, due to their rich structural assets and pleiotropic mode of action, are found to be suitable candidates for modulating and halting the phases of carcinogenesis and are thus considered as effective cancer chemotherapeutic or chemopreventive molecules.

CONFLICT OF INTEREST

The authors declare no conflict of interest, financial or otherwise.

ACKNOWLEDGEMENTS

Zahoor A. Wani thanks Science and Engineering Research Board (SERB), New Delhi for awarding National Post-Doctoral Fellowship (N-PDF) at CSIR-CIMAP, Lucknow.

REFERENCES

[1] Yerragunta V, Kumaraswamy T, Suman D, Anusha V, Patil P, Samhitha T. A review on chalcones and its importance. PharmaTutor 2013; 1(2): 54-9.

[2] Koran K, Özen F, Biryan F, Demirelli K, Görgülü AO. Eu+ 3-doped chalcone substituted cyclotriphosphazenes: Synthesis, characterizations, thermal and dielectrical properties. Inorg Chim Acta 2016; 450: 162-9.
[http://dx.doi.org/10.1016/j.ica.2016.05.043]

[3] Zhuang C, Zhang W, Sheng C, Zhang W, Xing C, Miao Z. Chalcone: A privileged structure in medicinal chemistry. Chem Rev 2017; 117(12): 7762-810.
[http://dx.doi.org/10.1021/acs.chemrev.7b00020] [PMID: 28488435]

[4] Katsori A-M, Hadjipavlou-Litina D. Recent progress in therapeutic applications of chalcones. Expert Opin Ther Pat 2011; 21(10): 1575-96.
[http://dx.doi.org/10.1517/13543776.2011.596529] [PMID: 21711087]

[5] Madhavi S, Sreenivasulu R, Yazala JP, Raju RR. Synthesis of chalcone incorporated quinazoline derivatives as anticancer agents. Saudi Pharm J 2017; 25(2): 275-9.
[http://dx.doi.org/10.1016/j.jsps.2016.06.005] [PMID: 28344479]

[6] Bhale PS, Chavan HV, Dongare SB, *et al.* Synthesis of extended conjugated indolyl chalcones as potent anti-breast cancer, anti-inflammatory and antioxidant agents. Bioorg Med Chem Lett 2017; 27(7): 1502-7.
[http://dx.doi.org/10.1016/j.bmcl.2017.02.052] [PMID: 28258796]

[7] Cai C-Y, Rao L, Rao Y, *et al.* Analogues of xanthones-Chalcones and bis-chalcones as α-glucosidase inhibitors and anti-diabetes candidates. Eur J Med Chem 2017; 130: 51-9.
[http://dx.doi.org/10.1016/j.ejmech.2017.02.007] [PMID: 28242551]

[8] Hawash MM, Kahraman DC, Eren F, Cetin Atalay R, Baytas SN. Synthesis and biological evaluation of novel pyrazolic chalcone derivatives as novel hepatocellular carcinoma therapeutics. Eur J Med Chem 2017; 129: 12-26.
[http://dx.doi.org/10.1016/j.ejmech.2017.02.002] [PMID: 28219046]

[9] Ramaiah MJ, Pushpavalli S, Krishna GR, *et al.* Chalcone-imidazolone conjugates induce apoptosis through DNA damage pathway by affecting telomeres. Cancer Cell Int 2011; 11(1): 11.
[http://dx.doi.org/10.1186/1475-2867-11-11] [PMID: 21518433]

[10] Kamal A, Kumar GB, Vishnuvardhan MV, *et al.* Synthesis of phenstatin/isocombretastatin-chalcone conjugates as potent tubulin polymerization inhibitors and mitochondrial apoptotic inducers. Org Biomol Chem 2015; 13(13): 3963-81.
[http://dx.doi.org/10.1039/C4OB02606C] [PMID: 25721862]

[11] Khan SR. Boronic chalcone derivatives and uses thereof. US7514579, 2009.

[12] Boumendjel A, McLeer-Florin A, Champelovier P, *et al.* A novel chalcone derivative which acts as a microtubule depolymerising agent and an inhibitor of P-gp and BCRP in *in vitro* and *in vivo* glioblastoma models. BMC Cancer 2009; 9(1): 242.
[http://dx.doi.org/10.1186/1471-2407-9-242] [PMID: 19619277]

[13] Makita H, Tanaka T, Fujitsuka H, *et al.* Chemoprevention of 4-nitroquinoline 1-oxide-induced rat oral carcinogenesis by the dietary flavonoids chalcone, 2-hydroxychalcone, and quercetin. Cancer Res 1996; 56(21): 4904-9.
[PMID: 8895742]

[14] Almasan A, Ashkenazi A. Apo2L/TRAIL: Apoptosis signaling, biology, and potential for cancer therapy. Cytokine Growth Factor Rev 2003; 14(3-4): 337-48.
[http://dx.doi.org/10.1016/S1359-6101(03)00029-7] [PMID: 12787570]

[15] Wu GS. TRAIL as a target in anti-cancer therapy. Cancer Lett 2009; 285(1): 1-5.
[http://dx.doi.org/10.1016/j.canlet.2009.02.029] [PMID: 19299078]

[16] Zhang L, Fang B. Mechanisms of resistance to TRAIL-induced apoptosis in cancer. Cancer Gene Ther 2005; 12(3): 228-37.
[http://dx.doi.org/10.1038/sj.cgt.7700792] [PMID: 15550937]

[17] Szliszka E, Czuba ZP, Mazur B, Sedek L, Paradysz A, Krol W. Chalcones enhance TRAIL-induced apoptosis in prostate cancer cells. Int J Mol Sci 2009; 11(1): 1-13.
[http://dx.doi.org/10.3390/ijms11010001] [PMID: 20161998]

[18] Kamal A, Dastagiri D, Ramaiah MJ, *et al.* Synthesis of imidazothiazole-chalcone derivatives as anticancer and apoptosis inducing agents. ChemMedChem 2010; 5(11): 1937-47.
[http://dx.doi.org/10.1002/cmdc.201000346] [PMID: 20836120]

[19] Ilango K, Valentina P, Saluja G. Synthesis and *in vitro* anticancer activity of some substituted chalcones derivatives. Res J Pharm Biol Chem Sci 2010; 1(2): 354-9.

[20] Anderson GL, Kaimari TAR. Adamantyl chalcones for the treatment of proliferative disorders. US8450377, 2013.

[21] Lin CN, Tu HY, Huang AM, Hoar TC, Yang SC, Pu YS. Synthesis and biological evaluation of 2′, 5′-dimethoxychalcone derivatives as microtubule-targeted anticancer agents. US20110306775, 2011.

[22] Rose SD, Hartman RF. Modified chalcone compounds as antimitotic agents. US7714025, 2010.

[23] Liu X, Go M-L. Antiproliferative activity of chalcones with basic functionalities. Bioorg Med Chem 2007; 15(22): 7021-34.
[http://dx.doi.org/10.1016/j.bmc.2007.07.042] [PMID: 17804245]

[24] Wani ZA, Guru SK, Rao AV, *et al.* A novel quinazolinone chalcone derivative induces mitochondrial dependent apoptosis and inhibits PI3K/Akt/mTOR signaling pathway in human colon cancer HCT-116 cells. Food Chem Toxicol 2016; 87: 1-11.
[http://dx.doi.org/10.1016/j.fct.2015.11.016] [PMID: 26615871]

[25] Shi H-B, Zhang S-J, Ge Q-F, Guo D-W, Cai C-M, Hu W-X. Synthesis and anticancer evaluation of thiazolyl-chalcones. Bioorg Med Chem Lett 2010; 20(22): 6555-9.
[http://dx.doi.org/10.1016/j.bmcl.2010.09.041] [PMID: 20888764]

[26] Kimura Y, Taniguchi M, Baba K. Antitumor and antimetastatic activities of 4-hydroxyderricin isolated from *Angelica keiskei* roots. Planta Med 2004; 70(3): 211-9.
[http://dx.doi.org/10.1055/s-2004-815537] [PMID: 15114497]

[27] Nishimura R, Tabata K, Arakawa M, *et al.* Isobavachalcone, a chalcone constituent of *Angelica keiskei*, induces apoptosis in neuroblastoma. Biol Pharm Bull 2007; 30(10): 1878-83.
[http://dx.doi.org/10.1248/bpb.30.1878] [PMID: 17917255]

[28] Kamal A, Kashi Reddy M, Viswanath A. The design and development of imidazothiazole-chalcone derivatives as potential anticancer drugs. Expert Opin Drug Discov 2013; 8(3): 289-304.
[http://dx.doi.org/10.1517/17460441.2013.758630] [PMID: 23317445]

[29] Kamal A, Dudekula D, Jonnala SR, Earla VB. Imidazothiazole-chalcone derivatives as potential anticancer agents and process for the preparation thereof. WO2011045646, 2011.

[30] Konieczny M, Skladanowski A, Lemke K, Pieczykolan J. Novel chalcone derivatives with cytotoxic activity. WO2011009826, 2011.

[31] Mielcke TR, Mascarello A, Filippi-Chiela E, *et al.* Activity of novel quinoxaline-derived chalcones on *in vitro* glioma cell proliferation. Eur J Med Chem 2012; 48: 255-64.
[http://dx.doi.org/10.1016/j.ejmech.2011.12.023] [PMID: 22209415]

[32] Kamal A, Reddy JS, Ramaiah MJ, Dastagiri D, Bharathi EV, Sagar MV, *et al.* Design, synthesis and biological evaluation of imidazopyridine/pyrimidine-chalcone derivatives as potential anticancer agents. MedChemComm 2010; 1(5): 355-60.
[http://dx.doi.org/10.1039/c0md00116c]

[33] Yang J-Y, Della-Fera MA, Rayalam S, Baile CA. Effect of xanthohumol and isoxanthohumol on 3T3-L1 cell apoptosis and adipogenesis. Apoptosis 2007; 12(11): 1953-63.
[http://dx.doi.org/10.1007/s10495-007-0130-4] [PMID: 17874298]

[34] Monteghirfo S, Tosetti F, Ambrosini C, *et al.* Antileukemia effects of xanthohumol in Bcr/Abl-transformed cells involve nuclear factor-kappaB and p53 modulation. Mol Cancer Ther 2008; 7(9): 2692-702.
[http://dx.doi.org/10.1158/1535-7163.MCT-08-0132] [PMID: 18790751]

[35] Erker T, Brunhofer G, Jäger U, Vanura K, Dirsch V, Heiss E. Vinylogous chalcone derivatives and their medical use. US20130123367, 2013.

[36] Chaudhuri B. Chalcone derivatives and their use in treating cancer. WO2015166040, 2016.

[37] Vanura K, Jager U, Erker T, Brunhofer-Bolzer G. Heteroaromatic chalcone derivatives and their medical use . WO2016030510, 2016.

[38] Sashidhara KV, Kumar A, Kumar M, Sarkar J, Sinha SK. Coumarin-chalcones as anticancer agents. US8815940, 2014.

[39] Christian F, Smith EL, Carmody RJ. The regulation of NF-κB subunits by phosphorylation. Cells

2016; 5(1): 12.
[http://dx.doi.org/10.3390/cells5010012] [PMID: 26999213]

[40] Mi X-G, Song Z-B, Sun L-G, *et al.* Cardamonin inhibited cell viability and tumorigenesis partially through blockade of testes-specific protease 50-mediated nuclear factor-kappaB signaling pathway activation. Int J Biochem Cell Biol 2016; 73: 63-71.
[http://dx.doi.org/10.1016/j.biocel.2016.02.001] [PMID: 26855338]

[41] Moon D-O, Choi YH, Moon S-K, Kim W-J, Kim G-Y. Butein suppresses the expression of nuclear factor-kappa B-mediated matrix metalloproteinase-9 and vascular endothelial growth factor in prostate cancer cells. Toxicol In Vitro 2010; 24(7): 1927-34.
[http://dx.doi.org/10.1016/j.tiv.2010.08.002] [PMID: 20696233]

[42] Srinivasan B, Johnson TE, Lad R, Xing C. Structure-activity relationship studies of chalcone leading to 3-hydroxy-4,3′,4′,5′-tetramethoxychalcone and its analogues as potent nuclear factor kappaB inhibitors and their anticancer activities. J Med Chem 2009; 52(22): 7228-35.
[http://dx.doi.org/10.1021/jm901278z] [PMID: 19883086]

[43] Shen KH, Chang JK, Hsu YL, Kuo PL. Chalcone arrests cell cycle progression and induces apoptosis through induction of mitochondrial pathway and inhibition of nuclear factor kappa B signalling in human bladder cancer cells. Basic Clin Pharmacol Toxicol 2007; 101(4): 254-61.
[http://dx.doi.org/10.1111/j.1742-7843.2007.00120.x] [PMID: 17845507]

[44] Ropero S, Esteller M. The role of histone deacetylases (HDACs) in human cancer. Mol Oncol 2007; 1(1): 19-25.
[http://dx.doi.org/10.1016/j.molonc.2007.01.001] [PMID: 19383284]

[45] Kuo M-H, Allis CD. Roles of histone acetyltransferases and deacetylases in gene regulation. BioEssays 1998; 20(8): 615-26.
[http://dx.doi.org/10.1002/(SICI)1521-1878(199808)20:8<615::AID-BIES4>3.0.CO;2-H] [PMID: 9780836]

[46] Orlikova B, Schnekenburger M, Zloh M, Golais F, Diederich M, Tasdemir D. Natural chalcones as dual inhibitors of HDACs and NF-κB. Oncol Rep 2012; 28(3): 797-805.
[http://dx.doi.org/10.3892/or.2012.1870] [PMID: 22710558]

[47] Li J, Ba D, Zhou S, Yang Z. Chalcone compound and its preparation method and application of the formulation having anticancer activity. CN106831376, 2017.

[48] Shi H, Hu W. Thiazoline substituted chalcones, preparation methods and application for preparing the antineoplastic. CN106674149, 2017.

[49] Lee H, Trivedi P, Karthikeyan C, Lindamulage IK. Quinolone chalcone compounds and their uses. WO2017083979, 2017.

[50] Chow LMC, Chan TH, Chan KF, Wong ILK, Law MC. Alkyne-, azide- and triazole-containing flavonoids as modulators for multidrug resistance in cancers. US20170044141, 2017.

[51] Zhao Q, Fan Y, Xu Y, Zhou H. Chalcone and flavone derivatives adopted as aurora kinase inhibitor. CN106543155, 2017.

[52] Li Z, Zhong J, Guo P, *et al.* Extraction method of deoxydihydroxanthoangelol H chalcone suitable to serve as liver cancer targeted drug . CN105669630, 2016.

[53] Fang Z, Zhang T. Dihydrochalcone compound based on C-glycoside synthesis and synthetic method thereof. CN106478560, 2017.

[54] Hu D, Wan Z, Song B, *et al.* Novel method for preparing chalcone derivatives and quinazoline application containing sulfide. CN104592132, 2017.

[55] Ling Y, Wang X, Wang Z, *et al.* Comprising the chalcone skeleton, and farnesyl thiosalicylic acid analogs preparation and use. CN104292140, 2016.

[56] Bu X, Zhu CG, Yue X, Zuo YL, Chen Y, Wen G. O-phenyl chalcone compounds and preparation

method and use thereof. US20160333033, 2017.

[57] Wan M, Li L, Li AL, Zhang L. Isoxazolyl aryl chalcone derivatives, methods for their preparation and their application. CN103896932, 2014.

[58] Ling YW, Zhiqiang W, Caixia X, *et al.* Farnesylated thioether-substituted chalcone derivative, preparation method and purpose thereof. CN104292139, 2015.

[59] Cao S, Xu X, Liao T, Ding P, Ma L, Zhang J T. Chalcone analogs containing 2-methyl-4-oxoquinazolin-6-yl, and methods and methods for their preparation and use. CN104803927, 2015.

[60] Wu Z, Fang MJ, Zhou Q, *et al.* A class of chalcone derivatives and their preparation and use thereof. CN103755541, 2015.

[61] Zhang C, Cui D, Xia Y, Zhang S. Pharmaceutical application of chalcone compound containing piperazine ring . CN103102331, 2015.

[62] Zhang C, Cui D, Xia Y, Qi J, Zhang H S. Chalcone compound containing piperazine ring and preparation and application thereof. CN103102332, 2015.

[63] Zhang D. Application of licochalcone A to prepare anticancer medicines or health-care products. CN103768042, 2014.

[64] Rose SD, Hartman RF. Modified chalcone compounds as antimitotic agents. US8552066, 2013.

[65] Brunhofer G, Dirsch V, Erker T, Hei E, Jager U, Vanura K. Vinylogous chalcone derivatives and their medical use. WO2012013725, 2012.

[66] Baeriswyl V, Christofori G. The angiogenic switch in carcinogenesis. Semin Cancer Biol 2009; 19(5): 329-37.
[http://dx.doi.org/10.1016/j.semcancer.2009.05.003] [PMID: 19482086]

[67] Bergers G, Benjamin LE. Tumorigenesis and the angiogenic switch. Nat Rev Cancer 2003; 3(6): 401-10.
[http://dx.doi.org/10.1038/nrc1093] [PMID: 12778130]

[68] Bowen JP, Robinson TP, Ehlers T, Goldsmith D, Arbiser J. Chalcone and its analogs as agents for the inhibition of angiogensis and related disease states. US6462075, 2002.

[69] Zhu X, Liu Z, Xie B, *et al.* Use of 2′,4′-dihydroxy-6′-methoxy-3′,5 ′-dimethyl chalcone for preparing anticancer medicine. CN1454895, 2003.

[70] Achanta G, Modzelewska A, Feng L, Khan SR, Huang P. A boronic-chalcone derivative exhibits potent anticancer activity through inhibition of the proteasome. Mol Pharmacol 2006; 70(1): 426-33. [PMID: 16636137]

[71] Zilfou JT, Lowe SW. Tumor suppressive functions of p53. Cold Spring Harb Perspect Biol 2009; 1(5): a001883.
[http://dx.doi.org/10.1101/cshperspect.a001883] [PMID: 20066118]

[72] Lane DP, Cheok CF, Lain S. p53-based cancer therapy. Cold Spring Harb Perspect Biol 2010; 2(9): a001222.
[http://dx.doi.org/10.1101/cshperspect.a001222] [PMID: 20463003]

[73] Modzelewska A, Pettit C, Achanta G, Davidson NE, Huang P, Khan SR. Anticancer activities of novel chalcone and bis-chalcone derivatives. Bioorg Med Chem 2006; 14(10): 3491-5.
[http://dx.doi.org/10.1016/j.bmc.2006.01.003] [PMID: 16434201]

[74] Lawrence NJ, McGown AT. The chemistry and biology of antimitotic chalcones and related enone systems. Curr Pharm Des 2005; 11(13): 1679-93.
[http://dx.doi.org/10.2174/1381612053764733] [PMID: 15892668]

[75] Rao YK, Fang S-H, Tzeng Y-M. Synthesis and biological evaluation of 3′,4′,5′-trimethoxychalcone analogues as inhibitors of nitric oxide production and tumor cell proliferation. Bioorg Med Chem 2009; 17(23): 7909-14.

[http://dx.doi.org/10.1016/j.bmc.2009.10.022] [PMID: 19875299]

[76] Seelig A, Landwojtowicz E. Structure-activity relationship of P-glycoprotein substrates and modifiers. Eur J Pharm Sci 2000; 12(1): 31-40. [http://dx.doi.org/10.1016/S0928-0987(00)00177-9] [PMID: 11121731]

[77] Romagnoli R, Baraldi PG, Carrion MD, *et al.* Design, synthesis, and biological evaluation of thiophene analogues of chalcones. Bioorg Med Chem 2008; 16(10): 5367-76. [http://dx.doi.org/10.1016/j.bmc.2008.04.026] [PMID: 18440234]

[78] Katsori A-M, Hadjipavlou-Litina D. Chalcones in cancer: Understanding their role in terms of QSAR. Curr Med Chem 2009; 16(9): 1062-81. [http://dx.doi.org/10.2174/092986709787581798] [PMID: 19275612]

[79] Ducki S, Forrest R, Hadfield JA, *et al.* Potent antimitotic and cell growth inhibitory properties of substituted chalcones. Bioorg Med Chem Lett 1998; 8(9): 1051-6. [http://dx.doi.org/10.1016/S0960-894X(98)00162-0] [PMID: 9871706]

[80] Xia Y, Yang Z-Y, Xia P, Bastow KF, Nakanishi Y, Lee K-H. Antitumor agents. Part 202: Novel 2′-amino chalcones: design, synthesis and biological evaluation. Bioorg Med Chem Lett 2000; 10(8): 699-701. [http://dx.doi.org/10.1016/S0960-894X(00)00072-X] [PMID: 10782667]

[81] Dimmock JR, Jha A, Zello GA, *et al.* Cytotoxic 4′-aminochalcones and related compounds. Pharmazie 2003; 58(4): 227-32. [PMID: 12749401]

[82] Shimiz K, Kondo R, Sakai K, Buabarn S, Dilokkunanant U. A geranylated chalcone with 5α-reductase inhibitory properties from *Artocarpus incisus.* Phytochemistry 2000; 54(8): 737-9. [http://dx.doi.org/10.1016/S0031-9422(00)00187-4] [PMID: 11014257]

[83] Jayasinghe L, Rupasinghe GK, Hara N, Fujimoto Y. Geranylated phenolic constituents from the fruits of *Artocarpus nobilis.* Phytochemistry 2006; 67(13): 1353-8. [http://dx.doi.org/10.1016/j.phytochem.2006.04.011] [PMID: 16730769]

[84] Ivanova Y, Momekov G, Petrov O, Karaivanova M, Kalcheva V. Cytotoxic Mannich bases of 6-(3-aryl-2-propenoyl)-2(3H)-benzoxazolones. Eur J Med Chem 2007; 42(11-12): 1382-7. [http://dx.doi.org/10.1016/j.ejmech.2007.02.019] [PMID: 17459529]

[85] Mahapatra DK, Asati V, Bharti SK. Chalcones and their therapeutic targets for the management of diabetes: structural and pharmacological perspectives. Eur J Med Chem 2015; 92: 839-65. [http://dx.doi.org/10.1016/j.ejmech.2015.01.051] [PMID: 25638569]

[86] Mahapatra DK, Bharti SK, Asati V. Anti-cancer chalcones: Structural and molecular target perspectives. Eur J Med Chem 2015; 98: 69-114. [http://dx.doi.org/10.1016/j.ejmech.2015.05.004] [PMID: 26005917]

[87] Mahapatra DK, Bharti SK, Asati V. Chalcone scaffolds as anti-infective agents: Structural and molecular target perspectives. Eur J Med Chem 2015; 101: 496-524. [http://dx.doi.org/10.1016/j.ejmech.2015.06.052] [PMID: 26188621]

[88] Batovska DI, Todorova IT. Trends in utilization of the pharmacological potential of chalcones. Curr Clin Pharmacol 2010; 5(1): 1-29. [http://dx.doi.org/10.2174/157488410790410579] [PMID: 19891604]

[89] Meng CQ, Ni L, Worsencroft KJ, *et al.* Carboxylated, heteroaryl-substituted chalcones as inhibitors of vascular cell adhesion molecule-1 expression for use in chronic inflammatory diseases. J Med Chem 2007; 50(6): 1304-15. [http://dx.doi.org/10.1021/jm0614230] [PMID: 17323940]

[90] Mathiesen L, Malterud KE, Sund RB. Hydrogen bond formation as basis for radical scavenging activity: A structure-activity study of C-methylated dihydrochalcones from *Myrica gale* and structurally related acetophenones. Free Radic Biol Med 1997; 22(1-2): 307-11.

[http://dx.doi.org/10.1016/S0891-5849(96)00277-8] [PMID: 8958155]

[91] Kim J-Y, Park SJ, Yun K-J, Cho Y-W, Park H-J, Lee K-T. Isoliquiritigenin isolated from the roots of Glycyrrhiza uralensis inhibits LPS-induced iNOS and COX-2 expression via the attenuation of NF-kappaB in RAW 264.7 macrophages. Eur J Pharmacol 2008; 584(1): 175-84. [http://dx.doi.org/10.1016/j.ejphar.2008.01.032] [PMID: 18295200]

[92] Gerhauser C, Alt A, Heiss E, *et al.* Cancer chemopreventive activity of Xanthohumol, a natural product derived from hop. Mol Cancer Ther 2002; 1(11): 959-69. [PMID: 12481418]

[93] Jandial DD, Blair CA, Zhang S, Krill LS, Zhang Y-B, Zi X. Molecular targeted approaches to cancer therapy and prevention using chalcones. Curr Cancer Drug Targets 2014; 14(2): 181-200. [http://dx.doi.org/10.2174/1568009614666140122160515] [PMID: 24467530]

CHAPTER 5

Regulation/Inhibition of Human Lactate Dehydrogenase A: An Innovative and Potential Approach for Anti-Cancer Drugs Development

Vinit Kumar[1], **Atul Kumar**[2] and **Reshma Rani**[3,*]

[1] *Amity Institute of Molecular Medicine and Stem Cell Research, Amity University, Noida 201313, India*

[2] *Amity Institute of Engineering & Technology, Amity University, Greater Noida 201313, India*

[3] *Amity Institute of Biotechnology, Amity University, Noida 201313, India*

Abstract: Human lactate dehydrogenase (*h*LDH-A), a glycolytic enzyme responsible for the conversion of pyruvate to lactate coupled with oxidation of NADH to NAD^+, plays a crucial role in the promotion of glycolysis in invasive tumor cells. *h*LDH-A has been considered a vital therapeutic target for invasive cancers therefore, *h*LDH-A inhibition reflects a valuable attempt in the development of innovative anticancer strategies. Reagents that regulate or inhibit *h*LDH-A enzyme/ gene can play a role in the prevention and treatment of various cancers and related diseases. In fact, selective inhibition of *h*LDH-A using small molecules holds potential prospects for the treatment of cancer. Consequently, significant progress has been made in the discovery of small-molecules, the selective inhibitors of *h*LDH-A displaying remarkable inhibitory potency. The LDH-based approaches in the development of anticancer therapy and treatment of related diseases are worthwhile because of the existence of LDH enzyme at the end of glycolytic pathway. In this book chapter, 59 review and research articles, and 15 patents filed on LDH and its application are discussed. Latest contributions in regulation/inhibition of the LDH-A enzyme by various agents are summarized in this book chapter.

Keywords: Aerobic glycolysis, anaerobic glycolysis, anti-inflammatory activity, anti-proliferative activity, cancer cell metabolism, cancer cell proliferation, epileptic treatment, FDG-PET, FRET, glycolytic pathway, gossypol, human lactate dehydrogenase A, human lactate dehydrogenase B, isostere of pyruvate, metabolic switch, mitochondrial dysfunction, $NADH/NAD^+$, nanosensor, *N*-hydroxy-indole, pyruvate dehydrogenase complex, selective *h*LDH5 inhibitors, tumor glycolysis, warburg effect.

* **Corresponding author Reshma Rani:** Amity Institute of Biotechnology, Amity University, Noida 201313, India; Tel: +91 1204392721; E-mails: reshudcy@gmail.com, rrani@amity.edu

Atta-ur-Rahman and Khurshid Zaman (Eds.)

1. INTRODUCTION

Cancer is one major cause among the leading causes of morbidity and mortality worldwide. According to the World Health Organization (WHO) approximately 14 million new cases of cancers and 8.2 million cancer related deaths were reported in 2012 worldwide and among them, most common causes of cancer death are cancers of lung (1.59 million deaths), liver (745 000 deaths), stomach (723 000 deaths), colorectal (694 000 deaths), breast (521 000 deaths) and oesophageal cancer (400 000 deaths) [1]. This data reflect the serious threats of cancer posed to human health, and the development of promising anticancer agents is, therefore, urgently required. WHO launched the global action plan in 2013, for the prevention, control and treatment of non-communicable diseases during 2013-2020 by aiming to reduce premature mortality from cancers. Common conventional approaches that are clinically used for the treatment of cancers, including surgery, chemo- and radiation therapy have some limitations due to serious side effects [2]. Various research studies confirm that cancer is a complex process and many enzymes including glycolytic enzymes are involved in initiation, maintenance and survival of various human cancers and some of them are thus considered as innovative targets for the development of anticancer agents [3]. Significant inhibition as well as reduction of enzyme activity involved in cancer by means of small molecules or other agents is a current and significant approach for drug development. Great efforts have been dedicated to design and develop 'drug-like' small molecules by following target-, structure- and fragment-based approaches for selective enzyme inhibition for the treatment of cancers [4].

2. CANCER CELL METABOLISM

The metabolic properties of cancer cells differ significantly from those of the normal cells. Unlike normal cells, most cancer cells rely on the enhanced rate of glycolysis that tends to ferment glucose into lactate, even under aerobic conditions. In fact, cancer cells are abnormally dependent on aerobic glycolysis for energy production at higher rate for maintenance of cancers [5]. It is hard to discuss the cancer cell metabolism without first mentioning the German scientist "Otto Warburg" who made a striking discovery in the 1920's. For the first time, he observed that the cancer cells hold the metabolic switch from oxidative phosphorylation (OXPHOS) towards aerobic glycolysis (Warburg effect) and thus, established a link between cancer and the peculiar glucose metabolism in cancer cells [6]. Since then "Warburg effect" has been validated in various human tumors and the parallel increase in enhanced glucose uptake has been exploited clinically for the diagnosis, staging, and monitoring of various cancers, including nonHodgkins lymphoma (NHL) by using fluorodeoxyglucose positron emission tomography (FDG-PET). It is a useful and sensitive modality for assessing disease activity in thyroid lymphoma and in cancer metastasis. In this technique, the biologically active molecule, an analogue of glucose i.e. fluorodeoxyglucose (FDG), is used for PET where the concentration of FDG tracer indicates metabolic activity of the tissue that corresponds to the regional glucose uptake [7]. Besides tumor imaging, Warburg effect can be exploited for drug designing to treat human cancers. Initially, Warburg hypothesized that the metabolic alteration specific to cancer cells is caused by a mitochondrial defect where complete oxidation of glucose is lost; however, it was later proven that this metabolic alteration is from oncogene-directed metabolic reprogramming, not from mitochondrial dysfunction [8 - 10]. The unique characteristic of tumor glycolysis of being highly functional is accompanied by high glucose consumption due to lower efficiency in energy production that ensures an adequate and rapid energy supply and biosynthetic intermediates for rapidly growing cancer cells [10 - 12]. In essence, cancer cells are hungrier for nutrients than normal cells are; thus, tumor glycolysis provides selective advantages to tumor cells for survival and proliferation. Succinctly, cancer is a metabolic disease and can be targeted by the following two facts (i) to produce enough energy to survive when supplies and waste disposal are limited, and (ii) to distract abundant metabolic intermediates to the biosynthetic pathways supporting cell proliferation. Recently, keen research interest in tumor glycolysis has emerged due to the strong metabolic dependencies of cancer cells. Despite various key factors (enzymes and transporters) that are intricate, tumor glycolysis is thus considered a promising target [10, 12].

3. GLYCOLYSIS AND LDHA

Glycolysis is a metabolic process, which comprises ten successive steps catalyzed by specific enzymes in the cytoplasm of the cells. At the end of glycolysis, two pyruvate molecules are formed by the catabolism of one glucose molecule with concurrent generation of two ATP molecules and two NADH (Nicotinamide Adenine Reduced Dinucleotide) molecules. Glycolysis can take place in both conditions; i) in the presence of oxygen i.e. aerobic condition and, ii) in the absence of oxygen i.e. anaerobic condition [13]. Although, in both the situations, the final products viz. two molecules of pyruvate, two molecules of ATP and two molecules of NADH are the same but depending upon the presence or absence of oxygen, further pyruvate can follow two different pathways. In aerobic (normoxia) condition, two molecules of pyruvate are transported into mitochondrial matrix where these molecules are decarboxylated and then enter into Krebs cycle (TCA; tricarboxylic acid) cycle to produce 36 molecules of ATP, carbon dioxide and water by oxidative phosphorylation (Fig. **1A**). In normal cells under normoxia, glycolysis and oxidative phosphorylation are tightly coupled processes. In contrast, in an anaerobic (hypoxia) condition pyruvate is red-

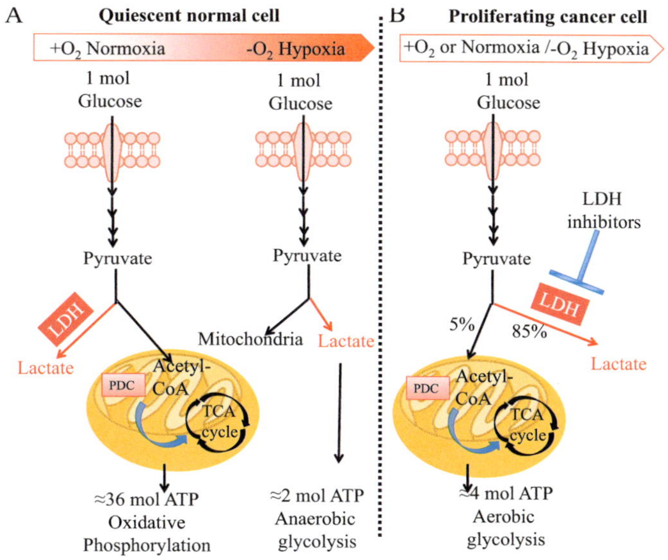

Fig. (1). Schematic representation of metabolic pathway in normal and cancer cells.

uced into lactate catalyzed by LDH and two molecules of ATP are produced in normal cells (Fig. **1A**). Concisely, in normal cells, glucose is metabolized into pyruvate and then CO_2 and acetyl-Co-A for entry into citric acid cycle under normoxia while under hypoxic conditions, OXPHOS remains inactive and LDH catalyzes the conversion of pyruvate into lactate coupled to the oxidation of the cofactor NADH to NAD^+ (Fig. **1A**). In addition, cancer cells adopted a distinguished metabolic pathway in which pyruvate is reduced into lactate even in aerobic condition (Fig. **1B**) for energy production. Abruptly, energetics of cancer cells is much less efficient than normal cells (Fig. **1**), and thus cancer cells are starving for glucose consumption for proliferation, maintenance and survival. Pyruvate is placed at a hub between different metabolic pathways including malate oxidation in proliferating cells [14]. Pyruvate serves as the main fuel of the TCA cycle for energy production, the precursor of alanine in a reversible transamination reaction involving glutamate as the nitrogen donor, and the substrate of a reversible oxidation-reduction reaction generating lactate in cancer cells. Among glycolytic enzymes, LDH is one of the key enzymes involved in the metabolic switch, where glucose is preferentially catabolized into pyruvate and finally into lactate catalyzed by LDH in cancer cells (Fig. **1B**). The LDH is thought to be a major molecular mediator of the Warburg effect and plays a central role in tumor glycolysis. Recent scientific advances proved that *h*LDH occupies an optimal checkpoint at the 'pyruvate bifurcation point' in the glycolytic pathway where pyruvate is directed towards lactate fermentation in cancer cells and differentiates the normal cells towards oxidative phosphorylation. The lactate dehydrogenase enzyme (LDH) has attracted significant attention for drug development against cancer.

4. ISOFORM OF LDH

Structurally, LDH is a tetrameric enzyme composed of two important major subunits (-35kDa each): LDH M (largely present in skeletal muscle and liver) and LDH H (mainly present in heart, spleen, kidney, brain and erythrocytes). These two subunits LDHM (or LDH-A) and LDHB (or LDH H) are encoded by two separate genes, *ldhA* and *ldhB*, respectively (Fig. **2**). These two subunits, LDH-A and LDH-B, combine into five different possible combinations in the following ways: *h*LDH1 = LDH-B4, *h*LDH2 = LDH-AB3, *h*LDH3 = LDH-A2B2, *h*LDH4 = LDH-A3B, *h*LDH5 = LDH-A4 (Fig. **2**). In humans, LDH exists in five main isoforms (*h*LDH1-5) mainly located in the cytosol. Two of the resulting isoform i.e. the homotetramer LDH5 (A4), simply called as LDH-A is assembled only from subunit A and is predominately found in skeletal muscle, whereas LDH1 (B4) recognized as LDH-B formed from only subunit B, primarily exists in heart muscle and other oxygenated tissues. The remaining three isoforms LDH2 (A1B3), LDH3 (A2B2) and LDH4 (A3B1) are hybrid tetramers (Fig. **2**) [15]. The additional sixth isoform of LDH subunit known as LDH-X or LDH-C4 has been found in human testis and sperm, and plays an important role in male fertility [16]. Probable side effects due to *h*LDH-A inhibition might be expected in people with hereditary deficiency of the *ldh-a* gene, leading to a complete lack of the LDHA subunit or patient with decreased *h*LDH-A activity in muscles. They showed myoglobinuria only after intense anaerobic exercise due to muscle damage, without showing any side effects under ordinary circumstances [17]. Thus, *h*LDH-A has been considered as a safe and innovative target in drug development.

5. LDH ACTIVE SITE

The X-ray crystal structure of LDH disclosed that it constitutes two essential domains: i) cofactor binding domain and, ii) substrate binding domain. The larger (cofactor binding) domain is formed by residues 20-162 and 248-266 while the smaller mixed α/β substrate binding domain is composed of residues 163-247 and 267-331. The co-factor (NADH) binds to LDH at one end of the central β-sheet with residues His195, Asp168, Arg171, and Thr246 in an extended conformation and its nicotinamide group partially overlaps the substrate-binding site [18]. In LDH-A subunit of *h*LDH5 the active site is located in rather a deep position within the protein and accessibility of it to substrate and cofactor or their surrogates, is narrow. This binding cavity is quite polar and rich in cationic residues (arginine). Analysis of a ternary complex (NADH-LDH-oxamate, Fig. (**3A**) [18, 19] indicated that oxamate (substrate) interacts with residues Gln99, Arg105, Asn137, Arg168, His192 and Thr247 via hydrogen bonding, whereas Leu164 and Ala237 are engaged in hydrophobic contacts. The side chain of Arg168 interacts with the carboxylate group of the ligand. The closure of a mobile loop (residues 96-107; numbering refers to *h*LDHA in PDB 1I10), in which the conserved Arg105 could stabilize the transition state in the hydride-transfer reaction, is indispensible for catalytic activity. A different ternary complex (NADH-LDH-pyruvate, Fig. (**3B**) [20] also showed similar kinds of bonding and confirmed the importance of Arg169, Thr248, and His193 for the ligand interactions. For example, the ternary complex depicted significant interaction of Arg169, Thr248 with carboxylate group of pyruvate as well with the carbonyl oxygen of the substrate [19, 20].

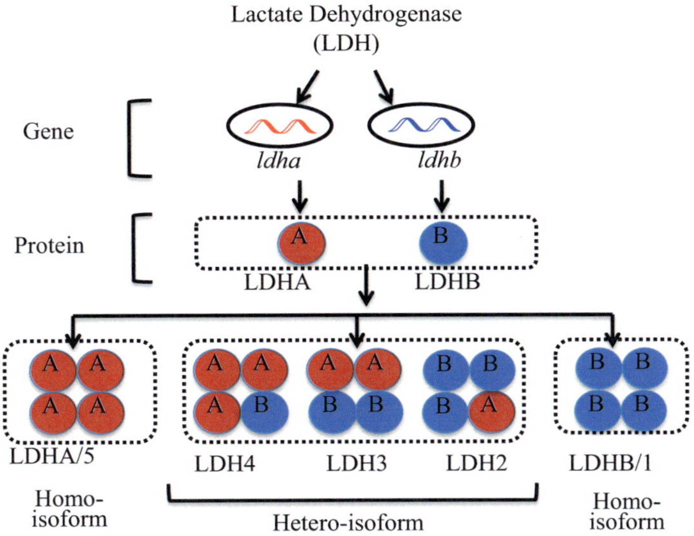

Fig. (2). Lactate dehydrogenase (LDH); LDH isoforms, homo-isoform and hetero-isoforms.

A docking analysis of some of the most potent inhibitors into the X-ray crystal structure of the LDH-A subunit of *h*LDH5 [PDB code: 1i10] displayed the most significant interactions with the enzyme active site and further confirmed that residues Arg169, Thr248 and His193 all play a fundamental role in the catalytic activity of *h*LDHA (Fig. **3**). The potential LDH inhibitors discovered so far have carboxylates functional group and hydroxyl or a carbonyl oxygen atom. Additionally, these chemical moieties (-COOH, -OH/-CO) are often in close proximity, which is consistent with the natural LDH substrates. An α-hydroxyacid (lactate) or an α-ketoacid (pyruvate) are thus mimicked by the LDH inhibitors.

These co-crystal structures of oxamate and pyruvate with LDH (Fig. **3A** & **3B**) enabled the rational design of chemical structures possessing potential inhibitory activities. The astonishing functional and structural diversity of the various chemical classes of *h*LDHA inhibitors involving natural and synthetic molecules are discovered so far. Therefore, prospective inhibitors possessing deprotonatable groups such as COOH are generally preferred for an efficient interaction with the active site of the enzyme.

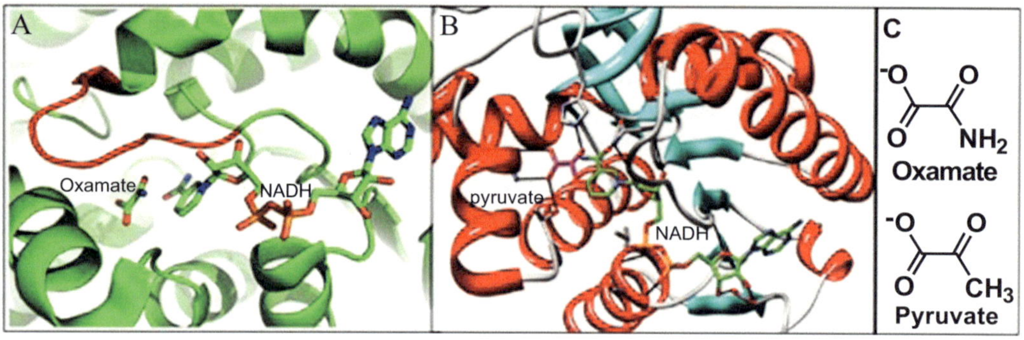

Fig. (3). (A) Represenative example of hLDHA-NADH-Oxamate (PDB 1I10); (B) LDH-NADH (green)-pyruvate (purple) (1.80Å resolution, PDB code: 3D4P). (C) Structure of substrate oxamate and pyruvate. Reproduced with permission ref [18, 20].

5. LDH CATALYTIC MECHANISM

The accepted catalytic mechanism of the conversion of pyruvate to lactate catalyzed by LDH is rather simple but reasonably complex, which starts with the initial binding of cofactor NADH to the active site of LDH enzyme, followed by binding of the substrate pyruvate. This comprises a ternary complex "LDH-NADH-pyruvate" which then undergoes a rate-limiting conformational change by which a substrate specific loop closes to form the desolvated ternary complex essentially in order to bring the amino acid Arg109 (a catalytic residue) into the active site where it polarizes the ketone functionality of substrate pyruvate, thus promoting hydride and proton transfer to the substrate. Apart from catalytic residues, other important amino acids such as Gln102, Arg171, and Thr246, are also involved in substrate discrimination and recognition, together with the catalytic residues Arg109, Asp168, and His195, which are highly conserved in all LDHs. In fact, amino acid residues Gln102, Arg109 and Thr246 are occupied at the substrate (pyruvate) recognition site by enclosing the methyl side chain of the native substrate, which is in fact oriented towards these residues. The catalytic mechanism comprises a direct and stereospecific transfer of a hydride ion (H^-) from the C4 carbon of the dihydronicotinamide ring of NADH (cofactor) to the carbonyl carbon of ketone group of the substrate (pyruvate), simultaneously with proton (H^+) transfer from the catalytic diad Asp168/His195 to the carbonyl oxygen of pyruvate, eventually resulting into the final product lactate. In this mechanism, His195 residue of catalytic diad Asp168/His195 play a unique role that is the imidazole ring of His195 act as proton donor/acceptor in this reaction and it also helps in orientation of the substrate (pyruvate) in the appropriate position so that it can easily interact with the C4 carbon of the dihydronicotinamide of cofactor. Amino acid Asp168 of catalytic diad Asp168/His195, interacts with His195 to stabilize the protonated/cationic form of its imidazole ring via formation of hydrogen bonding between the side chain carboxylic group of Asp168 and NH of imidazole ring of His195 residue. Further, the catalytic residue Arg171 impart in the fixing of the substrate through a strong two-point interaction between its amidine side chain and the carboxylate of pyruvate (Fig. **4**). Moreover, it is noteworthy that the hydrophobic side chain of Ile250 offered a hydrophobic environment which is favorable for the nicotinamide ring of NADH [21, 22]. LDH catalyzes the reduction of lactate to pyruvate by consuming NADH and this reaction equilibrium is shifted towards the formation of lactate.

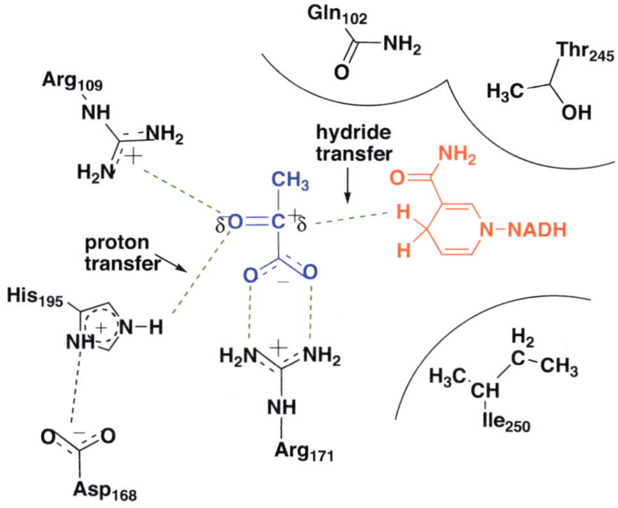

Fig. (4). Systematic representation of catalytical mechanism of conversion of pyruvate to lactate catalyzed by LDH, LDH binding pocket (black), substrate (red) and cofactor (blue).

The high concentration of lactate and NAD^+ facilitates oxidation of lactate to pyruvate. This reaction is reversible which is catalyzed by LDH in both directions, but like all the enzymes do not affect the position of the chemical equilibrium. The enzyme catalysis suggests that the homo-isoform of human LDH, *h*LDH-A has a higher affinity and higher V_{max} for pyruvate reduction than does *h*LDH-B, thus becomes more efficient for anaerobic metabolism and pyruvate reduction such as in hypoxic tumors. Conversely, *h*LDH-B favors the reverse reaction and is concerned more with aerobic oxidation of pyruvate [15]. Analysis in several human tumors as well as adjacent normal tissues confirms the higher concentration of LDH M subunits in the tumors than normal tissues [23]. In fact, there is a marked increase in concentration of LDH M subunits in cancerous tissues (thyroid and colon) compare to H subunits [23]. Therefore, *h*LDH-A plays a central role in the reprogramming of tumor cell metabolism, suggesting that it might be required for the maintenance and survival of tumor cells. In addition, *h*LDH-A can be exploited in drug design and development for anticancer agents whereas *h*LDH-B and *h*LDHC for anti- cardiovascular and anti-infertility agents, respectively.

6. *H*LDH-A AND ITS LINK WITH TUMORIGENESIS

The *h*LDH-A has been overexpressed in highly glycolytic human cancers [24 - 29] and is considered as prognostic factor such as gastric cancer [30], pancreatic cancer [31], colorectal cancer [32], non small cell lung cancer [33, 34] oral squamous cell carcinoma [35], endometrial cancer tissues [36], melanoma [37], squamous head and neck cancer [38], esophageal squamous cell carcinoma [39] etc. *h*LDHA is transcriptionally upregulated by various transcriptional factors responsible for hypoxic adaptation [24 - 28] and it has been identified as a direct target of hypoxia inducible factor 1 (HIF-1) [24 - 28], c-Myc [25 - 28] and the HER2/neu [28] oncogene and was found to be correlated with aggressive phenotypes, cell proliferation and poor prognosis in several tumors In fact, up-regulation of *h*LDHA is directly associated with both HIF-1a and HIF2a accumulation. Additionally, HIF1a is linked with VEGF, extramural invasion and metastases. The high concentration of *h*LDHA is linked with up-regulated HIF pathway and various aggressive phenotype in various cancers. Overexpression of *h*LDH-A level in serum and in plasma is induced by malignant tumor phenotypes, therefore can be indication of presence of cancer. c-Myc is able to increase the expression of LDH-A directly at the transcriptional level and transactivates the LDH-A promotor [40]. Further, glucose deprivation or glucose antimetabolite 2-deoxyglucose (2-DG) treatment causes nontrasformed cells to arrest G1 phase of cell cycle. When glycolysis is blocked, LDH-A mediate the apoptotic effect of c-Myc which is confirmed by the fact that in Rat1a fibroblast, overexpression of LDH-A alone is sufficient to stimulate apoptosis induced by glucose deprivation to increase production of lactate and is responsible to Warburg effect in tumors. The time course of serum induction of c-Myc followed by LDH-A expression in fibroblasts and direct induction of LDH-A expression by the Myc-ER fusion protein further confirms that LDH-A is a direct c-Myc responsive target gene. Moreover, both c-Myc transformed and LDH-A ectopically expressing Rat1a cells produce more lactate than control stably transfected Rat1a cells, again proved that the Warburg effect induced in fibroblasts by c-Myc is largely due to deregulated expression of LDH-A [40]. Furthermore LDH-A is necessary for c-Myc mediated anchorage independent growth of Rat1a cells, although LDHA overexpression alone is insufficient to induce the growth of c-Myc transformed Rat1a cells. With glucose deprivation, nontransformed Rat1a cells displayed minimal apoptotic cell death; in contrast 19% of the c-Myc transformed showed apoptosis. On exposures of 2-DG, Burkitt's lymphoma cells (Ramos and DW 6 cell lines) displayed apoptosis but not the ST486 lymphoma cells having overexpression of c-Myc and LDHA. However, Bcl-2 level is highly elevated in ST486 lymphoma cells in contrast to the Ramos and DW 6 cell lines might be due to the ST486 resist 2-DG induced apoptosis. In fibroblast cells, serum stimulate expression of c-Myc at 2-3 hour followed by expression of LDH-A at 4-6 hour, thus confirmed the LDH-A being a target of c-Myc. Moreover, overexpression of c-Myc is directly associated with elevated level of LDH-A in c-Myc transformed fibroblast, lymphoblastoid, lung cells and in Burkitt's lymphoma cells [40]. In 2014, Cui *et al.* reported that the increased expression of forkhead box protein 1 (FOXM1) upregulated *h*LDH-A expression by direct binding of FOXM1 with the promoter region of *h*LDH-A, causing increased LDH activity, lactate production, and glucose utilization in pancreatic cancer cell growth. In fact, FOXM1 markedly change the expression of phosphoglycerate kinase 1 (PGK-1) and LDH-A without affecting most glycolytic enzymes. Both, FOXM1 and LDH-A were found overexpressed concurrently in pancreatic tumors and cancer cell lines. Therefore, elevated FOXM1-LDHA signaling increased the pancreatic cancer cell growth and metastasis [29]. Collectively, several genetic studies provide proof-o--concept that *h*LDH-A expression is directly linked with the dysregulated expression and activation of various oncogenes and confirmed the involvement of *h*LDH-A in tumorigenesis. Moreover, overexpression of *h*LDH-A resulted higher lactate production, which triggered increased extracellular acidosis, resulting in a low pH and facilitating tumor invasion and metastasis [41] and viability of tumor cells [23]. In fact, the silencing of *h*LDH-A expression by means of shRNA demonstrated a reduction in the ability of tumors to proliferate under hypoxic conditions, markedly delayed tumor formation, stimulated mitochondrial respiration [26, 28, 42] and reduced tumor growth, even in the background of fumarate hydratase-deficient cells in a renal cancer xenograft mouse model [43]. The knockdown of *h*LDH-A directly by lysine-5 acetylation of *h*LDH-A and stimulating chaperone-mediated autophagy-regulated degradation of *h*LDH-A confirms that lysine-5 acetylation is inversely correlated in pancreatic cancer initiation and further established the role of *h*LDH-A in the regulation of cell growth [44]. Additionally, *h*LDH is responsible for catalyzing the conversion of glyoxylate to oxalate in the mitochondrial/peroxisomal glycine metabolism pathway in the liver and pancreas. Increased production of glyoxylate facilitates accumulation of oxalate, which ultimately caused the Primary Hyperoxaluria Type 1 (PHI) disease in presence of LDH. PHI disease is a rare autosomal recessive inborn error of glyoxylate metabolism, caused by liver- specific enzyme alanine: glyoxylate aminotransferase (also named serine -pyruvate aminotransferase) deficiency. Thus, reduced expression of the LDHA gene via RNAi molecule, optionally a double stranded nucleic acid ("dsNA") or comprising a hairpin or a tetraloop structure, a single- stranded antisense oligonucleotide have been used for development of effective pathway for treating and preventing primary hyperoxaluria type 1 (PHI), primary hyperoxaluria type 2 (PH2) and primary hyperoxaluria type 3 (PH3). A dsNA consisting of a first strand (between 32 and 80 nucleic acid residues in length) possessed a tetraloop, and a second strand (of 19 to 30 nucleotides in length). The second strand of dsNA anneals to the first strand to form a duplex, wherein second oligonucleotide strand is complementary to a target LDH- mRNA sequence. When dsNA was introduced into a mammalian cell, it was revealed that the at least 15 nucleotides of oligonucleotide strand length was sufficient to reduce LDH target mRNA expression. Brown, *et al.* have been discovered the robust knockdown of LDH-A in liver reduces the deleterious elevation level of lactate in mice [45]. Recently, it has been discovered that LDH-A secreted by glioblastoma cells induces Natural Killer Group 2 member D (NKG2D) on monocytes isolated from healthy cells. Elevated level of LDH-A identified in glioblastoma multiforme (GBM) patients confirms a link between expressions of NKG2D ligand on circulating monocytes. LDH-A inhibitors such as antibody inhibited LDH-A binding / incorporation/ endocytosis to immune cells to prevent down regulation of immune responses by tumor cells. Further, only LDH-A (not lactate) induces IL-6 gene in glioblastoma cell lines U87 inveterate that LDH-A offered an additional advantage on immune response with respect to cytokines. Thus therapeutic binding agents that inhibited incorporation, internalization and binding cause downregulation on immune system by blocking of incorporation of LDH-A into tumor cells. The anti-LDH-A antibody specific for LDH-A blocks downregulation of immune system by binding to the receptor for LDH-A where anti-LDH-5 antibody is directed to amino terminus of LDH-A [46]. Overall, the knockdown of *h*LDH-A by shRNA or small molecules offered definite confirmation of the critical role of *h*LDH-A in tumor initiation, development, maintenance and chemoresistance therapy.

7. REGULATION/INHIBITION OF LACTATE DEHYDROGENASE

*h*LDH-A, being an attractive target, plays an important role in preventing, ameliorating or correct dysfunctions and cancer related diseases. Regulation/ inhibition of *h*LDH-A by small molecules or by binding of these small molecules to *h*LDH-A gene provide an interesting platform to treat cancer and cancer related diseases. RNA based knockdown therapies, antibodies, RNAi, double stranded nucleic acid (dsNA), comprising a hairpin or a tetraloop structure, a single-stranded antisense oligonucleotide are useful in clinics and for this purpose *h*LDH-A is considered an attractive target [47]. The inhibition of *h*LDH-A by small molecules reduces ATP levels and increases oxygen consumption, thus leading to increased production of mitochondrial reactive oxygen species (ROS) and oxidative stress resulting in cell death [28]. Recently, small molecules, as potential inhibitors of *h*LDH-A, proved to be effective in hypoxic pancreatic cancer cell lines and exhibited synergistic cytotoxic activity with gemcitabine by attacking the key mechanisms involved in the proliferation, cell-cycle control, apoptosis and migration of pancreatic cancer cells [31]. The combination of paclitaxel and trastuzumab, separately, with oxamate, a structural isostere of pyruvate and a well-known pyruvate-competitive inhibitor of *h*LDH-A (K_i = 136μM) and *h*LDH-B (K_i = 94.4μM) [48], shows a synergistic inhibitory effect on taxol- and trastuzumab-resistant breast cancer cells by promoting cellular apoptosis, thus confirming the correlation of *h*LDH5 with resistance to chemotherapy [49, 50].

8. SMALL MOLECULES AS *H*LDHA INHIBITORS

Co-crystal structures of LDH-A with substrate or substrate mimicked structures enabled the rational design of chemical structures possessing selective potential inhibitory activity against *h*LDH-A. Astonishing functional and structural diversity of the potential *h*LDH-A inhibitors including natural and synthetic molecules have been discovered so far. A very few successful attempts to selectively inhibit *h*LDH-A enzyme by means of small organic "drug-like" molecules have been reported with the purpose of blocking glycolysis in cancer cells [51, 52]. Moreover, with the aim of maintenance of potential activities with improved selectivity toward *h*LDH-A, many efforts are still going on because only few clinical applications were so far envisioned. Very simple molecule oxamate (**1**), a structural isostere of pyruvate (**2**) and a well-known pyruvate-competitive inhibitor of *h*LDH-A possessing K_i value of 136μM however it also showed *h*LDH-B inhibitory activity with K_i = 94.4μM [48] thus showed mild selectivity towards *h*LDH-A. Additionally, It shows a synergistic inhibitory effect on taxol- and trastuzumab-resistant breast cancer cells by promoting cellular apoptosis [49, 50]. Gossypol (**3**) is a polyphenolic binaphthyl disesquiterpene is a natural product which is originally isolated from the cotton seeds of gossypium. It presented a complex and broad spectrum of promising biological activities, such as antitumor, antioxidant, antiviral, and antiparasitic activities (Fig. **5**) [53]. It exists in two enantiomeric forms, (*R*) and (*S*), via restricted rotation around the 2-2′ carbon-carbon single bond and, the (*R*) - (−) form of gossypol showed higher activity than the (*S*) - (+) isomer of gossypol [54]. For dose-dependent cytotoxic activity, (*R*)-(−) form of **1** showed mean IC_{50} values of 20μM in melanoma, lung cancer, breast cancer, cervical cancer, and leukemia cell lines [54]. Some natural products based on polyphenolic scaffolds (such as **4**; morin, **5**; epigallocatechin, **6**; galloflavin) were found to be potential anticancer agents due to their inhibitory activity against *h*LDH-A (Fig. **5**) [55]. The structure of epigallocatechin (**5**) (Fig. **5**) isolated from an aqueous extract of *Spatholobus suberectus*, inhibited both *h*LDH-A and HIF-1α expression. It showed significant inhibition of breast cancer growth (MCF-7, MDA-MB-231), triggered apoptosis without eliciting any toxic effect [56]. A tricyclic flavone-like molecule Galloflavin (**6**) (Fig. **5**), however, exhibited strong inhibitory activity against *h*LDH-A (Ki value of 5.46μM vs. pyruvate and 56.0μM vs. NADH) but in nonselective manner. It also showed inhibitory activity against *h*LDH-B (Ki = 15.1μM vs. pyruvate; 23.2μM vs. NADH) and was identified as a potent, nonselective *in vivo* antitumor agent [57]. In fact, compound **6** completely blocked the enzymatic activities of both LDH isoforms, endowed 60% inhibition of cell growth, and exerted comparable growth inhibition effects (IC_{50} values in the 90-150μM range) in breast cancer cell lines (MCF-7, MDA-MB-231, and MCF-Tam cells). It showed low cytotoxicity in healthy cells and the promising pharmacological effects in aggressive tumors; this encourages the further exploration of compound **6** [58].

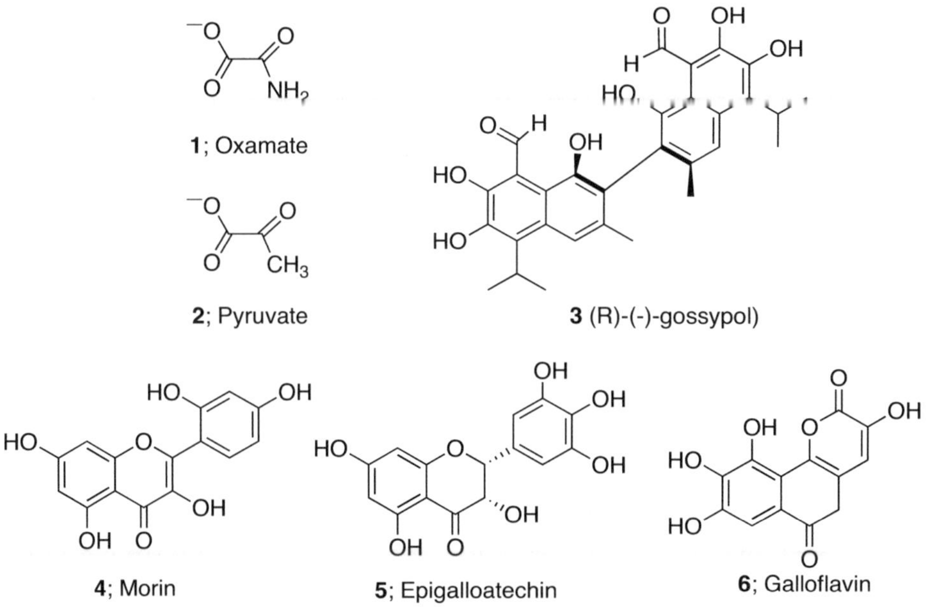

Fig. (5). Oxamate (**1**), pyruvate (**2**) and natural *h*LDHA inhibitors (**3-6**).

9. SYNTHETIC LDHA INHIBITORS

Dang *et al*. discovered the half analogue of gossypol, known as FX11 (**7**; Fig. **6**) which was found to inhibit neoplasia characterized by glycolytic metabolism including lymphomas, leukemias, brain cancer, breast cancer, colon and pancreatic cancer via inhibition of LDHA. FX11 seems to be effective in the inhibition of proliferation and survival in neoplasia. FX11 may be used alone or in combination with nicotinamide phosphoribosyltransferase (NAMPT) inhibitor of NAD^+ synthesis [59]. In search of drug like *h*LDH-A inhibitors, Minutolo *et al.* discovered a distinguished class of *h*LDHA inhibitors with potential therapeutic applications, represented by the *N*-hydroxyindole (NHIs) derivatives (**8**, **9**) (Fig. **6**) [60 - 63]. These NHIs comprise the central indole scaffold in which a hydroxyl group was occupied in the nitrogen atom in the 1-position and a carboxyl group in the 2-position of the indole moiety, whereas benzene ring of indole was substituted by various aryl, heteroaryl, electron-withdrawing group. These NHIs showed inhibitory activity in the competition with both the cofactor NADH and the substrate pyruvate, with Ki values in the low micromolar range against *h*LDHA. Structure activity relationship revealed that the inhibitory efficiency of NHIs might be relying on the "OH-COOH" pharmacophore motif because this type of structural motif partially resembles the structure of the natural substrates of LDH, i.e., an α -keto acid (pyruvate) or α -hydroxy acid (lactate). These NHIs derivatives exhibited *h*LDHA inhibitory activity in low micromolar range with significant selectivity of towards *h*LDHA over *h*LDHB.

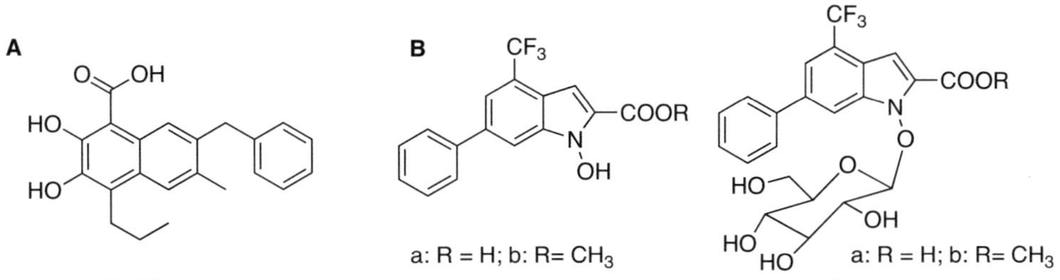

7; FX-11 8 9

Fig. (6). LDHA inhibitors; **A**: FX-11 (**1**) and **B**: NHIs derivatives.

Interestingly, representative molecule of this series **8a** also most active NHI derivative, exhibited marked selectivity for *h*LDHA over *h*LDHB. In fact, the insertion of an electron-withdrawing group (trifluoromethyl) in the 4-position of **8a** demonstrated more potency than **8b**, a methyl ester derivative of **8a**. Compound **8a** showed Ki values of 8.9μM in competition with NADH and 4.7μM in competition with pyruvate, whereas its methyl ester derivative **8b** displayed a slightly lower Ki value of 5.1μM in the NADH competition assay. Specific binding of **8a** to *h*LDH5 was further supported by 2D NMR analysis depicting Kd value of approximately 9μM (in NADH competition); however, BIAcore studies showed nonspecific binding [60]. Moreover, in combination with other drug like molecule, both NHI derivatives **8a** and **8b** showed marked improvement in potency towards *h*LDHA. Both these molecules displayed a synergistic cytotoxic effect in combination with gemcitabine under hypoxic conditions and also inhibited spheroid growth, cell migration, and invasion in pancreatic cancer cells [31]. Later same research group discovered glucose derived compounds of NHIs where -OH group present on 1 position of NHIs was conjugated with glucose moiety. These glucose conjugated NHI derivatives (Glu-NHIs) such as compounds **9a** and **9b** favor the accessibility of compound to the cancer cells and *in vivo*. Although compounds **9a** and **9b** presented weaker inhibitory activity than parent compounds against *h*LDHA, exhibiting Ki values of 19.5 and 37.8μM, respectively, in the NADH competition assay, they exhibited more efficacy than their N-OH analogs in cell-based assays [61 - 63]. Both compounds **9a** and **9b** (methylester derivative of **9a**) efficiently reduced dose-dependent lactate production in the HeLa cancer cell line and compromised cell proliferation in several cancer cell lines. Compound **9b** showed better cell permeability and reduced lactate production and antiproliferative activity [64]. With the aim of discovery of potential *h*LDH-A inhibitors, a series of *h*LDH-A inhibitors based on central scaffold quinoline was patented by GlaxoSmithKline (Brentford, UK) in 2012, for the treatment of cancer and diseases associated with tumor cell metabolism. The structural features of the compounds of this series are different from other *h*LDH-A inhibitors, where 3 and 4 position of central quinoline scaffold is substituted via various functional groups. An amide or sulfonamide group is inserted in the 3-position, and the 4-position of the quinoline is occupied by a carboxyl moiety bearing an aromatic ring conjugated through the NH group, and finally, the 7-position is substituted by various aromatic or heteroaromatic rings illustrated by structure **10**. Compound **10** demonstrated excellent inhibitory activities against *h*LDHA displaying a pIC_{50} value of 7.2 (IC_{50} = 63.1nM). The structure of these molecules suggests that the COOH group on the aniline pendant ring may competently mimic the substrate (pyruvate/lactate), and consequently bind the enzyme in the substrate-binding region. Unlike other *h*LDH-A inhibitors where a carboxylic acid group occupied an adjacent position or at least in the close proximity of a hydroxyl group, or a carbonyl-type oxygen atom, the structural features of molecules of this class are quite different where pyridine ring is substituted with the amide/ sulfonamide group, closely resemble the structure of the nicotinamide portion of cofactor $NADH/NAD^+$, whereas the COOH group on the aniline moiety may efficiently mimic the substrate (pyruvate/lactate), and can bind the enzyme in the substrate-binding region [65]. Further, similar kind of quinoline derivatives **11**, **12** have been reported by insertion of cyclopentyl group in 5 position of benzoic acid functionality and *N*-cyclopropylsulfamoyl group in 3 position of quinoline. Compound **11** showed significant improvement against in *h*LDH-A inhibitory activity possessing IC_{50} values of 16nM with 13-fold selectivity over *h*LDHB (IC_{50} of 220nM). For further improvement of potency of small molecules towards *h*LDHA, cyclopentyl group was replaced by 3,5-difluorophenoxy moiety in 5 position of benzoic acid functionality of the central scaffold of compound **11** resulting compound **12** exhibiting IC_{50} values of 1.9nM with 16 fold selectivity for *h*LDH-A over *h*LDH-B (IC_{50} of 43nM). Both compounds **11** and **12** were most potent selective *h*LDH-A inhibitors possessing inhibitory activity in low nanomolar range discovered so far. Currently, compound **12** is available for marketing for research purposes under agreement from GlaxoSmithKline claiming IC_{50} values of 1.9 and 14nM for LDH-A and LDH-B respectively [66, 67]. Further, the most active compound **12** reduced glucose consumption and inhibited cell proliferation and cell survival in the highly glycolytic Snu398 and HEPG2 human hepatocellular carcinoma cells. At a concentration of 10μM, compound **12** displayed an increased oxygen consumption rate and ROS activity, altered metabolic intermediates concentrations, and reduced the rate of formation of tumor spheres in A549 cells. These molecules were endowed with promising *h*LDHA inhibitory activities, although they showed poor pharmacokinetic properties that caused limitations for the further use of these molecules in *in vivo* experiments [67]. In addition to the *h*LDH-A inhibitors, Maloney *et al.* invented small molecules based on central scaffold "pyrazolyl-thiazole" in which carboxylate moiety is present at 4 position of thiazole ring attached to "N" of pyrazole ring in 1 position where as various aryl and heteroaryl groups are present in 3 and 4 position while trifluoromethyl (-CF_3) moiety is inserted at position 5 of pyrazole ring exemplified by compound **13** and **14** (Fig. **7**). They claimed compound **13** presented inhibitory activity in nanomolar range, and this compound and its ester derivatives as prodrug (**14**) could be useful for the development of pharmaceutically acceptable salt for treatment of cancer [68].

Apart from anticancer agents, small molecules of LDH inhibitory activity also utilized in drug design for epileptic treatment. Analogs of isosafrole (**15-17**) and their stereoisomeric forms are revealed to have the inhibitory effect of LDH, thus observed that compounds having isosafrole the central scaffold exhibited LDH-A inhibitory activity (Fig. **8**). For example, suchiripentoru (**15**) is an isosafrole where 3-position of propene group is occupied by a hydroxy group and a tertiary butyl group exhibited antiproliferative activity at lower concentrations. The 300mg/kg administration of Suchiripentoru suppressed the epilepsy wave. Thus, it is consistent with the use of an anti-epileptic drug for children epilepsy in Dravet syndrome [69, 70].

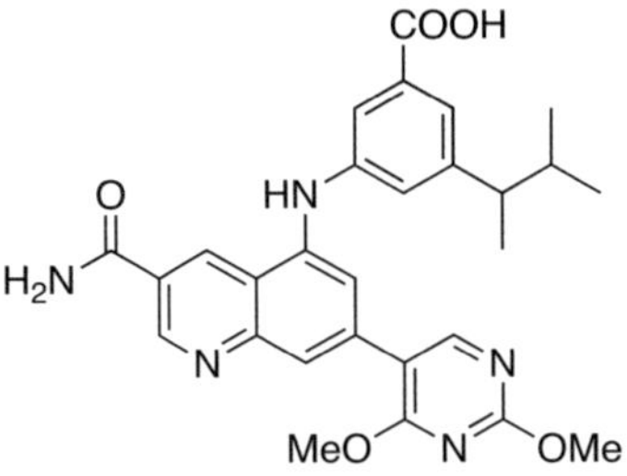

10

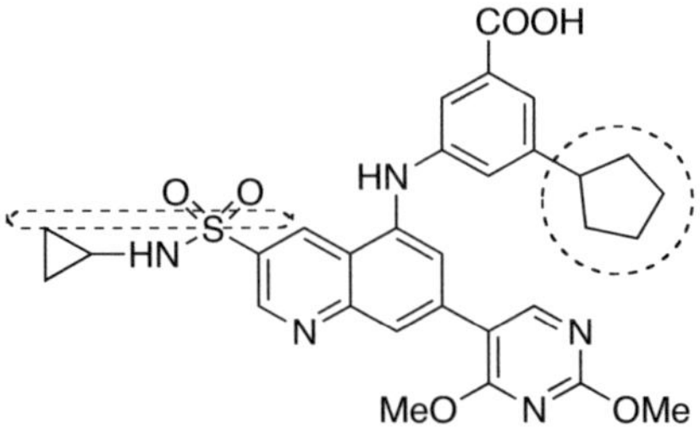

11

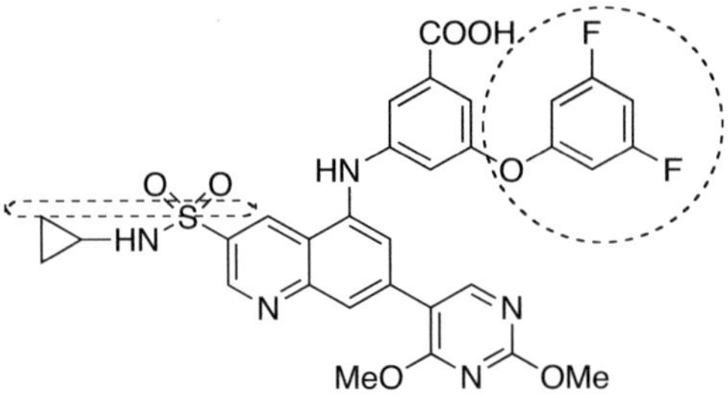

12

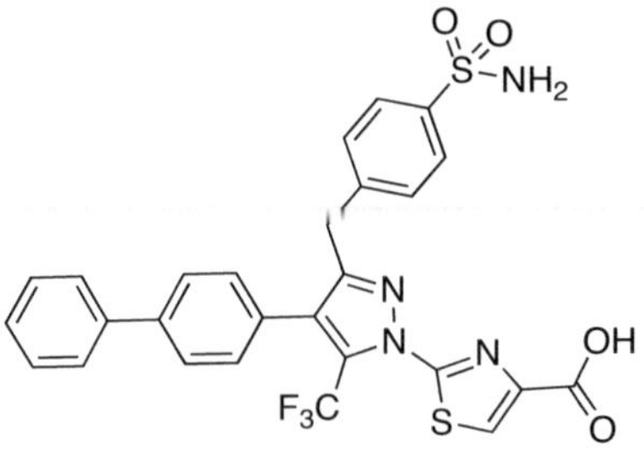

13

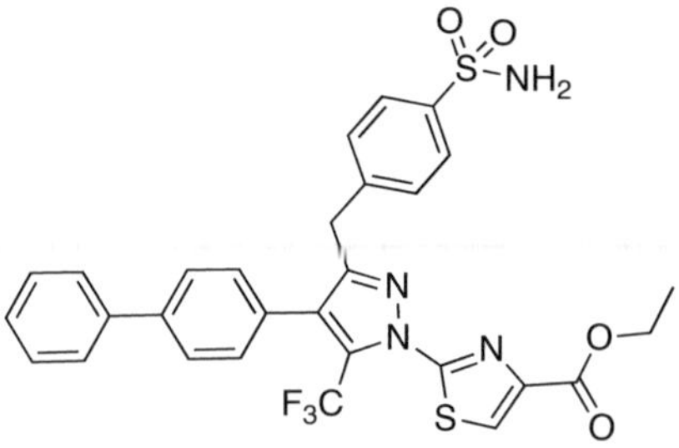

14

Fig. (7). Quinoline (**10-12**) and pyrazolyl-thiazole (**13, 14**) based hLDH-A inhibitors.

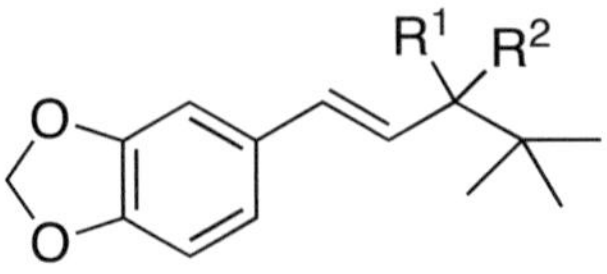

15

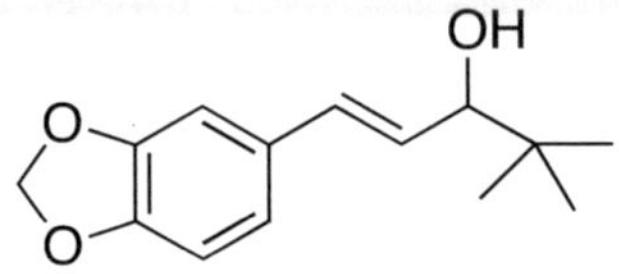

16

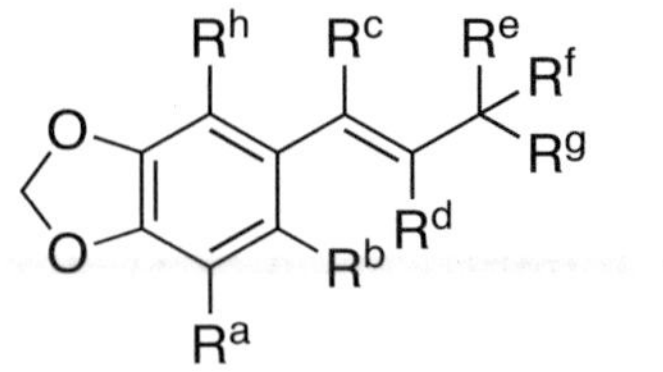

17

Fig. (8). LDH inihibitors for epileptic treatment.

10. NANOPARTICLE BASED DELIVERY FOR *H*LDH-A INHIBITION

The knockdown of *h*LDH-A by using dsRNAs with lipid nanoparticles and GalNac conjugates offered a therapeutic benefit in chronic kidney disease and pyruvate dehydrogenase complex deficiency. The LNP-mediated oligonucleotide and their therapeutic delivery for potential LDH-A inhibitory activity at the site of optimal target organs or cancers have been reported. LNP-mediated RNAi delivery system offered an innovative method for treating neoplasia and related diseases. Initially, in absence of valid evidences, the knockdown of robust level of LDHA achieved by RNAi agents have been predicted to be harmful to the patients. Although, therapeutic potential of RNA-based approach and its therapeutic modalities have been well established not only as effective approach but also well tolerated [45].

11. LDH IN OTHER DISEASES

LDH-A is not only useful in treatment of cancer and cancer related diseases but also useful in diseases related to cutaneous tissues such as skin cells, hair follicle and nails acquired glucose preferentially form the blood for skin cell proliferation, a process of growth and repair which decreases with ageing and photodamage. Bartolone *et al.* [71] postulated that with increased skin cell proliferation and collagen synthesis caused improved skin condition and appearance of skin and that can be attained by synergistic effect of LDH inhibitor in specific combination with a carboxylic acid. LDH inhibitors such as tartronic acid, pyruvic acid, alkyl ester of pyruvic acid oxalic acid etc. have been used in combination in amount of 0.001% to 20% by weight of composition, although maximum efficacy is attained by 4 to 8% by weight of composition existing preferable pH range near about 3.5 to 4.5 [71].

12. DETERMINATION AND QUANTIFICATION OF LDH

*h*LDHA enzyme has prominent involvement in many glycolytic cancers, cancer invasion and metastasis. It offered additional advantages to treat various disease and also considered as biomarkers therefore, determination and quantification of LDH is salient task and urgent in development of new innovative medical tools. Takagahara *et al.* [72] disclosed a method for fractional quantitative determination of isoenzyme of LDH by using LDH inhibitor 1,6-dihydronicotinamide adenine dinucleotide (**15**, 1,6-DHNAD) (Fig. **9**). 1,6-DHNAD inhibits both LDHA and LDHB isoforms but the degree of inhibition against LDHB considerably differ from LDHA isoform.

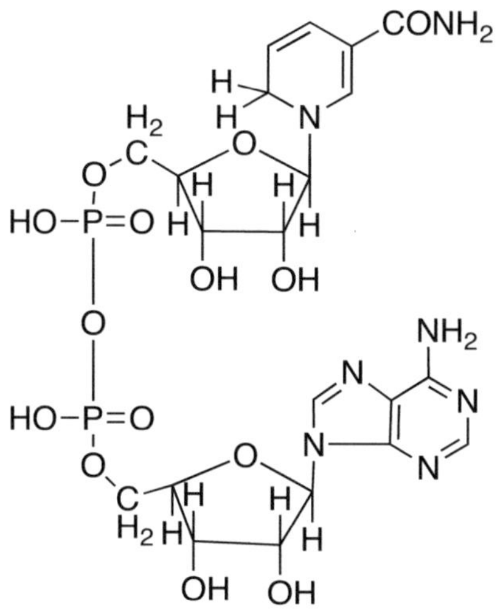

1,6-DHNAD

18

Fig. (9). Structure of 1,6-DHNAD.

The ratio of LDHA and LDHB in serum can be measured by utilizing the difference of inhibition degree by following equation (I)

$$P = (P_H - P_M)R_H + R_M \quad \textbf{(1)}$$

where in R_H equals the ratio of H-type LDH activity (LDHB activity) to total LDH activity when 1,6 DHNAD is absent.

P_H equals the ratio of H-type LDH activity (LDHB activity) when 1,6 DHNAD is present to H-type LDH activity (LDHB activity) when 1,6 DHNAD is absent.

P_M equals the ratio of M-type LDH activity (LDHA activity) when 1,6 DHNAD is present to M-type LDH activity (LDHA activity) when 1,6 DHNAD is absent.

P is the ratio of total LDH activity when 1,6 DHNAD is present to total LDH activity when 1,6 DHNAD is absent.

In this method, the determination agent was employed in measurement of LDH activity by using pyruvic acid as a substrate with respect to the sample. Further LDH activity was determined by using 1, 6-DHNAD inhibitor, whereas total LDH activity was measured by using only reduced NAD without using 1,6-DHNAD, then ratio of the former LDH activity to the total LDH activity has been calculated. Therefore, so obtained ratio can be compared with standard values whose inhibitory degree of isoenzyme previously reported and amount of isoenzyme can be easily determined by fractional quantitative determination. The 1,6-DHNAD displayed constant inhibition against LDHA and stable inhibition in LDHB and this method involving 1,6-DHNAD offered an excellent analytical method for analysis of LDH isoenzymes [72]. Later, Felipe *et al.* reported a nanosensor for detecting and quantifying lactate in wide range of samples, including different type of tissues, intra-cellular and even in subcellular compartments with in four orders of concentration magnitude presenting high spatial and temporal resolution [73]. This nanosensor could be useful in the quantification of i) lactate transporters activity, ii) rates of cellular lactate production and cellular lactate consumption, and iii) rate of mitochondrial pyruvate consumption. Along with these, authors also disclosed i) a system to enumerate the energy metabolism transformation that differentiate the cancer cells with single-cell resolution and ii) a method to recognize the interference of drugs candidate with mitochondrial energetics. The Forster Resonance Energy Transfer (FRET)-based lactate nanosensor further based on a bacterial transcription regulator LldR has been developed for detection and quantification of lactate in various samples. The LldR genes were selected from *Corynebacterium glutamicum* and from *Escherichia coli*. This FRET-based lactate nanosensor consisting of two modules, one is lactate-binding/regulatory domain and second is DNA-binding domain.

This nanosensor exhibited a biphasic dose response curve with dissociation constants of 8mM and 800mM for lactate, which allows high spatial and temporal resolution and quantitation of lactate in the range 10^{-6} to 10^{-2}M which indicate four orders of magnitude, and differs from all existing FRET metabolite nanosensors. The sensor showed a modest sensitivity to pH in the physiological range. This nanosensor offered new insight for the quantification of the i) activity of lactate transporters, ii) rates of cellular lactate production and cellular lactate consumption, and iii) rate of mitochondrial pyruvate consumption. This probe also covers a method to quantify the transformation in energy metabolism that exemplifies cancer cells with single-cell resolution and to discover interference of mitochondrial energetics with the effect of drug candidates [73]. In Table **1**, recent patents involving detection and identification of LDH and uses of LDH inhibitors in cancer diagnosis, prognosis and treatment have been discussed.

Table 1. Recent Patents Involving Detection and Identification of LDH and Uses of LDH inhibitors in Cancer Diagnosis, Prognosis and Treatment.

References	Inventors	Patent Number	Title
[40]	Dang, C.V., Shim, H.	WO9836774	Method of treating A lactate dehydrogenase-A (LDH-A)- associated disorder
[45]	Brown, B.D., Dudek, H.T., Lai, C.	WO2016057932	Therapeutic inhibition of lactate dehydrogenase and agents therefor
[46]	Courtney, C.	WO2015157299	Inhibition of Lactate dehydrogenase 5 (LDH-5), binding incorporation, internalization and/or endocytosis to immune cells
[47]	Liou, J.-R.	WO2003048350	Regulation of human lactate dehydrogenase
[55]	Mazzio, E., Soliman, K.	WO2006017494	Inhibition of anaerobic glucose metabolism and corresponding natural composition as a non-toxic approach to cancer treatment
[59]	Dang, C.V., Le Q.H., Dinavahi, R.,	US20120003156	Methods for treating neoplasia by inhibiting lactate dehydrogenase and/or nicotinamide phosphoribosyltransferase
[61]	Minutolo, F., Macchia, M., Granchi, C., Di Bussolo, V., Giannaccini, G., Lucacchini, A., Hergenrother, P.J., Calvaresi, E.C.	WO2013092735	Indole derivatives inhibitors of enzyme lactate dehydrogenase (LDH)
[62]	Minutolo. F., Macchia, M., Granchi, C., Di Bussolo, V., Giannaccini, G., Lucacchini, A., Hergenrother, P.J., Calvaresi, E.C.	US20140343001	Indole derivatives inhibitors of enzyme lactate dehydrogenase (LDH)
[65]	Chai, D., Colon, M., Dodson, C., Duffy, K.J., Nicholas, A.	WO2012061557	Preparation of substituted quinoline derivatives as lactate dehydrogenase A inhibitors
[68]	Maloney, D.J., Jadhav, A., Bantukallu, G.R., Brimacombe, K.R., Mott, B.T., Yang, S.M., Urban, D.J., Hu, X., Simeonov, A., Kouznetsova, J.L., Waterson, A.G., Sulikowski, G.A., Kim, K., Christov, P., Jana, S.	WO2016109559	Small molecule inhibitors of lactate dehydrogenase and methods of use thereof
[69]	Inoue, T. Yoshida, N., Otsuki, T., Lee, S.	WO2014115764	Lactic acid dehydrogenase inhibitor and pharmaceutical preparation containing same
[70]	Inoue, T., Nagisa, S.	WO2016129583	Lactate dehydrogenase inhibitor and antiepileptic drug containing same

(Table 1) contd.....

References	Inventors	Patent Number	Title
[71]	Bartolone, J.B., Penksa, C.M., Santhanam, C.M., Lang, B.D.	US5595730	Lactate dehydrogenase inhibitor and antiepileptic drug containing same
[72]	Takagahara, I., Yamauti, J., Yoshimura, S., Fujii, K., Horio, T.	US4258131	Method of fractional quantitative determination of isoenzyme of lactic dehydrogenase
[73]	Luis Felipe, B.O., Alejandro, S.M., Sebastian, C.C., Wolf, B.F.	WO2013154587	Genetically encoded probe for quantification of lactate, and methods for quantifying metabolic rates and lactate transport

CURRENT AND FUTURE DEVELOPMENTS

For scientific community, development of new approaches for the treatment of cancer without disturbing healthy tissues is still a challenging task. Mostly, cancer cells classified with an altered metabolism involving a shift to aerobic glycolysis with lactate production coupled with a higher uptake of glucose as the main source of energy. This metabolic shift toward aerobic glycolysis linked with amplified glucose uptake by cancer cell and lactate production, is largely considered as a key metabolic hallmark of cancer cells. Thus, selective advantages of the metabolic dependencies of tumor cells can be exploited for cancer treatment because either directly or indirectly, metabolism is a vital need in everything a cell does. *h*LDHA catalyzes a reversible reaction which involves the reduction of pyruvate to lactate coupled with oxidation of NADH to NAD^+, thus determining the availability of NAD^+ to maintain the continuity of glycolysis. The *h*LDHA isoform occupies a unique place in the list of promising targets for cancer treatment because of some interesting facts such as:

i. *h*LDHA plays a critical role in metabolic checkpoint in the cancer glycolytic pathway.
ii. It is considered as a direct target of oncogenes and its associations in activation of proto-oncogenes, cancer cell proliferation, maintenance and survival, and also in the maintenance of invasiveness and metastatic potential.
iii. *h*LDHA is associated with resistance to chemo- and radiotherapy of cancer cells.

Consideration of *h*LDH5 as a vital hallmark in cancer cell and its link with transcriptional factors makes it a prominent target for the discovery of drug-like molecules. Although substantial research efforts have been made from both academics and pharmaceutical companies to discover LDH inhibitors, but it seems a tough challenge to discover drug like inhibitors. However, it has been considered a challenging target due to its highly polar nature and small size of its natural substrate (pyruvate), along with the relatively large and open active site but its existence at the 'pyruvate bifurcation point' in the glycolytic pathway makes it a safe and innovative target. Since the discovery of *h*LDH5, significant progress has been made in understanding the biology and function of *h*LDH-A in various human cancers and in development of cancer drugs from *h*LDH5 inhibitors. Till date, various *h*LDH-A inhibitors have been discovered but very few *h*LDH-A inhibitors have progressed to the preclinical stage and into clinical trials. The *h*LDH-A attracts great interest to discover both synthetic and natural compounds that endowed significant *h*LDH-A inhibitory activity. Very recently, inhibitory potency of saffron extracts towards *h*LDH-A enzymes has been reported [74]. The crocetin, an important component of saffron, was found to inhibit LDH (IC_{50} = 54.9 $\pm$ 4.7μM). Various biological results obtained by small *h*LDH-A inhibitors as well as genetic proof suggested that promising molecules of selective inhibitory activity towards *h*LDH-A have been identified and tested in preclinical studies. Development of *h*LDH-A inhibitor that can enter into clinical trial is not easy, nevertheless is not impossible [75]. A better and deeper understanding of the molecular mechanisms may solve the question; why cancer cells are more dependent on some specific pathways and may offer new insight to target altered metabolic sites more selectively.

CONFLICT OF INTEREST

The authors declare no conflict of interest, financial or otherwise.

ACKNOWLEDGEMENTS

Authors are thankful to Amity University Noida. Reshma Rani is thankful to DST-SERB (Grant no. ECR/2017/000548) for financial assistance. Reshma Rani is also thankful to Prof. Filippo Minutolo (University of Pisa, Italy).

LIST OF ABBREVIATIONS

LDH	Lactate Dehydrogenase
***h*LDH5**	human Lactate Dehydrogenase
NADH	Nicotinamide Adenine Dinucleotide
OXPHOS	Oxidative Phosphorylation
FDG-PET	Fluorodeoxyglucose Positron Emission Tomography
NHL	NonHodgkins Lymphoma
ATP	Adenosine Triphosphate
TCA	Tricarboxlic Acid
ROS	Reactive Oxygen Species
HIF	Hypoxia Inducible Factor

HER2	Human Epidermal Growth Factor
FOXM1	Forhead Box Protein 1
PGK-1	Phosphoglycerate Kinase-1; Primary Hyperoxaluria Type 1
PGK-2	Primary Hyperoxaluria Type 2
PGK-3	Primary Hyperoxaluria Type 3
NKG2D	IL-6, NAMPT, LNP, Lipid Nanoparticle
GalNac	1,6-DHNAD, 1,6-dihydronicotinamide Adenine Dinucleotide
FRET	Forster Resonance Energy Transfer
LldR	Bacterial Transcription Regulator Gene

REFERENCES

[1] McGuire S. World Cancer Report 2014. Geneva, Switzerland: World Health Organization, International Agency for Research on Cancer, WHO Press, 2015. Adv Nutr 2016; 7(2): 418-9. [http://dx.doi.org/10.3945/an.116.012211] [PMID: 26980827]

[2] Casanovas O. Cancer: Limitations of therapies exposed. Nature 2012; 484(7392): 44-6. [http://dx.doi.org/10.1038/484044a] [PMID: 22481354]

[3] Hanahan D, Weinberg RA. Hallmarks of cancer: The next generation. Cell 2011; 144(5): 646-74. [http://dx.doi.org/10.1016/j.cell.2011.02.013] [PMID: 21376230]

[4] Cantor JR, Sabatini DM. Cancer cell metabolism: One hallmark, many faces. Cancer Discov 2012; 2(10): 881-98. [http://dx.doi.org/10.1158/2159-8290.CD-12-0345] [PMID: 23009760]

[5] Seyfried TN. Energetics of normal cells and cancer cells in cancer as a metabolic disease: On the origin management amd the prevention of cancer. Hoboken, NJ, USA: A Jhon wiley & Sons 2012; pp. 55-7.

[6] Warburg O. On the origin of cancer cells. Science 1956; 123(3191): 309-14. [http://dx.doi.org/10.1126/science.123.3191.309] [PMID: 13298683]

[7] Bénard F, Turcotte E. Imaging in breast cancer: Single-photon computed tomography and positron-emission tomography. Breast Cancer Res 2005; 7(4): 153-62. [http://dx.doi.org/10.1186/bcr1201] [PMID: 15987467]

[8] Kroemer G, Pouyssegur J. Tumor cell metabolism: Cancer's Achilles' heel. Cancer Cell 2008; 13(6): 472-82. [http://dx.doi.org/10.1016/j.ccr.2008.05.005] [PMID: 18538731]

[9] Ward PS, Thompson CB. Metabolic reprogramming: A cancer hallmark even warburg did not anticipate. Cancer Cell 2012; 21(3): 297-308. [http://dx.doi.org/10.1016/j.ccr.2012.02.014] [PMID: 22439925]

[10] Koppenol WH, Bounds PL, Dang CV. Otto Warburg's contributions to current concepts of cancer metabolism. Nat Rev Cancer 2011; 11(5): 325-37. [http://dx.doi.org/10.1038/nrc3038] [PMID: 21508971]

[11] Vander Heiden MG, Cantley LC, Thompson CB. Understanding the Warburg effect: The metabolic requirements of cell proliferation. Science 2009; 324(5930): 1029-33. [http://dx.doi.org/10.1126/science.1160809] [PMID: 19460998]

[12] Fiume L, Manerba M, Vettraino M, Di Stefano G. Inhibition of lactate dehydrogenase activity as an approach to cancer therapy. Future Med Chem 2014; 6(4): 429-45. [http://dx.doi.org/10.4155/fmc.13.206] [PMID: 24635523]

[13] Jones W, Bianchi K. Aerobic glycolysis: Beyond proliferation. Front Immunol 2015; 6: 227. [http://dx.doi.org/10.3389/fimmu.2015.00227] [PMID: 26029212]

[14] DeBerardinis RJ, Lum JJ, Hatzivassiliou G, Thompson CB. The biology of cancer: Metabolic reprogramming fuels cell growth and proliferation. Cell Metab 2008; 7(1): 11-20. [http://dx.doi.org/10.1016/j.cmet.2007.10.002] [PMID: 18177721]

[15] Dawson DM, Goodfriend TL, Kaplan NO. Lactic dehydrogenases: Functions of the two types. Rates of synthesis of the two major forms can be correlated with metabolic differentiation. Science 1964; 143(3609): 929-33. [http://dx.doi.org/10.1126/science.143.3609.929] [PMID: 14090142]

[16] Blanco A, Zinkham WH. Lactic dehydrogenases in human testes. Science 1963; 139(3555): 601-2. [http://dx.doi.org/10.1126/science.139.3555.601] [PMID: 17788300]

[17] Kanno T, Sudo K, Maekawa M, Nishimura Y, Ukita M, Fukutake K. Lactate dehydrogenase M-subunit deficiency: A new type of hereditary exertional myopathy. Clin Chim Acta 1988; 173(1): 89-98. [http://dx.doi.org/10.1016/0009-8981(88)90359-2] [PMID: 3383424]

[18] Read JA, Winter VJ, Eszes CM, Sessions RB, Brady RL. Structural basis for altered activity of M- and H-isozyme forms of human lactate dehydrogenase. Proteins 2001; 43(2): 175-85. [http://dx.doi.org/10.1002/1097-0134(20010501)43:2<175::AID-PROT1029>3.0.CO;2-#] [PMID: 11276087]

[19] Shi Y, Pinto BM. Human lactate dehydrogenase a inhibitors: A molecular dynamics investigation. PLoS One 2014; 9(1): e86365. [http://dx.doi.org/10.1371/journal.pone.0086365] [PMID: 24466056]

[20] Granchi C, Roy S, Giacomelli C, *et al.* Discovery of N-hydroxyindole-based inhibitors of human lactate dehydrogenase isoform A (LDH-A) as starvation agents against cancer cells. J Med Chem 2011; 54(6): 1599-612. [http://dx.doi.org/10.1021/jm101007q] [PMID: 21332213]

[21] Clarke AR, Wigley DB, Chia WN, Barstow D, Atkinson T, Holbrook JJ. Site-directed mutagenesis reveals role of mobile arginine residue in lactate dehydrogenase catalysis. Nature 1986; 324(6098): 699-702. [http://dx.doi.org/10.1038/324699a0] [PMID: 3796734]

[22] Masterson JE, Schwartz SD. The enzymatic reaction catalyzed by lactate dehydrogenase exhibits one dominant reaction path. Chem Phys 2014; 442(17): 132-6. [http://dx.doi.org/10.1016/j.chemphys.2014.02.018] [PMID: 25368440]

[23] Goldman RD, Kaplan NO, Hall TC. Lactic dehydrogenase in human neoplastic tissues. Cancer Res 1964; 24: 389-99. [PMID: 14147812]

[24] Koukourakis MI, Giatromanolaki A, Simopoulos C, Polychronidis A, Sivridis E. Lactate dehydrogenase 5 (LDH5) relates to up-regulated hypoxia inducible factor pathway and metastasis in colorectal cancer. Clin Exp Metastasis 2005; 22(1): 25-30. [http://dx.doi.org/10.1007/s10585-005-2343-7] [PMID: 16132575]

[25] Semenza GL. Oxygen-dependent regulation of mitochondrial respiration by hypoxia-inducible factor 1. Biochem J 2007; 405(1): 1-9. [http://dx.doi.org/10.1042/BJ20070389] [PMID: 17555402]

[26] Fantin VR, St-Pierre J, Leder P. Attenuation of LDH-A expression uncovers a link between glycolysis, mitochondrial physiology, and tumor maintenance. Cancer Cell 2006; 9(6): 425-34. [http://dx.doi.org/10.1016/j.ccr.2006.04.023] [PMID: 16766262]

[27] Shim H, Dolde C, Lewis BC, *et al.* c-Myc transactivation of LDH-A: implications for tumor metabolism and growth. Proc Natl Acad Sci USA 1997; 94(13): 6658-63.

[http://dx.doi.org/10.1073/pnas.94.13.6658] [PMID: 9192621]

[28] Le A, Cooper CR, Gouw AM, *et al.* Inhibition of lactate dehydrogenase A induces oxidative stress and inhibits tumor progression. Proc Natl Acad Sci USA 2010; 107(5): 2037-42. [http://dx.doi.org/10.1073/pnas.0914433107] [PMID: 20133848]

[29] Cui J, Shi M, Xie D, *et al.* FOXM1 promotes the warburg effect and pancreatic cancer progression via transactivation of LDHA expression. Clin Cancer Res 2014; 20(10): 2595-606. [http://dx.doi.org/10.1158/1078-0432.CCR-13-2407] [PMID: 24634381]

[30] Kolev Y, Uetake H, Takagi Y, Sugihara K. Lactate dehydrogenase-5 (LDH-5) expression in human gastric cancer: Association with hypoxia-inducible factor (HIF-1α) pathway, angiogenic factors production and poor prognosis. Ann Surg Oncol 2008; 15(8): 2336-44. [http://dx.doi.org/10.1245/s10434-008-9955-5] [PMID: 18521687]

[31] Maftouh M, Avan A, Sciarrillo R, *et al.* Synergistic interaction of novel lactate dehydrogenase inhibitors with gemcitabine against pancreatic cancer cells in hypoxia. Br J Cancer 2014; 110(1): 172-82. [http://dx.doi.org/10.1038/bjc.2013.681] [PMID: 24178759]

[32] Koukourakis MI, Giatromanolaki A, Sivridis E, *et al.* Prognostic and predictive role of lactate dehydrogenase 5 expression in colorectal cancer patients treated with PTK787/ZK 222584 (vatalanib) antiangiogenic therapy. Clin Cancer Res 2011; 17(14): 4892-900. [http://dx.doi.org/10.1158/1078-0432.CCR-10-2918] [PMID: 21632858]

[33] Koukourakis MI, Giatromanolaki A, Sivridis E, *et al.* Tumour and Angiogenesis Research Group. Lactate dehydrogenase-5 (LDH-5) overexpression in non-small-cell lung cancer tissues is linked to tumour hypoxia, angiogenic factor production and poor prognosis. Br J Cancer 2003; 89(5): 877-85. [http://dx.doi.org/10.1038/sj.bjc.6601205] [PMID: 12942121]

[34] Kayser G, Kassem A, Sienel W, *et al.* Lactate-dehydrogenase 5 is overexpressed in non-small cell lung cancer and correlates with the expression of the transketolase-like protein 1. Diagn Pathol 2010; 5: 22-32. [http://dx.doi.org/10.1186/1746-1596-5-22] [PMID: 20385008]

[35] Grimm M, Alexander D, Munz A, Hoffmann J, Reinert S. Increased LDH5 expression is associated with lymph node metastasis and outcome in oral squamous cell carcinoma. Clin Exp Metastasis 2013; 30(4): 529-40. [http://dx.doi.org/10.1007/s10585-012-9557-2] [PMID: 23184277]

[36] Giatromanolaki A, Sivridis E, Gatter KC, Turley H, Harris AL, Koukourakis MI. Lactate dehydrogenase 5 (LDH-5) expression in endometrial cancer relates to the activated VEGF/VEGFR2(KDR) pathway and prognosis. Gynecol Oncol 2006; 103(3): 912-8. [http://dx.doi.org/10.1016/j.ygyno.2006.05.043] [PMID: 16837029]

[37] Zhuang L, Scolyer RA, Murali R, *et al.* Lactate dehydrogenase 5 expression in melanoma increases with disease progression and is associated with expression of Bcl-XL and Mcl-1, but not Bcl-2 proteins. Mod Pathol 2010; 23(1): 45-53. [http://dx.doi.org/10.1038/modpathol.2009.129] [PMID: 19838163]

[38] Koukourakis MI, Giatromanolaki A, Winter S, Leek R, Sivridis E, Harris AL. Lactate dehydrogenase 5 expression in squamous cell head and neck cancer relates to prognosis following radical or postoperative radiotherapy. Oncology 2009; 77(5): 285-92. [http://dx.doi.org/10.1159/000259260] [PMID: 19923867]

[39] Yao F, Zhao T, Zhong C, Zhu J, Zhao H. LDHA is necessary for the tumorigenicity of esophageal squamous cell carcinoma. Tumour Biol 2013; 34(1): 25-31. [http://dx.doi.org/10.1007/s13277-012-0506-0] [PMID: 22961700]

[40] Dang CV, Shim H. Method of treating A lactate dehydrogenase-A (LDHA)- associated disorder. WO9836774, 1998.

[41] Neri D, Supuran CT. Interfering with pH regulation in tumours as a therapeutic strategy. Nat Rev Drug Discov 2011; 10(10): 767-77.
[http://dx.doi.org/10.1038/nrd3554] [PMID: 21921921]

[42] Wang ZY, Loo TY, Shen JG, *et al.* LDH-A silencing suppresses breast cancer tumorigenicity through induction of oxidative stress mediated mitochondrial pathway apoptosis. Breast Cancer Res Treat 2012; 131(3): 791-800.
[http://dx.doi.org/10.1007/s10549-011-1466-6] [PMID: 21452021]

[43] Xie H, Valera VA, Merino MJ, *et al.* LDH-A inhibition, a therapeutic strategy for treatment of hereditary leiomyomatosis and renal cell cancer. Mol Cancer Ther 2009; 8(3): 626-35.
[http://dx.doi.org/10.1158/1535-7163.MCT-08-1049] [PMID: 19276158]

[44] Zhao D, Zou SW, Liu Y, *et al.* Lysine-5 acetylation negatively regulates lactate dehydrogenase A and is decreased in pancreatic cancer. Cancer Cell 2013; 23(4): 464-76.
[http://dx.doi.org/10.1016/j.ccr.2013.02.005] [PMID: 23523103]

[45] Brown BD, Dudek HT, Lai C. Therapeutic inhibition of lactate dehydrogenase and agents thererfor. WO2016057932, 2016.

[46] Courtney C. Inhibition of Lactate dehydrogenase 5 (LDH-5), binding incorporation, internalization and/or endocytosis to immune cells. WO2015157299, 2015.

[47] Liou J-R. Regulation of human lactate dehydrogenase. WO2003048350, 2003.

[48] Choi SR, Beeler AB, Pradhan A, *et al.* Generation of oxamic acid libraries: Antimalarials and inhibitors of *Plasmodium falciparum* lactate dehydrogenase. J Comb Chem 2007; 9(2): 292-300.
[http://dx.doi.org/10.1021/cc060110n] [PMID: 17316052]

[49] Zhao Y, Liu H, Liu Z, *et al.* Overcoming trastuzumab resistance in breast cancer by targeting dysregulated glucose metabolism. Cancer Res 2011; 71(13): 4585-97.
[http://dx.doi.org/10.1158/0008-5472.CAN-11-0127] [PMID: 21498634]

[50] Zhou M, Zhao Y, Ding Y, Liu H, Liu Z, Fodstad O, *et al.* Warburg effect in chemosensitivity: Targeting lactate dehydrogenase-A re-sensitizes. Taxol-resistant cancer cells to Taxol Mol Cancer 2010; 9: 1-22.
[http://dx.doi.org/10.1186/1476-4598-9-33]

[51] Rani R, Kumar V. Recent update on human lactate dehydrogenase enzyme 5 (*h*LDH5) inhibitors: A promising approach for cancer chemotherapy. J Med Chem 2016; 59(2): 487-96.
[http://dx.doi.org/10.1021/acs.jmedchem.5b00168] [PMID: 26340601]

[52] Allison SJ, Knight JR, Granchi C, Reshma R, Minutolo F, Milner J, *et al.* LDH-A/p53 regulate cancer cell NAD(H) enabling therapeutic access to cancer cell killing via LDH-A by both p53-dependent and p53-independent pathways. Oncogenesis 2014; 3: e102.
[http://dx.doi.org/10.1038/oncsis.2014.16] [PMID: 24819061]

[53] Vander Jagt DL, Deck LM, Royer RE. Gossypol: prototype of inhibitors targeted to dinucleotide folds. Curr Med Chem 2000; 7(4): 479-98.
[http://dx.doi.org/10.2174/0929867003375119] [PMID: 10702620]

[54] Shelley MD, Hartley L, Fish RG, *et al.* Stereo-specific cytotoxic effects of gossypol enantiomers and gossypolone in tumour cell lines. Cancer Lett 1999; 135(2): 171-80.
[http://dx.doi.org/10.1016/S0304-3835(98)00302-4] [PMID: 10096426]

[55] Mazzio E, Soliman K. Inhibition of anaerobic glucose metabolism and corresponding natural composition as a non-toxic approach to cancer treatment. WO2006017494, 2006.

[56] Wang Z, Wang D, Han S, *et al.* Bioactivity-guided identification and cell signaling technology to delineate the lactate dehydrogenase A inhibition effects of *Spatholobus suberectus* on breast cancer. PLoS One 2013; 8(2): e56631.
[http://dx.doi.org/10.1371/journal.pone.0056631] [PMID: 23457597]

[57] Manerba M, Vettraino M, Fiume L, *et al.* Galloflavin (CAS 568-80-9): A novel inhibitor of lactate dehydrogenase. ChemMedChem 2012; 7(2): 311-7.
[http://dx.doi.org/10.1002/cmdc.201100471] [PMID: 22052811]

[58] Farabegoli F, Vettraino M, Manerba M, Fiume L, Roberti M, Di Stefano G. Galloflavin, a new lactate dehydrogenase inhibitor, induces the death of human breast cancer cells with different glycolytic attitude by affecting distinct signaling pathways. Eur J Pharm Sci 2012; 47(4): 729-38.
[http://dx.doi.org/10.1016/j.ejps.2012.08.012] [PMID: 22954722]

[59] Dang CV, Le QH, Dinavahi R. Methods for treating neoplasia by inhibiting lactate dehydrogenase and/or nicotinamide phosphoribosyltransferase. US20120003156, 2012.

[60] Ward RA, Brassington C, Breeze AL, *et al.* Design and synthesis of novel lactate dehydrogenase A inhibitors by fragment-based lead generation. J Med Chem 2012; 55(7): 3285-306.
[http://dx.doi.org/10.1021/jm201734r] [PMID: 22417091]

[61] Minutolo F, Macchia M, Granchi C, *et al.* Indole derivatives inhibitors of enzyme lactate dehydrogenase (LDH). WO2013092735, 2013.

[62] Minutolo F, Macchia M, Granchi C, *et al.* Indole derivatives inhibitors of enzyme lactate dehydrogenase (LDH). US20140343001, 2014.

[63] Granchi C, Calvaresi EC, Tuccinardi T, *et al.* Assessing the differential action on cancer cells of LDH-A inhibitors based on the N-hydroxyindole-2-carboxylate (NHI) and malonic (Mal) scaffolds. Org Biomol Chem 2013; 11(38): 6588-96.
[http://dx.doi.org/10.1039/c3ob40870a] [PMID: 23986182]

[64] Calvaresi EC, Granchi C, Tuccinardi T, *et al.* Dual targeting of the Warburg effect with a glucose-conjugated lactate dehydrogenase inhibitor. ChemBioChem 2013; 14(17): 2263-7.
[http://dx.doi.org/10.1002/cbic.201300562] [PMID: 24174263]

[65] Chai D, Colon M, Dodson C, Duffy KJ, Shaw AN. Preparation of substituted quinoline derivatives as lactate dehydrogenase A inhibitors. WO2012061557, 2012.

[66] Billiard J, Dennison JB, Briand J, *et al.* Quinoline 3-sulfonamides inhibit lactate dehydrogenase A and reverse aerobic glycolysis in cancer cells. Cancer Metab 2013; 1(1): 19.
[http://dx.doi.org/10.1186/2049-3002-1-19] [PMID: 24280423]

[67] Xie H, Hanai J, Ren JG, *et al.* Targeting lactate dehydrogenase-a inhibits tumorigenesis and tumor progression in mouse models of lung cancer and impacts tumor-initiating cells. Cell Metab 2014; 19(5): 795-809.
[http://dx.doi.org/10.1016/j.cmet.2014.03.003] [PMID: 24726384]

[68] Maloney DJ, Jadhav A, Bantukallu GR, *et al.* Small molecule inhibitors of lactate dehydrogenase and methods of use thereof. WO2016109559, 2016.

[69] Inoue T, Yoshida N, Otsuki T, Lee S. Lactic acid dehydrogenase inhibitor and pharmaceutical preparation containing same. WO2014115764, 2014.

[70] Inoue T, Nagisa S. Lactate dehydrogenase inhibitor and antiepileptic drug containing same. WO2016129583, 2016.

[71] Bartolone JB, Penksa CM, Santhanam CM, Lang BD. Lactate dehydrogenase inhibitors in cosmetic composition. US5595730, 1997.

[72] Takagahara I, Yamauti J, Yoshimura S, Fujii K, Horio T. Method of fractional quantitative determination of isoenzyme of lactic dehydrogenase. US4258131, 1981.

[73] Luis Felipe BO, Alejandro SM, Sebastian CC, Wolf BF. Genetically encoded probe for quantification of lactate, and methods for quantifying metabolic rates and lactate transport. WO2013154587, 2013.

[74] Granchi C, Fortunato S, Meini S, *et al.* Characterization of the saffron derivative crocetin as an inhibitor of human lactate dehydrogenase 5 in the antiglycolytic approach against cancer. J Agric Food

Chem 2017; 65(28): 5639-49.
[http://dx.doi.org/10.1021/acs.jafc.7b01668] [PMID: 28643510]

[75] Rani R, Kumar V. When will small molecule lactate dehydrogenase inhibitors realize their potential in the cancer clinic? Future Med Chem 2017; 9(11): 1113-5.
[http://dx.doi.org/10.4155/fmc-2017-0082] [PMID: 28722474]

CHAPTER 6

Cancer Chemo-Immunotherapeutics

Muzammal Hussain[a,b,*] and **Jiancun Zhang**[a,*]

[a] *State Key Laboratory of Respiratory Disease, Guangzhou Institutes of Biomedicine and Health, Chinese Academy of Sciences, 190 Kaiyuan Avenue, Science Park, Guangzhou, 510530, P.R. China*

[b] *University of Chinese Academy of Sciences, Beijing, 100049, P.R. China*

Abstract: Cancer chemo-immunotherapeutics has evolved with a strategic slogan - 'marrying chemotherapy with immunotherapy' - in order to optimize the chance for cure. The ultimate goal is to execute a 'two hit' impact, able on the one hand to mount a robust anti-tumour immune response, and on the other hand, selectively eradicate tumour growth and progression. Tremendous progress has been, and being, made in this regard by testing various 'chemotherapy-immunotherapy' drug combinations in the clinic, and also implementing multiple pharmacological and biological interventions against fundamental regulatory pathways involved in tumour development, progression, and tumour immune escape mechanisms. This chapter discusses the current 'chemotherapy-immunotherapy' combinations in clinical studies/trials, as well as the pharmacological manipulation of host-tumour cell interactions mapping the road ahead to a novel trend/concept of 'two hit' chemo-immunotherapeutics. At the end, we also discuss the patents issued and recent patent applications stating the novel chemo-immunotherapy methods with diverse interventional combinations, some of which produce synergistic anti-tumour effects, to treat multiple advanced cancers.

Keywords: ARG, Cancer, Chemotherapy, Chemo-immunotherapy, Cancer vaccines, CIK cells, CTLA4, Cytokine, FOLFOX, GVAX, IDO, Immune suppression, Immuno-oncology, Kinase inhibition, mAbs, mTOR, MAPK, PKA, R-CHOP, TroVax®.

1. INTRODUCTION

Cancer chemo-immunotherapeutics implements treatment regimens that both maximize tumour regression and the anti-tumour immune response for the long

* **Corresponding author Muzammal Hussain:** Guangzhou Institutes of Biomedicine and Health, Chinese Academy of Sciences, 190 Kaiyuan Avenue, Science Park, Guangzhou, 510530, P.R. China; University of Chinese Academy of Sciences, Beijing, 100049, P.R. China; Tel: +86 020 32015323; E-mail: muzammal@gibh.ac.cn

* **Corresponding author Jiancun Zhang:** Guangzhou Institutes of Biomedicine and Health, Chinese Academy of Sciences, 190 Kaiyuan Avenue, Science Park, Guangzhou, 510530, P.R. China; Tel: +86 020 32015323; E-mail: zhang_jiancun@gibh.ac.cn

Atta-ur-Rahman and Khurshid Zaman (Eds.)

term clinical benefit of cancer patients [1]. Although cancer chemotherapy has historically been considered as immunosuppressive, emerging evidence indicates that certain chemotherapies can augment tumour immunity through multiple mechanisms including induction of immunogenic cell death and by disrupting strategies that tumours use to evade immune recognition [2 - 4]. This dual role, cytotoxicity and immune activation, from chemotherapy has prompted the scientific community to call for a radical but strategic shift in the way tumours are treated in order to achieve better clinical outcomes [1]. To this regard, cancer chemo-immunotherapeutics has evolved with a strategic slogan - 'marrying chemotherapy with immunotherapy' - in order to optimize the chance for cure [5, 6]. The ultimate goal is to execute a 'two hit' impact, able on the one hand to mount a robust anti-tumour immune response, and on the other hand, selectively eradicate tumour growth and progression. Tremendous progress has been, and being, made in this regard by implementing multiple chemotherapy-immunotherapy drug combinations with complimentary mechanisms of action to attain additive or synergistic anti-tumour effects [7, 8]. Apart from this, the complex interactions between host and tumour cells within the tumour microenvironment may lead to 'tumour-associated immune suppression', which is characterized by diverse mechanisms of oncogenic signaling pathways that play critical roles in tumour initiation, progression, and immunoescape [9]. Emerging data indicate that small-molecule based therapeutic interventions against such signaling pathways may have the potential to provide a 'two-hit' chemo-immunotherapeutic opportunity: direct killing of tumour cells, and the rescuing of endogenous anti-tumour immunity [10 - 12]. The purpose of this chapter is to discuss the clinical significance of current chemo- and immuno-therapy drug combinations, as well as highlight the 'two hit' chemo-immunotherapeutic potential of targeting the oncogenic signaling pathways that play crucial roles in tumour growth and progression, and in tumour-associated immune suppression. Moreover, we also discuss patents issued and recent patent applications demonstrating novel chemo-immunotherapeutic methods/formulations for the treatment of cancer.

2. CURRENT CHEMO-IMMUNOTHERAPEUTIC DRUG COMBINATIONS IN CLINICAL STUDIES

In recent decades, a general trend of harnessing endogenous anti-tumour immunity by modifying the diverse mechanisms of immunosuppressive tumour immune microenvironment has provided the knowledge and techniques to develop novel immunotherapeutic approaches for the treatment of cancer [7]. These include:

a. Antibodies, such as monoclonal antibody drugs (mAbs) and the recent immune checkpoint-modulating antibodies;
b. Vaccines, such as tumour cell-based autologous vaccines and dendritic cell (DC)-based vaccines; and
c. Immunostimulatory cytokines, and cytokine-induced killer (CIK) cells.

Several combinations of these immunotherapeutics with traditional chemotherapy are in various phases of clinical trials (Table **1**). In addition, superior clinical benefits of chemotherapy-immunotherapy combinations have also been convincingly demonstrated in the settings of large randomized trials.

Table 1. Summary of Currently Ongoing Clinical Trials Involving Cancer Chemo-Immunotherapy.

Chemo-Immunotherapy	**Target of the Listed Antibody**	**Type of Cancer**	**Phase**	**Reference (NCT ID)**
Chemotherapy-mAbs Combinations				
Doxorubicin, vincristine, cytarabine, etoposide, cyclophosphamide, methotrexate, leucovorin, filgrastim, epratuzumab	CD22	Acute lymphoblastic leukemia	Phase I/II	NCT00098839
Bendamustine, lenalidomide, rituximab	CD20	Chronic lymphocytic leukemia; Small lymphocytic lymphoma	Phase II	NCT01754857
Cyclophosphamide, fludarabine, ofatumumab	CD20	B-cell lymphoid leukemia	Phase II	NCT01762202
Bendamustine + ofatumumab	CD20	Mantle cell lymphoma	Phase II	NCT01437709
Carboplatin, paclitaxel, oregovomab	CA125	Ovarian neoplasms	Phase II	NCT01616303
Cisplatin, docetaxel, cetuximab	EGF receptor	Lung cancer	Phase II	NCT01059188
Fludarabine, cyclophosphamide, ofatumumab	CD20	Chronic lymphocytic leukemia; Small lymphocytic lymphoma	Phase II	NCT01145209
Paclitaxel, lapatinib, trastuzumab	HER2/neu	Breast carcinoma	Phase II	NCT01891357
Cyclophosphamide, fludarabine, rituximab	CD20	Multiple leukemias and lymphomas	Phase III	NCT02048813
CHOP chemotherapy (cyclophosphamide, hydroxydaunorubicin, vincristine, prednisone) plus G-CSF, combined with alemtuzumab	CD52	T-cell lymphoma	Phase III	NCT00646854
Fludarabine, rituximab	CD20	Chronic lymphocytic leukemia	Phase III	NCT00513747

(Table 1) contd.....

Chemo-Immunotherapy	Target of the Listed Antibody	Type of Cancer	Phase	Reference (NCT ID)
CHOP chemotherapy (cyclophosphamide, hydroxydaunorubicin, vincristine, prednisone) + rituximab	CD20	Non-Hodgkin's lymphoma	Phase III	NCT00278421
Chemotherapy-Immune Checkpoint Inhibitor Combinations				
Motolimod, pegylated liposomal doxorubicin, durvalumab	CD274	Ovarian cancer	Phase I/II	NCT02431559
Paclitaxel, capecitabine, pembrolizumab	PD-1	Triple negative breast cancer	Phase I/II	NCT02734290
Oxaliplatin, capecitabine, durvalumab, tremelimumab	CTLA-4	Esophageal cancer	Phase I/II	NCT02735239
Chemotherapy-Vaccine Combinations				
Imiquimod + Tumour lysate vaccine	N/A	Grade II glioma	Phase 0	NCT01678352
Cyclophosphamide, CRS-207 (Listeria monocytogenes)	N/A	Malignant pleural mesothelioma	Phase I	NCT01675765
Gemcitabine, TG01/GM-CSF	N/A	Pancreatic cancer	Phase I/II	NCT02261714
Platinum/pemetrexed + WT1-targeted DC vaccination	N/A	Malignant pleural mesothelioma	Phase I/II	NCT02649829
Temozolomide chemotherapy + WT1-targeted DC vaccination	N/A	Glioblastoma multiforme of brain	Phase I/II	NCT02649582
Docetaxel, DCVAC/PCa	N/A	Prostate cancer	Phase II	NCT02105675
Paclitaxel or topotecan or doxorubicin, DCVAC/OvCa	N/A	Epithelial ovarian carcinoma	Phase II	NCT02107378
Docetaxel + Sipuleucel-T	N/A	Prostate cancer	Phase II	NCT02793219
Pemetrexed and carboplatin + DCVAC/LuCa	N/A	Non-small cell lung cancer (NSCLC)	Phase II	NCT02669719
Docetaxel + Dendritic cells DCVAC	N/A	Metastatic castrate-resistant prostate cancer	Phase III	NCT02111577
Gemcitabine, carboplatin + Epstein-Barr Virus (EBV)-specific autologous cytotoxic T lymphocytes	N/A	Nasopharyngeal cancer	Phase III	NCT02578641
Chemotherapy-CIK Combinations				
Gemcitabine, cisplatin + D-CIK	N/A	NSCLC	Phase I/II	NCT02651441
FOLFOX (Oxaliplatin, leucovorin, 5-FU) + autologous tumour lysate pulsed D-CIK (Ag-D-CIK)	N/A	Gastrointestinal cancers/neoplasms	Phase II	NCT02215837

(Table 1) contd.....

Chemo-Immunotherapy	Target of the Listed Antibody	Type of Cancer	Phase	Reference (NCT ID)
Paclitaxel, cisplatin, DC-CIK	N/A	Esophageal neoplasms	Phase II	NCT02644863
Cisplatin + paclitaxel + CIK cells	N/A	Lung cancer	Phase II/III	NCT01631357
Chemotherapy-Oncolytic Immunotherapy Combinations				
Temozolomide + DNX-2401 (oncolytic adenovirus)	N/A	Glioblastoma	Phase I	NCT01956734
Pemetrexed/cisplatin, Cyclophosphamide + ONCOS-102 (GM-CSF coding oncolytic adenovirus)	N/A	Mesothelioma	Phase I/II	NCT02879669
Gemcitabine, paclitaxel + LOAd703 (oncolytic adenovirus)	N/A	Pancreatic cancer	Phase I/II	NCT02705196
Paclitaxel + oncolytic Reovirus (Reolysin NSC # 729968)	N/A	Fallopian tube carcinoma ovarian carcinoma Primary peritoneal carcinoma	Phase II	NCT01199263
Sorafenib + Pexa Vec (vaccinia virus based oncolytic immunotherapy)	N/A	Hepatocellular carcinoma	Phase III	NCT02562755

N/A: Not applicable

2.1. Chemotherapy-mAbs Combinations

Anticancer mAbs directly target specific antigens expressed by cancer cells. More than a dozen of mAbs have been approved by the Food and Drug Administration (FDA) as standard treatment of several different cancers, including the prototypical rituximab for B-cell lymphoma and trastuzumab for breast cancer. Rituximab was approved in 1997 and has become a regular part of standard chemo-immunotherapeutic interventions aimed at resolving different types of leukemias and lymphomas [13, 14]. Chemo-immunotherapy regimens involving chemotherapy-rituximab combinations have shown improved treatment outcomes compared with chemotherapy alone [15 - 18]. Especially, front-line chemo-immunotherapy with R-CHOP (rituximab, cyclophosphamide, doxorubicin, vincristine, prednisone) and R-Flu (rituximab, fludarabine) regimens has achieved high rates of complete remission (CR) and minimal residual disease (MRD) negativity in Phases II and III clinical trials [19, 20]. Similarly, front-line chemo-immunotherapy with FCR (fludarabine, cyclophosphamide, rituximab) regimen has also induced long-term remissions and highly relevant improvement in overall survival (OS) in patients with chronic lymphocytic leukemia (CLL) and follicular lymphoma [17, 21]. In addition, several randomized Phase III trials have demonstrated superior clinical results when antibody is added to chemotherapy regimens in relapsed patients who have not previously been exposed to mAbs [22]. Many Phase II/III clinical studies of chemotherapy-rituximab combinations are currently ongoing (Table **1**), which have demonstrated improved response rates and prolonged progression-free survival (PFS) in patients with different types of leukemias or lymphomas.

2.2. Chemotherapy-Immune Checkpoint Inhibitor Combinations

Immune checkpoint inhibitors targeting checkpoints in the immune regulation cascade currently form the mainstay of cancer immunotherapy [23, 24]. The cytotoxic T lymphocyte antigen-4 (CTLA4) monoclonal antibody ipilimumab was the first checkpoint inhibitor approved by FDA. Similarly, nivolumab and pembrolizumab are the first mAbs against the immune checkpoint programmed death 1 (PD-1) receptor, which have been approved for clinical use [24, 25]. The evidence for the notable effects of immune checkpoint inhibitors in combination with chemotherapy has expanded in recent years, with numerous clinical studies underway or completed in a variety of solid tumours, including melanoma and non-small cell lung cancer (NSCLC) [23, 26]. One of the earliest combinations tested was ipilimumab and dacarbazine in two separate Phases II and III trials comparing dacarbazine alone to dacarbazine with ipilimumab in melanoma patients [27, 28]. These studies manifested that OS was significantly improved in the combination arm versus dacarbazine alone [27, 28]. Ipilimumab has also been combined with carboplatin and paclitaxel in two separate Phase II studies in NSCLC and SCLC, which demonstrated that phased ipilimumab plus paclitaxel and carboplatin may provoke superior immune responses, and thus enhance PFS [29, 30]. However, conflicting results regarding efficacy of ipilimumab combinations with etoposide and platinum (cisplatin or carboplatin) chemotherapy have been demonstrated in two recently reported Phases II and III trials conducted in patients with extensive-stage SCLC. In the Phase II study, despite a combination of ipilimumab with carboplatin and etoposide was proposed to benefit a subgroup of patients with extensive-stage SCLC, primary end point (1-year PFS) of the study was not met [31]. Similarly, the Phase III trial demonstrated that addition of ipilimumab to etoposide and platinum (cisplatin or carboplatin) did not result in a statistically significant improvement in OS versus chemotherapy alone in patients with newly diagnosed extensive-stage disease SCLC [32]. Although the rationale for these studies was derived from previous combinations of ipilimumab with carboplatin and dacarbazine, it remains elusive why ipilimumab did not confer additional benefit over etoposide and platinum. In addition, treatment-related toxicities, such as neurological toxicity, hepatotoxicity, etc., were substantially higher in both studies, which made the delivery of chemo-immunotherapy challenging. Ipilimumab has a well-defined toxicity profile, and its combination with chemotherapy have shown increased toxicity when compared with monotherapy [31, 32]. Looking from this perspective, newer agents such as anti-PD-1/PD-L1 drugs, with a more favorable toxicity profile might be easier to combine with chemotherapy. However, there are currently limited data for PD-1/PD-L1 combinations with chemotherapy. In a Phase I study, nivolumab in combination with three different chemotherapy regimens: cisplatin/ gemcitabine, cisplatin/pemetrexed, or carboplatin/paclitaxel, has demonstrated acceptable overall response rate (ORR), PFS, and 1-year OS rates in chemotherapy-naïve NSCLC patients, with a safety profile reflecting additive nivolumab and chemotherapy toxicities [33]. Similarly, a combination of pembrolizumab with doublet chemotherapy is being evaluated in a larger cohort of advanced NSCLC (NCT02039674).

2.3. Chemotherapy-Vaccine Combinations

Cancer vaccines can actively provoke endogenous anti-tumour immunity, in particular the T cell-mediated adaptive immune responses [34]. The first personalized therapeutic cancer vaccine, sipuleucel-T (Provenge), was approved in 2010 by FDA for the treatment of advanced prostate cancer. The combination of chemotherapy and cancer vaccines is viewed as potentially synergistic through different mechanisms, including: inhibition of T-regulatory cells (Tregs), release of tumour antigens, and modification of the biological milieu in tumours [35 - 39]. Armed with better understanding of the immune system, various vaccination approaches have now been developed, ranging from simple peptide to more complex engineered cellular vaccines, DC vaccines, virus vectored vaccines and oncolytic viral vaccines [34, 40 - 42]. Many of these approaches have been combined successfully with chemotherapy in recent years to harness the potential synergies for the benefits of cancer patients.

TG4010 (Transgene SA, Illkirch, France) belongs to a class of genetic vaccines and is based on a poxvirus (modified vaccinia virus Ankara) that codes for MUC1 tumour-associated antigen and interleukin (IL)-2. Combination of TG4010 with first-line chemotherapy has been found encouraging in patients with advanced NSCLC in two previously conducted separate Phase II studies. Initially, a multicenter, randomized Phase II study demonstrated the feasibility of TG4010 in combination with cisplatin and vinorelbine in advanced NSCLC with an ORR of 37% [43]. A MUC1-specific cellular immune response was observed in lymphocyte samples from all responding patients, which was found to be predictive of TG4010 efficacy. Later on, another Phase IIb study suggested that the addition of TG4010 to first-line chemotherapy (cisplatin and gemcitabine) for NSCLC is feasible and generally well tolerated. Several efficacy metrics showed a better outcome when the cancer vaccine was added, supporting the hypothesis of synergy between immunotherapy and chemotherapy [44]. This study also provided a rationale for a currently ongoing confirmatory Phase IIb/III TIME trial (NCT01383148). And, the most recent results from the Phase IIb part of TIME trial have further validated that TG4010 may enhance the effect of chemotherapy with significantly improved PFS [45]. Notably, no serious adverse event was related to the combination of TG4010 with chemotherapy.

Elpamotide is a peptide vaccine for vascular endothelial growth factor receptor 2. In recent Phase II/III trials, a combination of gemcitabine and elpamotide has been found tolerable with a moderate anti-tumour effect in patients with advanced solid tumours [46, 47]. Similarly, a five-peptide cancer vaccine in combination with cyclophosphamide has been found well tolerated with promising tumour-associated antigen (TAA)-specific T cell responses that were significantly associated with longer OS in advanced solid tumours [48]. Another Phase Ib study has recently demonstrated immunomodulating and anti-tumour activity with a better survival rate upon administration of a poly-epitope peptide vaccination to thymidylate synthase (TSPP) in combination with chemo-immunotherapy (poly-chemotherapy plus IL-2) in metastatic colorectal cancer patients [49]. Carboplatin-paclitaxel therapy has recently been shown to foster vigorous human papillomavirus type 16 (HPV16)-synthetic long peptides (SLP) vaccination-induced T cell responses when vaccination was given after chemotherapy in E6/E7-positive TC-1 mouse tumour model and in patients with advanced cervical cancer [50]. In addition, a recent Phase I/II study combining gemcitabine, the immune modulator Pegintron and p53 SLP vaccine in patients with platinum-resistant ovarian cancer patients has validated the development of combined chemo-immunotherapeutic regimens as a viable approach to treat cancer [51].

GVAX is a vaccine with allogeneic tumour cells that have been transfected with granulocyte and macrophage colony stimulating factor (GM-CSF). Improved efficacy of mitoxantrone has recently been described in patients with castration-resistant prostate cancer (CRPC) after vaccination with GVAX. The median PFS after mitoxantrone was significantly longer in vaccinated patients as compared to controls, which was proposed to be due to the immune-stimulating effect of mitoxantrone in patients with heightened anti-tumour immunity after GVAX [52]. In a Phase II trial involving patients with high-risk locally advanced prostate cancer, administration of GVAX two days after neoadjuvant docetaxel has been found safe and well tolerated combination with significant evidence of clinical benefit [53]. Also, GVAX has previously been combined with docetaxel in two Phase III trials (VITAL-1 and -2) involving patients with advanced prostate cancer; nevertheless, both trials were halted prematurely because of a lower OS with the vaccine (GVAX) regimen, as well as the futility (little chance to reach the primary end point i.e. improved survival) [54].

Furthermore, a possible synergy between sipuleucel-T and docetaxel has been suggested in a recent case report in which docetaxel was administered just before sipuleucel-T to a patient with metastatic CRPC [55]. Administration of docetaxel before immunotherapy enhanced the response to sipuleucel-T, although further trials are warranted to investigate the optimal sequencing and timing of sipuleucel-T with other conventional chemotherapeutic regimens.

2.4. Chemotherapy-Cytokine Combinations

Cytokines are proteins secreted by different immune cells, which regulate innate and adaptive immunity in autocrine and paracrine fashion. IL-2 was the first cytokine which demonstrated an anti-tumoural effect by activating LAK immune effector cells [56]. Several cytokines have therapeutic potential when delivered exogenously alone or in combination with chemotherapy.

INF-α and GM-CSF based chemo-immunotherapeutic combinations have been found promising in advanced metastatic cancers. In a previous Phase II study, combination of INF-α with 5-fluorouracil (5-FU) and cisplatin increased PFS in patients with advanced hepatocellular carcinoma (HCC) [57]. Similar findings in advanced HCC patients were also reported by another study evaluating a combination of 5-FU and pegylated interferon (PEG-IFN) α-2b [58]. GM-CS--based chemo-immunotherapy involving GM-CSF, rituximab, fludarabine, and cyclophosphamide or mitoxantrone has recently been demonstrated well-tolerated with an ORR of 87% in patients with indolent non-Hodgkin lymphoma (NHL) and CLL [59]. Administration of GM-CSF in combination with lenalidomide has also been demonstrated safe with modest evidence of anti-tumour activity in patients with CRPC [60]. Moreover, maintenance immunotherapy with GM-CSF within an intermittent chemotherapy framework of docetaxel with prednisone has been found feasible in a prospective Phase II trial involving metastatic CRPC [61]. More interestingly, the outcomes from a recent Phase III trial, GOLFIG-2, have provided a proof-of-principle that GOLFIG chemo-immunotherapy that comprises a combination of gemcitabine, oxaliplatin, levofolinate, 5-FU, GM-CSF, and IL-2 may represent a novel reliable option for first-line treatment of metastatic colorectal cancer (CRC) [62]. Although the study underwent early termination because of poor recruitment in the control arm, GOLFIG regimen showed superior outcomes in terms of PFS, response rate, and a trend to longer survival, that were probably because of enhanced anti-tumour immunity (increase in NK- and T-cells, while decrease in Treg cells) [62]. Similarly, a chemo-immunotherapeutic combination of gemcitabine and capecitabine together with concurrently administered GV1001 vaccine with adjuvant GM-CSF developed an immune response to GV1001, while reducing MDSCs in patients with advanced pancreatic cancer [63].

2.5. Chemotherapy-CIK Cells Combinations

CIK cells are a heterogeneous population of T cells featuring a mixed T- and NK cell-like phenotype, which can expand from incubation of peripheral blood mononuclear cells with certain cytokines [64]. They have emerged as a promising immunotherapy approach in oncology [64].

There is robust clinical rationale for the therapeutic effectiveness of chemotherapy-CIK cells combinations in advanced cancers. Autologous CIK cell immunotherapy in combination with chemotherapy (5-Fluorouridine, leucovorin and oxaliplatin [FOLFOX4] plan) has recently been found well tolerated with improved OS and an increasing trend towards PFS in metastatic CRC patients [65]. Similarly, the combinations of DC-CIK immunotherapy with different forms of chemotherapy have been found effective and safe in multiple advanced cancers, including gastric cancer [66, 67], multiple myeloma [68 - 71], cervical cancer [72], NSCLC [73, 74], CRC [75], and breast cancer [76]. These DC-CIK-chemotherapy combinations were found to improve the anti-tumour immune function, reduce the recurrence rate and prolong the survival time of the patients. Recent meta-analysis studies in multiple cancer types have also shown that the combination of CIK/DC-CIK therapy and chemotherapy may superiorly prolong the survival time, enhance anti-tumour immune function and alleviate the adverse events caused by chemotherapy [67, 77, 78]. Moreover, adjuvant chemotherapy combined with autologous CIK therapy has emerged as a promising modality for treating gastric cancer patients [79, 80].

Moreover, CIK immunotherapy and different forms of chemotherapy may potentially enhance the mutual effectiveness in clinical settings. Sequential CIK immunotherapy has been shown to enhance the efficacy of gemcitabine plus cisplatin chemotherapy in metastatic nasopharyngeal carcinoma patients [81]. Likewise, MDSCs-decreasing chemotherapy has been found to increase the efficacy of CIK immunotherapy in metastatic renal cell carcinoma and pancreatic cancer [82].

2.6. Chemotherapy-Oncolytic Immunotherapy Combinations

Oncolytic immunotherapy is an innovative class of cancer therapy that exploits both native and genetically modified viruses to promote anti-tumour immune responses through a dual mechanism: selectively kill tumour cells, while at the same time inducing systemic anti-tumour immunity [83]. T-Vec (talimogene laherparepvec) is the first-in-class oncolytic immunotherapy which has recently been approved by FDA for local treatment of advanced melanoma [84]. Oncolytic immunotherapy has entered clinical arena in recent years, and its combinations with conventional single-and multi-agent chemotherapy regimens have been found potentially highly synergistic in both preclinical and clinical studies [85, 86]. In addition, the emerging clinical data has also evidenced good safety, intriguing efficacy, and extended survival with different chemo- and oncolytic immuno-therapy combinations [87 - 90]. Currently, many Phases I to III trials are ongoing to further explore the potential synergy and efficacy of chemotherapy-oncolytic immunotherapy combinations in multiple advanced human cancers (Table **1**).

3. TUMOURAL INHIBITION OF HOST-TUMOUR CELL INTERACTIONS: MAPPING THE ROAD AHEAD TO 'TWO HIT' CHEMO-IMMUNOTHERAPEUTICS

Over the past decade, the host-tumour cells interactions have emerged as fundamental determinant of tumour development, progression and immunoescape mechanisms. They are also the major determinant of treatment outcomes for human malignancies [91 - 93].

Like other disease conditions, tumours are recognized by the immune system and their development can be stopped or controlled long term through a process known as 'tumour immunosurveillance'. It is a process whereby the immune system can recognize and destroy cancerous and/or pre-cancerous cells via recognition of tumour specific antigens [91, 93, 94]. The effector mechanisms of anti-tumour immune surveillance are driven by a complex and dynamic network of intercellular mediators (e.g. cytokines, chemokines, inflammatory enzymes, etc.) and cellular cross-talks involving both the innate (e.g. natural killer (NK) cells) and the adaptive (e.g. T cells) components of the immune system [94, 95]. However, it is well-established that tumours can paralyze these otherwise efficient immune attacks. They potentiate their own progression and survival by fostering a complex and highly dynamic microenvironment that privileges a variety of immune-suppressive regulators, rather than immune effectors [9, 94, 95]. The most particular immune-suppressive regulators include:

i. Tumour-associated macrophages and fibroblasts;
ii. Tregs and MDSCs, and
iii. Various immunoinhibitory mediators, including enzymes (e.g. indoleamine-2, 3-dioxygenase (IDO), arginase (ARG), etc.), small molecules (e.g. prostaglandin-E2 (PGE_2), extracellular adenosine, etc.) soluble factors and several cytokines and chemokines [9, 95].

All these immune-suppressive regulators are implicated in the complex network of stromal-immune-cancer cell interactions that suppress anti-tumour immunity, ultimately leading to tumour immune evasion/escape [95, 96]. The underlying mechanisms for this tumour immune evasion encompass a wide array of extrinsic and/or intrinsic signaling pathways induced by cells or mediators favoring tumour-associated immune suppression, and modulating tumour cell death. Among the several pathways stimulated by tumour-stroma-immune cell-derived mediators, the kinase signaling pathways such as cyclic adenosine mono-phosphate (cAMP)-dependent protein kinase A (PKA) pathway, phosphoinositide 3 kinase (PI3K) signaling pathway, and mitogen-activated protein kinase (MAPK) pathway, have particularly taken the center stage because of possessing dichotomous role - promote tumour growth/progression and aid tumour immunoescape - in the tumour microenvironment [10, 97, 98].

The identification of multiple mechanisms of tumour-associated immune suppression has provided a range of novel targets for small-molecule based therapeutic interventions to develop novel therapies. In particular, small-molecule interventions against oncogenic kinase signaling pathways possessing dichotomous role in the tumour microenvironment may offer opportunities to develop single-targeted 'two hit' cancer chemo-immunotherapeutics [11, 12]. It is relatively a new concept/trend in cancer treatment research that aims to harness the chemo-immunotherapeutic aspects of small-molecules that target 'dichotomous' oncogenic pathways at different levels, and thus have the potential to impart a 'two hit' impact: chemoprevention by direct killing of tumour cells, as well as enhanced anti-tumour immune responses.

3.1. 'Two Hit' Chemo-Immunotherapeutic Potential of Oncogenic Kinase Signaling Inhibition

Adenosine and PGE_2 signaling via the autocrine and paracrine activation of respective A2A/A2B and EP2/EP4 receptors converges on a common intracellular signaling pathway, the cAMP-PKAI pathway, in cancer and immune cells [10, 12]. There is strong preclinical and clinical evidence that implicates the aberrant regulation of cAMP-PKAI signaling in the development and progression, as well as the immune escape mechanisms of multiple advanced cancers [10, 12]. Mounting evidence from pre-clinical and clinical settings also indicate that pharmacological inhibition at different levels of adenosine-PGE_2/cAMP/PKAI nexus, either upstream or downstream, may have the potential to execute a 'two hit' impact in the tumour microenvironment [10, 12]. Especially, the recently reviewed experimental and pre-clinical data clearly indicate that pharmacological targeting downstream at effector level, i.e. PKAI inhibition, may provide opportunities to develop a more specific and effective form of single-targeted 'two hit' cancer chemo-immunotherapeutics [11, 12]. Selective antagonism/ inhibition of RIα subunit of PKAI (RI/PKA) not only provide multifaceted direct anti-tumour effects (such as growth arrest, tumour reversion, apoptosis induction, angiogenesis inhibition and chemoprevention), but also restore/potentiate the suppressed tumour microenvironment to mount a robust anti-tumour immune response [11, 12]. In addition, selective RI/PKA inhibition may also serve as an adjunctive couple to enhance the efficacy of different forms of current immunotherapy, as it may alleviate Tregs-derived immune suppressive mechanisms and enhance cytotoxic T cell-mediated anti-tumour immunity [11]. Rp-8-Br-cAMPS (Fig. **1**) is a selective PKAI antagonist that has shown chemopreventive and immune-rescuing potential in the tumour micro-environment.

PI3K is another most frequently deregulated kinase signaling pathway in cancer. Dysregulated PI3K/Akt/mTOR axis is a characteristic feature in the development of several malignant traits of cancer cells (such as leukemia, breast cancer, NSCLC, etc.), as well as their escape from anti-tumour immunity [99 - 103]. In recent years, it has been manifested that inhibition of different components of PI3K/Akt/mTOR pathway in tumour cells or immune cells may have the potential to provide 'two hit' chemo-immunotherapeutic opportunity [97]. In particular, Akt or mTOR inhibitors have been demonstrated to not only directly kill tumour cells, but also enhance anti-tumour immunity [104 - 107]. Moreover, Akt or mTOR inhibitors have been shown to reverse immune-resistant phenotypes of tumours and effectively sensitize them to different forms of immunotherapy by inducing or potentiating cytotoxic T cell-mediated immune responses [97, 104]. However, despite its critical involvement in cancer progression and immune escape, PI3K/Akt/mTOR signaling is also crucial for endogenous anti-tumour immune responses. These counteracting aspects of PI3K/Akt/mTOR signaling owe to different PI3K isoforms that could induce multiple mechanisms of intracellular signal transduction in cancer and immune cells [108]. Therefore, the prospective 'two hit' therapeutic manipulation of PI3K/Akt/mTOR signaling would need to be considered with deep care, as the function of single isoform can be dually involved in promoting both tumour progression and anti-tumour immune effector mechanisms. Looking from this perspective, mTOR in its two multiprotein complexes: mTOR complex-1 (mTORC1) and mTOR complex-2 (mTORC2), has emerged as a rational target in recent experimental and pre-clinical studies [109, 110]. To date, several mTOR kinase inhibitors capable of inhibiting both mTORC1/2 (e.g. AZD8055, INK/MLN-128, AZD2014 and CC-223) have entered patient trials [111 - 115]. Amongst these mTORC1/2 inhibitors, AZD8055 (Fig. **1**) may be a candidate of particular interest for prospective 'two hit' chemo-immunotherapeutic exploitation, as it has demonstrated promising direct anti-cancer as well as immune enhancing effects in several pre-clinical studies (Table **2**) [102, 116].

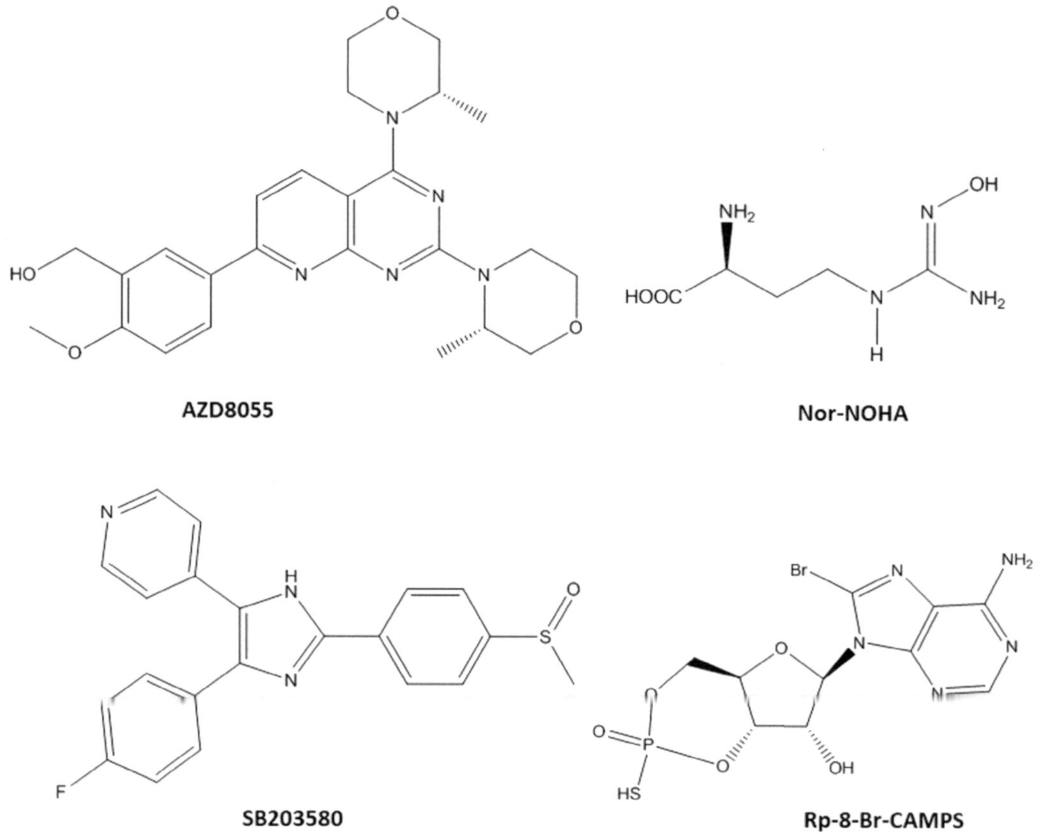

Fig. (1). Chemical structures of compounds with 'two hit' chemo-immunotherapeutic potential. The preclinical data indicate that there is huge potential of combining these compounds with conventional immunotherapeutic regimens to enhance anti-cancer immunity. In addition, they may also be considered as lead candidates for future development of single-target 'two-in-one' cancer chemo-immunotherapy.

Besides cAMP/PKAI and PI3K/mTOR signaling, p38 MAPK signaling has also emerged as crucial aspect of cancer development, progression, and immune escape mechanisms. Selective activation of p38 MAPK within the tumour microenvironment induces the production of cytokines that promote tumour growth, invasion, and metastasis [117, 118]. Similarly, tumour-induced p38 MAPK activation in DCs and then subsequent suppression of cytotoxic T lymphocyte responses is an effective means for tumours to escape immune control [119, 120]. More recently, tumour-secreted transforming growth factor (TGF)-β-mediated activation of p38 MAPK signaling has also been demonstrated to induce Tregs in ovarian cancer microenvironment, which ultimately was proposed to enhance tumour immune tolerance [121]. On the other hand, selective p38 MAPK inhibition has been manifested to induce direct anti-tumour effects (i.e. inhibition of tumour growth, invasion and migration) in multiple advanced cancers, such as breast cancer [122], pancreatic cancer [123] and cervical cancer [124]. Likewise, selective p38 MAPK inhibition in DCs has been evidenced to induce superior anti-tumour T effector cell immune responses and overcome Tregs-mediated immunosuppression [125 - 127]. In addition, p38 MAPK inhibition has been proposed as a promising approach for improving DC-based immunotherapy in human cancers [125]. Collectively, these findings clearly infer that selective inhibition of p38 MAPK signaling in the tumour microenvironment has the potential to be exploited as 'two hit' chemo-immunotherapeutics. Nevertheless, similar to that of PI3K, p38 MAPK also exists in different isoforms and appears to involve diverse and complex signal transduction mechanisms in tumour and immune cells [128]. Therefore, its prospective 'two hit' manipulation would definitely need the deep understanding of underneath signaling mechanisms. Looking from this perspective, SB203580 (Fig. **1**), a specific inhibitor of p38 MAPK, seems to be an attractive candidate. SB203580 has been demonstrated to inhibit tumour development and progression, and prevent the induction of immunosuppressive Tregs in the tumour microenvironment (Table **2**).

3.2. Does Tumoural Inhibition of ARG and IDO Possess 'Two Hit' Chemo-Immunotherapeutic Potential?

ARG and IDO are the two intracellular enzymes which catalyze the rate-limiting steps in the catabolism of two amino acids l-arginine and tryptophan, respectively. In the tumour microenvironment, both enzymes comprise a pivotal axis in tumour progression and immunoescape mechanisms via their respective amino acid catabolizing activities [129].

ARG (two isoforms: ARG-1 and ARG-2) is expressed by tumour cells, MDSCs and tumour-associated macrophages, and catabolizes the amino acid l-arginine to l-ornithine and urea [129]. Research over the past decade has provided compelling evidence for ARG-mediated catabolism of l-arginine to play pivotal role in tumorigenesis and tumour immune escape/tolerance (Table **2**) [129 - 151]. Ornithine, the downstream product of ARG-mediated l-arginine catabolism, serves as a precursor for biosynthesis of polyamines, which act as potent endogenous promoters of tumour growth and progression in multiple human cancers [129, 148]. In addition to direct effects on tumour proliferation, ARG catabolism of l-arginine has also been implicated in MDSCs-mediated suppression of anti-tumour T cell responses [150, 152, 153], as well as in IL-6-mediated DC-dependent CD4 (+) T cell dysfunction [154]. Therapeutically, nor-NOHA (N (omega)-hydroxy- nor-l-arginine) (Fig. **1**) - a compound well known for its potent inhibitory effect on ARG activity - have been demonstrated to inhibit *in vitro* proliferation of the high ARG-expressing tumour cells [147 - 149], as well as reverse the ARG-dependent T-cell immunosuppression in preclinical tumour models [151, 155].

Table 2. Exemplary Inhibitors with 'Two Hit' Chemo-Immunotherapeutic Potential [130 - 151].

Drug	**Target**	**Direct Anti-Tumor Effects**	**Anti-Tumor Immune Enhancing Effects**
Rp-8-Br-cAMPS	PKAI	• Reduces tumour development and progression [130, 131]	• Counteracts cAMP/PKAI-mediated suppression of NK cells and cytotoxic T lymphocytes [132 - 134] • Prevents Tregs-derived suppression of T cell immunity [135]
AZD8055	mTORC1/2	• Cytotoxic effects: suppresses tumour growth by inhibiting tumour cell proliferation and inducing cell death through mechanisms of apoptosis and autophagy [105, 106, 136 - 139] • Enhances cancer cells chemo-sensitivity and radio-sensitivity [140 - 142]	• Increases infiltration, activation and proliferation of CD8 (+) T cells and NK cells in the tumour microenvironment, and enhances the activity of cancer immunotherapy synergistically [104]
SB203580	p38 MAPK	• Inhibits tumour growth through apoptosis induction [143, 144] • Inhibits tumour cells migration and invasion, and prevents metastasis [118, 145] • Enhances sensitivity to chemotherapy [146]	• Can inhibit the induction of immunosuppressive Tregs in tumour microenvironment [121]
nor-NOHA	ARG-1/2	• Inhibits proliferation, migration and angiogenic capacity of tumour cells with high ARG activity [147 - 149]	• Can reverse ARG-mediated suppression of anti-tumour T-cell immunity [150, 151]

IDO (two isoforms: IDO-1 and IDO-2) is expressed by tumour cells, antigen presenting DCs and stromal cells, and mediates the catabolism of the essential amino acid tryptophan along the kynurenine pathway [129]. A complex relationship exists between IDO-mediated catabolism of tryptophan, tumour immunoescape/tolerance, and tumour progression [129]. Increased IDO activity inhibits cell proliferation and induces apoptosis in T cells and NK cells through tryptophan depletion and production of toxic tryptophan catabolites in the tumour microenvironment [129, 156, 157]. In addition, induction of Tregs activity by IDO contributes to the promotion of immune tolerance in cancer tissue [157]. On the other hand, the end product of IDO-mediated catabolism of tryptophan, nicotinamide adenine dinucleotide (NAD+), is highly consumed in the growth and development of tumour tissues [158]. Moreover, reduced expression of IDOs by gene silencing techniques has been demonstrated to inhibit tumour growth and progression, which further demonstrates the non-immune dependent role of IDO in tumorigenesis [158]. Therapeutically, several IDO inhibitors, including 1-methyl-tryptophan (1-MT), have shown promising anti-tumour immune enhancing effects, some of which nowadays have entered clinical evaluation [157, 159]. Nevertheless, it still remains elusive whether IDO inhibitors inhibit cancer cells proliferation/progression independent of their immune enhancing effects.

Collectively, the data discussed above clearly infer that selective ARG and IDO inhibition may hold 'two hit' chemo-immunotherapeutic potential in the tumour microenvironment, although the data still remains scarce in this direction. Particularly, studies ought to be endorsed to explore the direct anti-tumour effects of tumoural IDOs inhibition.

4. PATENTS ISSUED AND RECENT PATENT APPLLICATIONS IN CANCER CHEMO-IMMUNOTHERAPEUTICS

This section will shed light on patents issued and recent patent applications published in the field of cancer chemo-immunotherapy, which have identified several new approaches in terms of methods and formulations, demonstrating synergistic interventional combinations as well, to treat cancer (Tables **3** & **4**). Many of these approaches characterize the simultaneous, concurrent or separate (with a substantial gap) administrations of a wide variety of chemo- and immune-therapeutic regimens in suitable combinations, thereby, producing direct anti-tumour effects as well as enhancing anti-cancer immune responses. In this regard, Harrop *et al.* [160] have recently resented a method (US8133681B2) that relates to simultaneous or concurrent administration of a tumour-associated antigen (e.g. TroVax® vaccine), as well as chemotherapeutic agent(s) (e.g. FOLFOX) along with a pharmaceutically acceptable carrier, diluent or excipient. The method is based on a surprising finding that stimulating an immune response against an antigen by administering an antigen is enhanced by the treatment with a chemotherapeutic agent(s) [160].

Hadasit Medical Research Services previously presented a method involving sequential administrations of a therapeutically effective combination of a chemotherapeutic drug (e.g. doxorubicin) and an immunostimulating cytokine (e.g. IL-2), both encapsulated in liposomes [161]. The method produced significantly greater therapeutic effects (as evidenced by survival rate and tumour size) in tumour models of lung and colon carcinomas, than a combination of the effects produced by the free or liposome-encapsulated components administered individually [161]. Another pharmaceutical approach, comprising a combination of chemotherapy and immuno gene therapy with a polymer, implies administration of chemotherapeutic agent preferably prior to gene delivery (e.g. pIL-12/polymer) [162]. The inventors proposed that prior administration of chemotherapy may cause tumour destruction and release tumour antigens, which could be later used by the therapeutic gene (e.g. pIL-12/polymer) for eliciting highly specific and robust anti-tumour immune response against the target cancer [162]. Similarly, Weichselbaum *et al.* [163] have presented a transcriptional targeting method that relates to co-administration of a construct encoding a therapeutic polypeptide (e.g. TNF-α) and a chemotherapeutic agent to a subject, wherein the chemotherapeutic agent induces the expression of the polypeptide, thereby avoiding toxicity that may be associated with systemic administration. The authors proposed that combined treatment effect of the therapeutic polypeptide with chemotherapy may enhance the therapeutic response of the tumour cells to a greater extent than treatment with either therapy alone [163]. Apart from this, Salem *et al.* [164] have recently proposed a three-component chemo-immunotherapeutic formulation that comprises microparticles, a chemotherapeutic agent, and an immune adjuvant. According to this formulation, a microparticle carrier system, preferably a biodegradable polymeric material, is used for the easier co-delivery of chemo- and immuno-therapeutic agents. The microparticle-based approach ensures effective phagocytosis and also helps mitigate the toxic and immunosuppressive effects of chemotherapeutic agents by reduction in the dose and by providing controlled delivery of both therapeutic agents [164]. The method also allows for an easier co-delivery of agents that are difficult to co-deliver in the same solution [164].

The patented methods in combined chemo-immunotherapy also provide the ways to alleviate or reduce post-chemotherapy side-effects, and thus, improving the quality of life experienced by patients receiving chemotherapy. For instance, reduction in the severity of post-chemotherapeutic side effects was presented by a European patent (EP1357935) administering thymosin α1 (an immunomodulator that enhances T cell function) in conjunction with conventional chemotherapy [165]. The inventors proposed that thymosin α1's ability to block chemotherapy-induced vasoactive intestinal peptide (VIP) - one of the chemoreceptor trigger zone (CTZ) neurotransmitters that activate the vomiting center - provides an advantage to control the gastrointestinal adverse effects like nausea and vomiting, and thus may improve quality of life [165]. A recent method by Gevas *et al.* [166] emphasizes the use of anti-G17 immunization in combination with standard chemotherapy to lower the post-chemotherapeutic toxic effects on normal tissues. In particular, anti-G17 immunization/5-FU-leucovorin combination has been found more effective to increase the efficacy of colorectal cancer treatment. It is believed that anti-G17 antibody titers produced by immunization are effective in inhibiting G17-dependent tumour cell growth and, in turn, lower doses of chemotherapeutic agents may be required for treating the patient. This ultimately may improve patient's quality of life and also prolong the survival time [166]. Moreover, two patents (US6022538 and EP0980205) by Santoli *et al.* [167, 168] provided a chemo-immunotherapeutic method of treating drug-resistant cancer via co-administration of adoptive transfer therapy (non-MHC restricted cytotoxic cells) in combination with chemotherapy agents (adriamycin or cisplatin), which not only produce synergistic anti-tumour effects but also permit lower doses of the chemotherapeutic agents, ultimately resulting in the reduction of associated toxicities [167, 168].

Table 3. Patents in Chemo-Immunotherapy.

Patent Number	Title	Assignee
US8133681	Chemo-immunotherapy method	Oxford Biomedica (UK) Limited
US6787132	Combined chemo-immunotherapy with liposomal drugs and cytokines	Hadasit Medical Research Services and Development, Ltd.
US7964571	Combination of immuno gene therapy and chemotherapy for treatment of cancer and hyperproliferative diseases	Egen, Inc.
US8034791	Activation of Egr-1 promoter by DNA damaging chemotherapeutics	The University of Chicago, Dana-Farber Cancer Institute
EP1357935	Reducing side effects of chemotherapy in cancer patients	Sciclone Pharmaceuticals, Inc.
US8343930	Combination therapy for the treatment of tumors	Cancer Advances, Inc.
US6022538	Method of treating malignancies	The, Wistar Institute of Anatomy And Biology (Philadelphia, PA)
EP0980205	Use of a combination of TALL104 cells with adriamycin or cisplatin in the therapy of malignancies	The, Wistar Institute of Anatomy and Biology
US8344100	Polyepitope peptide derived from thymidylate synthase having immunological and antitumor activity	Universitá degli Studi di Siena
US8685394	Combination of anti-CTLA4 antibody with diverse therapeutic regimens for the synergistic treatment of proliferative diseases	Bristol-Myers Squibb Company
US7851599	Combination of an anti-ED-B fibronectin domain antibody-IL-2 fusion protein and gemcitabine	Philogen S.p.A.

There are also some patents which provide combinations of an anti-tumour peptide/antibody with conventional chemotherapy to treat advanced cancers. US patent 8344100 is a particular striking example of a chemo-immunotherapy that combines a poly-epitope peptide derived from TSPP with conventional fluoropyrimidine-based chemotherapy to treat gastroenteric, breast, and head and neck carcinomas [169]. TSPP possesses anti-tumour immunoprotective and/or immunotherapeutic activity and is capable of destroying tumour cells that over-express TS enzyme, via induction of CTL responses. Similarly, US patent 868539 refers to the combined use of an anti-CTLA4 antibody (e.g. ipilimumab or tremilimumab) with diverse chemotherapeutic regimens (such as tyrosine kinase inhibitors and microtubule-stabilizing agents) for the synergistic treatment of lung cancer, pancreatic cancer, colon cancer, prostate cancer, and leukemia [170]. In addition, US7851599B2 represent a specific form of chemo-immunotherapy that relates to a combination of anti-ED-B fibronectin domain antibody-IL-2 fusion protein and gemcitabine for the treatment of pancreatic cancer [171]. Furthermore, recent patent applications also state novel chemo-immunotherapy methods with diverse interventional combinations, some of which produce synergistic anti-tumour effects, to treat multiple advanced cancers (Table **4**) [164, 172 - 179].

Table 4. Recent Patent Applications in Combined Chemo-Immunotherapy.

Patent Application Number	Title	Interventional Combination	Applicants	Reference
US20140127253	Biodegradable particulate formulations	Doxorubicin + immune adjuvant CpG	University of Iowa Research Foundation	[164]
WO2016096577	Combined use of a chemotherapeutic agent and a cyclic dinucleotide for cancer treatment	Gemcitabine + STING agonist cyclic dinucleotide	Invivogen	[172]
US20160067322	Method of treating lung cancer by vaccination with MUC1 lipopeptide	Platinum-based chemotherapy + vaccination with a muc-1 lipopetide	Merck patent GmbH	[173]
WO2016061182	Combination therapy for use in cancer therapy	Mitomycin and fluorouracil (5-FU) + recombinant Listeria strain	The Trustees of the University of Pennsylvania	[174]
US20160074494	Cancer therapy	mTOR inhibitor + a non-pathogenic heat-killed *Mycobacterium*	Immodulon therapeutics	[175]
WO2016041014	Treatment of tumours using peptideprotein conjugates	Chemotherapy + LIGHT polypeptide conjugated to a tumourhoming peptide	The University of Western Australia	[176]

(Table 4) contd.....

Patent Application Number	Title	Interventional Combination	Applicants	Reference
WO2015095404	Methods of treating cancers using PD1 axis binding antagonists and taxanes	Paclitaxel/docetaxel + Nivolumab/lambrolizumab/pidilizumab	Genentech, Inc. F. HoffmannLA Roche AG	[177]
US20140056844	Methods of metabolic targeting cancer cells using chemo- and immunotherapy for treating cancer	Various chemotherapeutic agents + Immunologic agents (IFN-gamma, GM-CSF, IL-4 or TNF-α)	Cure cancer worldwide corporation	[178]
WO2008091643	Evaluating synergy of combinations comprising an antibody in immune suppressive pathways concurrent to immunotherapy	Gemcitabine or Topotecan + a monoclonal antibody + a cytokine + NOHA or 1-MT	Altarex medical corp. Schultes, Birgit, C. Noujaim, Antoine, A. Nicodemus, Christopher, F.	[179]

CURRENT AND FUTURE DEVELOPMENTS

Cancer chemo-immunotherapeutics is a rapidly evolving field that has the potential to deliver substantial benefits to patients with multiple advanced cancers. Although long considered as incompatible, owing to the immunosuppressive impact of conventional chemotherapeutic agents, the chemo- and immuno-therapy combinations have now started to deliver the translational breakthroughs into the clinic. In fact, many chemo- and immune-therapeutic regimens have emerged to hold genuine promise as potential partners, producing synergistic effects and, thereby, resulting in startling tumour regression in people with a range of different cancers. The preclinical and clinical data emerging over the last five years have revealed that chemotherapeutic regimens could enhance the efficacy of immunotherapy in different ways, such as overcoming parts of immuno-suppression, enhancing cross-presentation of tumour antigens, and supporting better penetration of tumour cells in tumour core [180]. Also, numerous chemo-immunotherapy drug combinations are currently being tested in clinical trials and are likely to be the best approach to improving patient outcomes (Table **1**). However, there is still much to be understood, as some recent clinical trials showed poor patient response and could not meet the primary end points [31, 32].

As such, more preclinical and clinical trials are needed to explore the optimal choice, the proper dose, and scheduling of the individual components in chemo-immunotherapy combinations. It will also be crucial to explore the immunomodulatory impact of different drugs or supplements - cancer patients often receive concomitantly for symptom management - for the implementation of chemo-immunotherapy efficient combinations [7, 181].

Apart from this, the success of chemo-immunotherapy also depends upon tumour-stroma-immune cell interactions that pave the route to tumour-associated immune suppression (discussed above). As our knowledge of tumour-associated immune suppression is increasing day by day, it is becoming clearly evident that these mechanisms may hinder or attenuate the efficacy of immunotherapeutic strategies [11]. Emerging data indicate that small-molecule based therapeutic approaches which target tumour-associated immune suppressive mechanisms (for instance, oncogenic signaling kinase inhibitors) may have the great potential to enhance anti-tumour immune responses, thereby optimizing the chance for cure. Such therapies/inhibitors can be regarded as potential partners for the growing suite of chemo-immunotherapy combinations in preclinical and clinical settings - acting to kick-start the suppressed tumour microenvironment to mount a robust anti-tumour immune response.

CONFLICT OF INTEREST

The author (editor) declares no conflict of interest, financial or otherwise.

ACKNOWLEDGEMENTS

Muzammal Hussain is supported by CAS-TWAS President's fellowship.

REFERENCES

[1] Emens LA. Chemoimmunotherapy. Cancer J 2010; 16(4): 295-303. [http://dx.doi.org/10.1097/PPO.0b013e3181eb5066] [PMID: 20693839]

[2] Zhang Z, Yu X, Wang Z, Wu P, Huang J. Anthracyclines potentiate anti-tumor immunity: A new opportunity for chemoimmunotherapy. Cancer Lett 2015; 369(2): 331-5. [http://dx.doi.org/10.1016/j.canlet.2015.10.002] [PMID: 26454214]

[3] Zitvogel L, Galluzzi L, Smyth MJ, Kroemer G. Mechanism of action of conventional and targeted anticancer therapies: Reinstating immunosurveillance. Immunity 2013; 39(1): 74-88. [http://dx.doi.org/10.1016/j.immuni.2013.06.014] [PMID: 23890065]

[4] Zitvogel L, Kepp O, Kroemer G. Immune parameters affecting the efficacy of chemotherapeutic regimens. Nat Rev Clin Oncol 2011; 8(3): 151-60. [http://dx.doi.org/10.1038/nrclinonc.2010.223] [PMID: 21364688]

[5] Hanoteau A, Henin C, Moser M. The interplay of immunotherapy and chemotherapy, a novel approach. Med Sci (Paris) 2016; 32(4): 353-61. [http://dx.doi.org/10.1051/medsci/20163204013] [PMID: 27137692]

[6] Muller AJ, Prendergast GC. Marrying immunotherapy with chemotherapy: Why say IDO? Cancer Res 2005; 65(18): 8065-8.
[http://dx.doi.org/10.1158/0008-5472.CAN-05-2213] [PMID: 16166276]

[7] Emens LA, Middleton G. The interplay of immunotherapy and chemotherapy: Harnessing potential synergies. Cancer Immunol Res 2015; 3(5): 436-43.
[http://dx.doi.org/10.1158/2326-6066.CIR-15-0064] [PMID: 25941355]

[8] Hanoteau A, Moser M. Chemotherapy and immunotherapy: A close interplay to fight cancer? OncoImmunology 2016; 5(7): e1190061.
[http://dx.doi.org/10.1080/2162402X.2016.1190061] [PMID: 27622046]

[9] Seliger B. Strategies of tumor immune evasion. BioDrugs 2005; 19(6): 347-54.
[http://dx.doi.org/10.2165/00063030-200519060-00002] [PMID: 16392887]

[10] Hussain M, Javeed A, Ashraf M, Yuzhu H, Mukhtar MM. Multilevel pharmacological manipulation of adenosine-prostaglandin E(2)/cAMP nexus in the tumor microenvironment: A two hit therapeutic opportunity. Pharmacol Res 2013; 73: 8-19.
[http://dx.doi.org/10.1016/j.phrs.2013.04.006] [PMID: 23619528]

[11] Hussain M, Shah Z, Abbas N, Javeed A, Mukhtar MM, Zhang J. Targeting tumor-associated immune suppression with selective protein kinase A type I (PKAI) inhibitors may enhance cancer immunotherapy. Med Hypotheses 2016; 86: 56-9.
[http://dx.doi.org/10.1016/j.mehy.2015.11.031] [PMID: 26804598]

[12] Hussain M, Tang F, Liu J, Zhang J, Javeed A. Dichotomous role of protein kinase A type I (PKAI) in the tumor microenvironment: A potential target for two-in-one cancer chemoimmunotherapeutics. Cancer Lett 2015; 369(1): 9-19.
[http://dx.doi.org/10.1016/j.canlet.2015.07.047] [PMID: 26276720]

[13] Grillo-López AJ. Rituximab: An insiders historical perspective. Semin Oncol 2000; 27(6) (Suppl 12): 9-16.
[PMID: 11226006]

[14] Weiner GJ. Rituximab: Mechanism of action. Semin Hematol 2010; 47(2): 115-23.
[http://dx.doi.org/10.1053/j.seminhematol.2010.01.011] [PMID: 20350658]

[15] Eichhorst B, Fink AM, Bahlo J, *et al.* international group of investigators; German CLL Study Group (GCLLSG). First-line chemoimmunotherapy with bendamustine and rituximab versus fludarabine, cyclophosphamide, and rituximab in patients with advanced chronic lymphocytic leukaemia (CLL10): An international, open-label, randomised, Phase III, non-inferiority trial. Lancet Oncol 2016; 17(7): 928-42.
[http://dx.doi.org/10.1016/S1470-2045(16)30051-1] [PMID: 27216274]

[16] Ferreri AJ, Cwynarski K, Pulczynski E, *et al.* International Extranodal Lymphoma Study Group (IELSG). Chemoimmunotherapy with methotrexate, cytarabine, thiotepa, and rituximab (MATRix regimen) in patients with primary CNS lymphoma: Results of the first randomisation of the International Extranodal Lymphoma Study Group-32 (IELSG32) Phase II trial. Lancet Haematol 2016; 3(5): e217-27.
[http://dx.doi.org/10.1016/S2352-3026(16)00036-3] [PMID: 27132696]

[17] Fischer K, Bahlo J, Fink AM, *et al.* Long-term remissions after FCR chemoimmunotherapy in previously untreated patients with CLL: Updated results of the CLL8 trial. Blood 2016; 127(2): 208-15.
[http://dx.doi.org/10.1182/blood-2015-06-651125] [PMID: 26486789]

[18] Li Z, Li F, Yi S, *et al.* Superior efficacy of rituximab-based chemoimmunotherapy as an initial therapy in newly diagnosed patients with B cell indolent lymphomas: Long-term results from a single center in China. BMC Cancer 2015; 15: 555.
[http://dx.doi.org/10.1186/s12885-015-1534-0] [PMID: 26219471]

[19] Nastoupil LJ, Sinha R, Byrtek M, *et al.* Comparison of the effectiveness of frontline chemoimmunotherapy regimens for follicular lymphoma used in the United States. Leuk Lymphoma 2015; 56(5): 1295-302.
[http://dx.doi.org/10.3109/10428194.2014.953144] [PMID: 25263322]

[20] Olszewski AJ, Shafqat H, Ali S. Disparate survival outcomes after front-line chemoimmunotherapy in older patients with follicular, nodal marginal zone and small lymphocytic lymphoma. Leuk Lymphoma 2015; 56(4): 942-50.
[http://dx.doi.org/10.3109/10428194.2014.936013] [PMID: 24956144]

[21] Cencini E, Fabbri A, Schiattone L, Bartalucci G, Bocchia M. Low-dose chemoimmunotherapy with fludarabine, cyclophosphamide, and rituximab in follicular lymphoma. Eur J Haematol 2015; 94(3): 277-8.
[http://dx.doi.org/10.1111/ejh.12428] [PMID: 25080977]

[22] Halwani AS, Link BK. Chemotherapy and antibody combinations for relapsed/refractory non-Hodgkins lymphoma. Expert Rev Anticancer Ther 2011; 11(3): 443-55.
[http://dx.doi.org/10.1586/era.11.9] [PMID: 21417857]

[23] Harris SJ, Brown J, Lopez J, Yap TA. Immuno-oncology combinations: Raising the tail of the survival curve. Cancer Biol Med 2016; 13(2): 171-93.
[http://dx.doi.org/10.20892/j.issn.2095-3941.2016.0015] [PMID: 27458526]

[24] Hoos A. Development of immuno-oncology drugs - from CTLA4 to PD1 to the next generations. Nat Rev Drug Discov 2016; 15(4): 235-47.
[http://dx.doi.org/10.1038/nrd.2015.35] [PMID: 26965203]

[25] Utriainen M, Rämet M. Immuno-oncologysilver bullets or mass destruction weapons? Duodecim 2016; 132(8): 721-8.
[PMID: 27244931]

[26] Scagliotti GV, Bironzo P, Vansteenkiste JF. Addressing the unmet need in lung cancer: The potential of immuno-oncology. Cancer Treat Rev 2015; 41(6): 465-75.
[http://dx.doi.org/10.1016/j.ctrv.2015.04.001] [PMID: 25936526]

[27] Hersh EM, ODay SJ, Powderly J, *et al.* A Phase II multicenter study of ipilimumab with or without dacarbazine in chemotherapy-naïve patients with advanced melanoma. Invest New Drugs 2011; 29(3): 489-98.
[http://dx.doi.org/10.1007/s10637-009-9376-8] [PMID: 20082117]

[28] Robert C, Thomas L, Bondarenko I, *et al.* Ipilimumab plus dacarbazine for previously untreated metastatic melanoma. N Engl J Med 2011; 364(26): 2517-26.
[http://dx.doi.org/10.1056/NEJMoa1104621] [PMID: 21639810]

[29] Lynch TJ, Bondarenko I, Luft A, *et al.* Ipilimumab in combination with paclitaxel and carboplatin as first-line treatment in stage IIIB/IV non-small-cell lung cancer: Results from a randomized, double-blind, multicenter Phase II study. J Clin Oncol 2012; 30(17): 2046-54.
[http://dx.doi.org/10.1200/JCO.2011.38.4032] [PMID: 22547592]

[30] Reck M, Bondarenko I, Luft A, *et al.* Ipilimumab in combination with paclitaxel and carboplatin as first-line therapy in extensive-disease-small-cell lung cancer: Results from a randomized, double-blind, multicenter Phase II trial. Ann Oncol 2013; 24(1): 75-83.
[http://dx.doi.org/10.1093/annonc/mds213] [PMID: 22858559]

[31] Arriola E, Wheater M, Galea I, *et al.* Outcome and biomarker analysis from a multicenter Phase II study of ipilimumab in combination with carboplatin and etoposide as first-line therapy for extensive-stage SCLC. J Thorac Oncol 2016; 11(9): 1511-21.
[http://dx.doi.org/10.1016/j.jtho.2016.05.028] [PMID: 27296105]

[32] Reck M, Luft A, Szczesna A, *et al.* Phase III randomized trial of ipilimumab plus etoposide and platinum versus placebo plus etoposide and platinum in extensive-stage small-cell lung cancer. J Clin

Oncol 2016; JCO676601
[http://dx.doi.org/10.1200/JCO.2016.67.6601] [PMID: 27458307]

[33] Antonia SJ, Brahmer JR, Gettinger S, *et al.* Nivolumab (anti-PD-1; BMS-936558, ONO-4538) in combination with platinum-based doublet chemotherapy (PT-DC) in advanced non-small cell lung cancer (NSCLC). ASCO annual meeting. Chicago, USA . 2014.

[34] Yaddanapudi K, Mitchell RA, Eaton JW. Cancer vaccines: Looking to the future. OncoImmunology 2013; 2(3): e23403.
[http://dx.doi.org/10.4161/onci.23403] [PMID: 23802081]

[35] Antonia SJ, Mirza N, Fricke I, *et al.* Combination of p53 cancer vaccine with chemotherapy in patients with extensive stage small cell lung cancer. Clin Cancer Res 2006; 12(3 Pt 1): 878-87.
[http://dx.doi.org/10.1158/1078-0432.CCR-05-2013] [PMID: 16467102]

[36] Arlen PM, Gulley JL, Parker C, *et al.* A randomized Phase II study of concurrent docetaxel plus vaccine versus vaccine alone in metastatic androgen-independent prostate cancer. Clin Cancer Res 2006; 12(4): 1260-9.
[http://dx.doi.org/10.1158/1078-0432.CCR-05-2059] [PMID: 16489082]

[37] Casares N, Pequignot MO, Tesniere A, *et al.* Caspase-dependent immunogenicity of doxorubicin-induced tumor cell death. J Exp Med 2005; 202(12): 1691-701.
[http://dx.doi.org/10.1084/jem.20050915] [PMID: 16365148]

[38] Obeid M, Tesniere A, Ghiringhelli F, *et al.* Calreticulin exposure dictates the immunogenicity of cancer cell death. Nat Med 2007; 13(1): 54-61.
[http://dx.doi.org/10.1038/nm1523] [PMID: 17187072]

[39] Kang TH, Mao CP, Lee SY, *et al.* Chemotherapy acts as an adjuvant to convert the tumor microenvironment into a highly permissive state for vaccination-induced antitumor immunity. Cancer Res 2013; 73(8): 2493-504.
[http://dx.doi.org/10.1158/0008-5472.CAN-12-4241] [PMID: 23418322]

[40] Aranda F, Vacchelli E, Eggermont A, *et al.* Trial watch: Peptide vaccines in cancer therapy. OncoImmunology 2013; 2(12): e26621.
[http://dx.doi.org/10.4161/onci.26621] [PMID: 24498550]

[41] Haniffa M, Collin M, Ginhoux F. Identification of human tissue cross-presenting dendritic cells: A new target for cancer vaccines. OncoImmunology 2013; 2(3): e23140.
[http://dx.doi.org/10.4161/onci.23140] [PMID: 23802067]

[42] Senovilla L, Vacchelli E, Garcia P, *et al.* Trial watch: DNA vaccines for cancer therapy. OncoImmunology 2013; 2(4): e23803.
[http://dx.doi.org/10.4161/onci.23803] [PMID: 23734328]

[43] Ramlau R, Quoix E, Rolski J, *et al.* A Phase II study of Tg4010 (Mva-Muc1-Il2) in association with chemotherapy in patients with stage III/IV Non-small cell lung cancer. J Thorac Oncol 2008; 3(7): 735-44.
[http://dx.doi.org/10.1097/JTO.0b013e31817c6b4f] [PMID: 18594319]

[44] Quoix E, Ramlau R, Westeel V, *et al.* Therapeutic vaccination with TG4010 and first-line chemotherapy in advanced non-small-cell lung cancer: A controlled Phase 2B trial. Lancet Oncol 2011; 12(12): 1125-33.
[http://dx.doi.org/10.1016/S1470-2045(11)70259-5] [PMID: 22019520]

[45] Quoix E, Lena H, Losonczy G, *et al.* TG4010 immunotherapy and first-line chemotherapy for advanced non-small-cell lung cancer (TIME): Results from the Phase IIb part of a randomised, double-blind, placebo-controlled, Phase IIb/III trial. Lancet Oncol 2016; 17(2): 212-23.
[http://dx.doi.org/10.1016/S1470-2045(15)00483-0] [PMID: 26727163]

[46] Matsuyama M, Ishii H, Furuse J, *et al.* Phase II trial of combination therapy of gemcitabine plus anti-angiogenic vaccination of elpamotide in patients with advanced or recurrent biliary tract cancer. Invest

New Drugs 2015; 33(2): 490-5.
[http://dx.doi.org/10.1007/s10637-014-0197-z] [PMID: 25502982]

[47] Yamaue H, Tsunoda T, Tani M, *et al.* Randomized Phase II/III clinical trial of elpamotide for patients with advanced pancreatic cancer: PEGASUS-PC Study. Cancer Sci 2015; 106(7): 883-90.
[http://dx.doi.org/10.1111/cas.12674] [PMID: 25867139]

[48] Murahashi M, Hijikata Y, Yamada K, *et al.* Phase I clinical trial of a five-peptide cancer vaccine combined with cyclophosphamide in advanced solid tumors. Clin Immunol 2016; 166-167: 48-58.
[http://dx.doi.org/10.1016/j.clim.2016.03.015] [PMID: 27072896]

[49] Correale P, Botta C, Martino EC, *et al.* Phase Ib study of poly-epitope peptide vaccination to thymidylate synthase (TSPP) and GOLFIG chemo-immunotherapy for treatment of metastatic colorectal cancer patients. OncoImmunology 2015; 5(4): e1101205.
[http://dx.doi.org/10.1080/2162402X.2015.1101205] [PMID: 27141384]

[50] Welters MJ, van der Sluis TC, van Meir H, *et al.* Vaccination during myeloid cell depletion by cancer chemotherapy fosters robust T cell responses. Sci Transl Med 2016; 8(334): 334ra52.
[http://dx.doi.org/10.1126/scitranslmed.aad8307] [PMID: 27075626]

[51] Dijkgraaf EM, Santegoets SJ, Reyners AK, *et al.* A Phase I/II study combining gemcitabine, Pegintron and p53 SLP vaccine in patients with platinum-resistant ovarian cancer. Oncotarget 2015; 6(31): 32228-43.
[PMID: 26334096]

[52] van Dodewaard-de Jong JM, Santegoets SJ, van de Ven PM, *et al.* Improved efficacy of mitoxantrone in patients with castration-resistant prostate cancer after vaccination with GM-CSF-transduced allogeneic prostate cancer cells. OncoImmunology 2015; 5(4): e1105431.
[http://dx.doi.org/10.1080/2162402X.2015.1105431] [PMID: 27141390]

[53] Vuky J, Corman JM, Porter C, Olgac S, Auerbach E, Dahl K. Phase II trial of neoadjuvant docetaxel and CG1940/CG8711 followed by radical prostatectomy in patients with high-risk clinically localized prostate cancer. Oncologist 2013; 18(6): 687-8.
[http://dx.doi.org/10.1634/theoncologist.2011-0234] [PMID: 23740935]

[54] Slovin SR. Toward maximizing immunotherapy in metastatic castration-resistant prostate cancer - rationale for combinatorial approaches using chemotherapy. Front Oncol 2012; 2: 43.
[http://dx.doi.org/10.3389/fonc.2012.00043] [PMID: 22662316]

[55] McNamara M, Berry W. Complete Biochemical response (prostate specific antigen) to sipuleucel-T in Metastatic castrate-resistant prostate cancer: A case report with docetaxel chemotherapy administered just before sipuleucel-T. Clin Genitourin Cancer 2015; 13(5): e361-4.
[http://dx.doi.org/10.1016/j.clgc.2015.02.004] [PMID: 25735199]

[56] Sone S, Ogura T. Local interleukin-2 therapy for cancer, and its effector induction mechanisms. Oncology 1994; 51(2): 170-6.
[http://dx.doi.org/10.1159/000227331] [PMID: 8196900]

[57] Yamashita T, Arai K, Sunagozaka H, *et al.* Randomized, Phase II study comparing interferon combined with hepatic arterial infusion of fluorouracil plus cisplatin and fluorouracil alone in patients with advanced hepatocellular carcinoma. Oncology 2011; 81(5-6): 281-90.
[http://dx.doi.org/10.1159/000334439] [PMID: 22133996]

[58] Kasai K, Ushio A, Kasai Y, *et al.* Therapeutic efficacy of combination therapy with intra-arterial 5-fluorouracil and systemic pegylated interferon α-2b for advanced hepatocellular carcinoma with portal venous invasion. Cancer 2012; 118(13): 3302-10.
[http://dx.doi.org/10.1002/cncr.26648] [PMID: 22072099]

[59] Cohen JB, Bucur S, Winton EF, *et al.* Combination of GM-CSF with fludarabine-containing regimens in chronic lymphocytic leukemia and indolent Non-Hodgkin Lymphoma. Clin Lymphoma Myeloma Leuk 2015; 15(9): 514-8.
[http://dx.doi.org/10.1016/j.clml.2015.06.009] [PMID: 26297176]

[60] Garcia JA, Elson P, Tyler A, Triozzi P, Dreicer R. Sargramostim (GM-CSF) and lenalidomide in castration-resistant prostate cancer (CRPC): Results from a Phase I-II clinical trial. Urol Oncol 2014; 32(1): 33 e11-7.
[http://dx.doi.org/10.1016/j.urolonc.2012.12.004] [PMID: 23510862]

[61] Aggarwal RR, Beer TM, Weinberg VK, *et al.* Intermittent chemotherapy as a platform for testing novel agents in patients with metastatic castration-resistant prostate cancer: A department of defense prostate cancer clinical trials consortium randomized Phase II trial of intermittent docetaxel with prednisone with or without maintenance GM-CSF. Clin Genitourin Cancer 2015; 13(3): e191-8.
[http://dx.doi.org/10.1016/j.clgc.2014.12.004] [PMID: 25557266]

[62] Correale P, Botta C, Rotundo MS, *et al.* Gemcitabine, oxaliplatin, levofolinate, 5-fluorouracil, granulocyte-macrophage colony-stimulating factor, and interleukin-2 (GOLFIG) versus FOLFOX chemotherapy in metastatic colorectal cancer patients: The GOLFIG-2 multicentric open-label randomized Phase III trial. J Immunother 2014; 37(1): 26-35.
[http://dx.doi.org/10.1097/CJI.0000000000000004] [PMID: 24316553]

[63] Annels NE, Shaw VE, Gabitass RF, *et al.* The effects of gemcitabine and capecitabine combination chemotherapy and of low-dose adjuvant GM-CSF on the levels of myeloid-derived suppressor cells in patients with advanced pancreatic cancer. Cancer Immunol Immunother 2014; 63(2): 175-83.
[http://dx.doi.org/10.1007/s00262-013-1502-y] [PMID: 24292263]

[64] Sangiolo D. Cytokine induced killer cells as promising immunotherapy for solid tumors. J Cancer 2011; 2: 363-8.
[http://dx.doi.org/10.7150/jca.2.363] [PMID: 21716717]

[65] Zhao H, Wang Y, Yu J, *et al.* Autologous cytokine-induced killer cells improves overall survival of metastatic colorectal cancer patients: Results from a Phase II clinical trial. Clin Colorectal Cancer 2016; 15(3): 228-35.
[http://dx.doi.org/10.1016/j.clcc.2016.02.005] [PMID: 27052743]

[66] Mu Y, Wang WH, Xie JP, Zhang YX, Yang YP, Zhou CH. Efficacy and safety of cord blood-derived dendritic cells plus cytokine-induced killer cells combined with chemotherapy in the treatment of patients with advanced gastric cancer: A randomized Phase II study. Onco Targets Ther 2016; 9: 4617-27.
[http://dx.doi.org/10.2147/OTT.S107745] [PMID: 27524915]

[67] Mu Y, Zhou CH, Chen SF, *et al.* Effectiveness and safety of chemotherapy combined with cytokine-induced killer cell /dendritic cell-cytokine-induced killer cell therapy for treatment of gastric cancer in China: A systematic review and meta-analysis. Cytotherapy 2016; 18(9): 1162-77.
[http://dx.doi.org/10.1016/j.jcyt.2016.05.015] [PMID: 27421742]

[68] Zhao X, Ding HF, Liu J, *et al.* Effect of immunotherapy of dendritic cells and cytokine-induced killer cells combined with chemotherapy on secreting function of T lymphocytes in patients with multiple myeloma. Zhongguo Shi Yan Xue Ye Xue Za Zhi 2015; 23(6): 1633-7.
[PMID: 26708885]

[69] Zhao X, Ding HF, Xu M, *et al.* Clinical efficacy of dendritic cells and cytokine-induced killer cells combined with chemotherapy for treating newly diagnosed multiple myeloma and their effect on function of CD4(+) CD25(+) T cells in peripheral blood. Zhongguo Shi Yan Xue Ye Xue Za Zhi 2016; 24(1): 122-6.
[PMID: 26913407]

[70] Zhao X, Ji CY, Liu GQ, *et al.* Immunomodulatory effect of DC/CIK combined with chemotherapy in multiple myeloma and the clinical efficacy. Int J Clin Exp Pathol 2015; 8(10): 13146-55.
[PMID: 26722513]

[71] Lu G, Xing J, Liu GQ, *et al.* Clinical efficacy of DC and CIK immunotherapy combined with chemotherapy and its impact on treg cells in newly diagnosed multiple myeloma. Zhongguo Shi Yan Xue Ye Xue Za Zhi 2015; 23(3): 737-41.

[PMID: 26117028]

[72] Chen B, Liu L, Xu H, Yang Y, Zhang L, Zhang F. Effectiveness of immune therapy combined with chemotherapy on the immune function and recurrence rate of cervical cancer. Exp Ther Med 2015; 9(3): 1063-7.
[PMID: 25667679]

[73] Zhu XP, Xu YH, Zhou J, Pan XF. A clinical study evaluating dendritic and cytokine-induced killer cells combined with concurrent radiochemotherapy for stage IIIB non-small cell lung cancer. Genet Mol Res 2015; 14(3): 10228-35.
[http://dx.doi.org/10.4238/2015.August.28.6] [PMID: 26345959]

[74] Li DP, Li W, Feng J, Chen K, Tao M. Adjuvant chemotherapy with sequential cytokine-induced killer (CIK) cells in stage IB non-small cell lung cancer. Oncol Res 2015; 22(2): 67-74.
[http://dx.doi.org/10.3727/096504014X14024160459168] [PMID: 25706393]

[75] Lin T, Song C, Chuo DY, Zhang H, Zhao J. Clinical effects of autologous dendritic cells combined with cytokine-induced killer cells followed by chemotherapy in treating patients with advanced colorectal cancer: A prospective study. Tumour Biol 2016; 37(4): 4367-72.
[http://dx.doi.org/10.1007/s13277-015-3957-2] [PMID: 26499782]

[76] Mao Q, Li L, Zhang C, Sun Y, Liu S, Cui S. Clinical effects of immunotherapy of DC-CIK combined with chemotherapy in treating patients with metastatic breast cancer. Pak J Pharm Sci 2015; 28(3) (Suppl.): 1055-8.
[PMID: 26051718]

[77] Zheng C, Yu G, Wang H, *et al.* Meta-analysis of chemotherapy and dendritic cells with cytokine-induced killer cells in the treatment of non-small-cell lung cancer. Int J Clin Exp Med 2015; 8(8): 14527-37.
[PMID: 26550444]

[78] Lan XP, Chen YG, Wang Z, *et al.* Immunotherapy of DC-CIK cells enhances the efficacy of chemotherapy for solid cancer: A meta-analysis of randomized controlled trials in Chinese patients. J Zhejiang Univ Sci B 2015; 16(9): 743-56.
[http://dx.doi.org/10.1631/jzus.B1500003] [PMID: 26365116]

[79] Chen Y, Guo ZQ, Shi CM, Zhou ZF, Ye YB, Chen Q. Efficacy of adjuvant chemotherapy combined with immunotherapy with cytokine-induced killer cells for gastric cancer after d2 gastrectomy. Int J Clin Exp Med 2015; 8(5): 7728-36.
[PMID: 26221323]

[80] Chen Y, Lin J, Guo ZQ, *et al.* MHC I-related chain a expression in gastric carcinoma and the efficacy of immunotherapy with cytokine-induced killer cells. Am J Cancer Res 2015; 5(10): 3221-30.
[PMID: 26693072]

[81] Li Y, Pan K, Liu LZ, *et al.* Sequential cytokine-induced killer cell immunotherapy enhances the efficacy of the gemcitabine plus cisplatin chemotherapy regimen for metastatic nasopharyngeal carcinoma. PLoS One 2015; 10(6): e0130620.
[http://dx.doi.org/10.1371/journal.pone.0130620] [PMID: 26098948]

[82] Wang Z, Liu Y, Zhang Y, Shang Y, Gao Q. MDSC-decreasing chemotherapy increases the efficacy of cytokine-induced killer cell immunotherapy in metastatic renal cell carcinoma and pancreatic cancer. Oncotarget 2016; 7(4): 4760-9.
[PMID: 26716894]

[83] Kaufman HL, Kohlhapp FJ, Zloza A. Oncolytic viruses: A new class of immunotherapy drugs. Nat Rev Drug Discov 2015; 14(9): 642-62.
[http://dx.doi.org/10.1038/nrd4663] [PMID: 26323545]

[84] Bommareddy PK, Patel A, Hossain S, Kaufman HL. Talimogene laherparepvec (T-VEC) and other oncolytic viruses for the treatment of melanoma. Am J Clin Dermatol 2017; 18(1): 1-15.
[http://dx.doi.org/10.1007/s40257-016-0238-9] [PMID: 27988837]

[85] Bourgeois-Daigneault MC, St-Germain LE, Roy DG, *et al.* Combination of Paclitaxel and MG1 oncolytic virus as a successful strategy for breast cancer treatment. Breast Cancer Res 2016; 18(1): 83. [http://dx.doi.org/10.1186/s13058-016-0744-y] [PMID: 27503504]

[86] Simpson GR, Relph K, Harrington K, Melcher A, Pandha H. Cancer immunotherapy via combining oncolytic virotherapy with chemotherapy: Recent advances. Oncolytic Virother 2016; 5: 1-13. [PMID: 27579292]

[87] Cerullo V, Diaconu I, Kangasniemi L, *et al.* Immunological effects of low-dose cyclophosphamide in cancer patients treated with oncolytic adenovirus. Mol Ther 2011; 19(9): 1737-46. [http://dx.doi.org/10.1038/mt.2011.113] [PMID: 21673660]

[88] Comins C, Spicer J, Protheroe A, *et al.* REO-10: A Phase I study of intravenous reovirus and docetaxel in patients with advanced cancer. Clin Cancer Res 2010; 16(22): 5564-72. [http://dx.doi.org/10.1158/1078-0432.CCR-10-1233] [PMID: 20926400]

[89] Karapanagiotou EM, Roulstone V, Twigger K, *et al.* Phase I/II trial of carboplatin and paclitaxel chemotherapy in combination with intravenous oncolytic reovirus in patients with advanced malignancies. Clin Cancer Res 2012; 18(7): 2080-9. [http://dx.doi.org/10.1158/1078-0432.CCR-11-2181] [PMID: 22316603]

[90] Lolkema MP, Arkenau HT, Harrington K, *et al.* A Phase I study of the combination of intravenous reovirus type 3 dearing and gemcitabine in patients with advanced cancer. Clin Cancer Res 2011; 17(3): 581-8. [http://dx.doi.org/10.1158/1078-0432.CCR-10-2159] [PMID: 21106728]

[91] McAllister SS, Weinberg RA. Tumor-host interactions: A far-reaching relationship. J Clin Oncol 2010; 28(26): 4022-8. [http://dx.doi.org/10.1200/JCO.2010.28.4257] [PMID: 20644094]

[92] Nakasone ES, Askautrud HA, Kees T, *et al.* Imaging tumor-stroma interactions during chemotherapy reveals contributions of the microenvironment to resistance. Cancer Cell 2012; 21(4): 488-503. [http://dx.doi.org/10.1016/j.ccr.2012.02.017] [PMID: 22516258]

[93] Tisdale MJ. Tumor-host interactions. J Cell Biochem 2004; 93(5): 871-7. [http://dx.doi.org/10.1002/jcb.20246] [PMID: 15449322]

[94] Finn OJ. Immuno-oncology: Understanding the function and dysfunction of the immune system in cancer. Ann Oncol 2012; 23 (Suppl. 8): i6-9. [http://dx.doi.org/10.1093/annonc/mds256] [PMID: 22918931]

[95] Whiteside TL. Inhibiting the inhibitors: Evaluating agents targeting cancer immunosuppression. Expert Opin Biol Ther 2010; 10(7): 1019-35. [http://dx.doi.org/10.1517/14712598.2010.482207] [PMID: 20415597]

[96] Ostman A, Pietras K. Introduction to tumor-stroma interactions. Exp Cell Res 2013; 319(11): 1595. [http://dx.doi.org/10.1016/j.yexcr.2013.05.026] [PMID: 25242505]

[97] Jiang Q, Weiss JM, Wiltrout RH. A matched couple: Combining kinase inhibitors with immunotherapy for cancer treatment. OncoImmunology 2012; 1(1): 115-7. [http://dx.doi.org/10.4161/onci.1.1.18036] [PMID: 22720229]

[98] Ott PA, Adams S. Small-molecule protein kinase inhibitors and their effects on the immune system: Implications for cancer treatment. Immunotherapy 2011; 3(2): 213-27. [http://dx.doi.org/10.2217/imt.10.99] [PMID: 21322760]

[99] Dituri F, Mazzocca A, Giannelli G, Antonaci S. PI3K functions in cancer progression, anticancer immunity and immune evasion by tumors. Clin Dev Immunol 2011; 2011: 947858. [http://dx.doi.org/10.1155/2011/947858]

[100] Wyszynski RW, Gibbs BF, Varani L, Iannotta D, Sumbayev VV. Interleukin-1 beta induces the expression and production of stem cell factor by epithelial cells: Crucial involvement of the PI-

3K/mTOR pathway and HIF-1 transcription complex. Cell Mol Immunol 2016; 13(1): 47-56. [http://dx.doi.org/10.1038/cmi.2014.113] [PMID: 25418470]

[101] Ma X, Guo P, Qiu Y, *et al.* Loss of AIM2 expression promotes hepatocarcinoma progression through activation of mTOR-S6K1 pathway. Oncotarget 2016; 7(24): 36185-97. [http://dx.doi.org/10.18632/oncotarget.9154] [PMID: 27167192]

[102] Lastwika KJ, Wilson W III, Li QK, *et al.* Control of PD-L1 expression by oncogenic activation of the AKT-mTOR pathway in non-small cell lung cancer. Cancer Res 2016; 76(2): 227-38. [http://dx.doi.org/10.1158/0008-5472.CAN-14-3362] [PMID: 26637667]

[103] Noh KH, Kang TH, Kim JH, *et al.* Activation of Akt as a mechanism for tumor immune evasion. Mol Ther 2009; 17(3): 439-47. [http://dx.doi.org/10.1038/mt.2008.255] [PMID: 19107122]

[104] Jiang Q, Weiss JM, Back T, *et al.* mTOR kinase inhibitor AZD8055 enhances the immunotherapeutic activity of an agonist CD40 antibody in cancer treatment. Cancer Res 2011; 71(12): 4074-84. [http://dx.doi.org/10.1158/0008-5472.CAN-10-3968] [PMID: 21540234]

[105] Risberg K, Redalen KR, Sønstevold L, Bjørnetrø T, Sølvernes J, Ree AH. Pro-survival responses to the dual inhibition of anti-apoptotic Bcl-2 family proteins and mTOR-mediated signaling in hypoxic colorectal carcinoma cells. BMC Cancer 2016; 16: 531. [http://dx.doi.org/10.1186/s12885-016-2600-y] [PMID: 27461218]

[106] Zhao L, Teng B, Wen L, *et al.* mTOR inhibitor AZD8055 inhibits proliferation and induces apoptosis in laryngeal carcinoma. Int J Clin Exp Med 2014; 7(2): 337-47. [PMID: 24600487]

[107] Thomson AW, Turnquist HR, Raimondi G. Immunoregulatory functions of mTOR inhibition. Nat Rev Immunol 2009; 9(5): 324-37. [http://dx.doi.org/10.1038/nri2546] [PMID: 19390566]

[108] Vanhaesebroeck B, Whitehead MA, Piñeiro R. Molecules in medicine mini-review: Isoforms of PI3K in biology and disease. J Mol Med 2016; 94(1): 5-11. [http://dx.doi.org/10.1007/s00109-015-1352-5] [PMID: 26658520]

[109] Berezhnoy A, Castro I, Levay A, Malek TR, Gilboa E. Aptamer-targeted inhibition of mTOR in T cells enhances antitumor immunity. J Clin Invest 2014; 124(1): 188-97. [http://dx.doi.org/10.1172/JCI69856] [PMID: 24292708]

[110] Coppock JD, Wieking BG, Molinolo AA, Gutkind JS, Miskimins WK, Lee JH. Improved clearance during treatment of HPV-positive head and neck cancer through mTOR inhibition. Neoplasia 2013; 15(6): 620-30. [http://dx.doi.org/10.1593/neo.13432] [PMID: 23730210]

[111] Owonikoko TK. Inhibitors of mTOR pathway for cancer therapy, moving on from rapalogs to TORKinibs. Cancer 2015; 121(19): 3390-2. [http://dx.doi.org/10.1002/cncr.29424] [PMID: 26177743]

[112] Naing A, Aghajanian C, Raymond E, *et al.* Safety, tolerability, pharmacokinetics and pharmacodynamics of AZD8055 in advanced solid tumours and lymphoma. Br J Cancer 2012; 107(7): 1093-9. [http://dx.doi.org/10.1038/bjc.2012.368] [PMID: 22935583]

[113] Ghobrial IM, Siegel DS, Vij R, *et al.* TAK-228 (formerly MLN0128), an investigational oral dual TORC1/2 inhibitor: A Phase I dose escalation study in patients with relapsed or refractory multiple myeloma, non-Hodgkin lymphoma, or Waldenströms macroglobulinemia. Am J Hematol 2016; 91(4): 400-5. [http://dx.doi.org/10.1002/ajh.24300] [PMID: 26800393]

[114] Basu B, Dean E, Puglisi M, *et al.* First-in-human pharmacokinetic and pharmacodynamic study of the dual m-TORC 1/2 inhibitor AZD2014. Clin Cancer Res 2015; 21(15): 3412-9.

[http://dx.doi.org/10.1158/1078-0432.CCR-14-2422] [PMID: 25805799]

[115] Bendell JC, Kelley RK, Shih KC, *et al.* A Phase I dose-escalation study to assess safety, tolerability, pharmacokinetics, and preliminary efficacy of the dual mTORC1/mTORC2 kinase inhibitor CC-223 in patients with advanced solid tumors or multiple myeloma. Cancer 2015; 121(19): 3481-90. [http://dx.doi.org/10.1002/cncr.29422] [PMID: 26177599]

[116] Cao G, Wang Q, Li G, *et al.* mTOR inhibition potentiates cytotoxicity of Vγ4 γδ T cells via up-regulating NKG2D and TNF-α. J Leukoc Biol 2016; 100(5): 1181-9. [http://dx.doi.org/10.1189/jlb.5A0116-053RR] [PMID: 27256566]

[117] Zhao M, Howard EW, Parris AB, Guo Z, Zhao Q, Yang X. Alcohol promotes migration and invasion of triple-negative breast cancer cells through activation of p38 MAPK and JNK. Mol Carcinog 2017; 56(3): 849-62. [http://dx.doi.org/10.1002/mc.22538] [PMID: 27533114]

[118] Zhao W, Lu M, Zhang Q. Chloride intracellular channel 1 regulates migration and invasion in gastric cancer by triggering the ROS-mediated p38 MAPK signaling pathway. Mol Med Rep 2015; 12(6): 8041-7. [PMID: 26497050]

[119] Wang S, Yang J, Qian J, Wezeman M, Kwak LW, Yi Q. Tumor evasion of the immune system: Inhibiting p38 MAPK signaling restores the function of dendritic cells in multiple myeloma. Blood 2006; 107(6): 2432-9. [http://dx.doi.org/10.1182/blood-2005-06-2486] [PMID: 16291589]

[120] Oosterhoff D, Lougheed S, van de Ven R, *et al.* Tumor-mediated inhibition of human dendritic cell differentiation and function is consistently counteracted by combined p38 MAPK and STAT3 inhibition. OncoImmunology 2012; 1(5): 649-58. [http://dx.doi.org/10.4161/onci.20365] [PMID: 22934257]

[121] Wu M, Chen X, Lou J, *et al.* TGF-β1 contributes to CD8+ Treg induction through p38 MAPK signaling in ovarian cancer microenvironment. Oncotarget 2016; 7(28): 44534-44. [PMID: 27322208]

[122] Wang J, Cui L, Feng L, *et al.* Isoalantolactone inhibits the migration and invasion of human breast cancer MDA-MB-231 cells via suppression of the p38 MAPK/NF-κB signaling pathway. Oncol Rep 2016; 36(3): 1269-76. [PMID: 27461575]

[123] Cao L, Chen X, Xiao X, Ma Q, Li W. Resveratrol inhibits hyperglycemia-driven ROS-induced invasion and migration of pancreatic cancer cells via suppression of the ERK and p38 MAPK signaling pathways. Int J Oncol 2016; 49(2): 735-43. [PMID: 27278736]

[124] Jin X, Mo Q, Zhang Y, *et al.* The p38 MAPK inhibitor BIRB796 enhances the antitumor effects of VX680 in cervical cancer. Cancer Biol Ther 2016; 17(5): 566-76. [http://dx.doi.org/10.1080/15384047.2016.1177676] [PMID: 27082306]

[125] Lu Y, Zhang M, Wang S, *et al.* p38 MAPK-inhibited dendritic cells induce superior antitumour immune responses and overcome regulatory T-cell-mediated immunosuppression. Nat Commun 2014; 5: 4229. [http://dx.doi.org/10.1038/ncomms5229] [PMID: 24957461]

[126] Cannon MJ, Goyne HE, Stone PJ, *et al.* Modulation of p38 MAPK signaling enhances dendritic cell activation of human CD4+ Th17 responses to ovarian tumor antigen. Cancer Immunol Immunother 2013; 62(5): 839-49. [http://dx.doi.org/10.1007/s00262-013-1391-0] [PMID: 23354626]

[127] Kühnöl C, Herbarth M, Föll J, Staege MS, Kramm C. CD137 stimulation and p38 MAPK inhibition improve reactivity in an *in vitro* model of glioblastoma immunotherapy. Cancer Immunol Immunother 2013; 62(12): 1797-809.

[http://dx.doi.org/10.1007/s00262-013-1484-9] [PMID: 24129764]

[128] Koul HK, Pal M, Koul S. Role of p38 MAP kinase signal transduction in solid tumors. Genes Cancer 2013; 4(9-10): 342-59.
[http://dx.doi.org/10.1177/1947601913507951] [PMID: 24349632]

[129] Muller AJ, Scherle PA. Targeting the mechanisms of tumoral immune tolerance with small-molecule inhibitors. Nat Rev Cancer 2006; 6(8): 613-25.
[http://dx.doi.org/10.1038/nrc1929] [PMID: 16862192]

[130] Brudvik KW, Paulsen JE, Aandahl EM, Roald B, Taskén K. Protein kinase A antagonist inhibits β-catenin nuclear translocation, c-Myc and COX-2 expression and tumor promotion in Apc(Min/+) mice. Mol Cancer 2011; 10: 149.
[http://dx.doi.org/10.1186/1476-4598-10-149] [PMID: 22168384]

[131] Timoshenko AV, Xu G, Chakrabarti S, Lala PK, Chakraborty C. Role of prostaglandin E2 receptors in migration of murine and human breast cancer cells. Exp Cell Res 2003; 289(2): 265-74.
[http://dx.doi.org/10.1016/S0014-4827(03)00269-6] [PMID: 14499627]

[132] Aandahl EM, Moretto WJ, Haslett PA, *et al.* Inhibition of antigen-specific T cell proliferation and cytokine production by protein kinase A type I. J Immunol 2002; 169(2): 802-8.
[http://dx.doi.org/10.4049/jimmunol.169.2.802] [PMID: 12097383]

[133] Raskovalova T, Lokshin A, Huang X, Jackson EK, Gorelik E. Adenosine-mediated inhibition of cytotoxic activity and cytokine production by IL-2/NKp46-activated NK cells: Involvement of protein kinase A isozyme I (PKA I). Immunol Res 2006; 36(1-3): 91-9.
[http://dx.doi.org/10.1385/IR:36:1:91] [PMID: 17337770]

[134] Raskovalova T, Lokshin A, Huang X, *et al.* Inhibition of cytokine production and cytotoxic activity of human antimelanoma specific CD8+ and CD4+ T lymphocytes by adenosine-protein kinase A type I signaling. Cancer Res 2007; 67(12): 5949-56.
[http://dx.doi.org/10.1158/0008-5472.CAN-06-4249] [PMID: 17575165]

[135] Yaqub S, Taskén K. Role for the cAMP-protein kinase A signaling pathway in suppression of antitumor immune responses by regulatory T cells. Crit Rev Oncog 2008; 14(1): 57-77.
[http://dx.doi.org/10.1615/CritRevOncog.v14.i1.40] [PMID: 19105570]

[136] Massey AJ, Stephens P, Rawlinson R, McGurk L, Plummer R, Curtin NJ. mTORC1 and DNA-PKcs as novel molecular determinants of sensitivity to Chk1 inhibition. Mol Oncol 2016; 10(1): 101-12.
[http://dx.doi.org/10.1016/j.molonc.2015.08.004] [PMID: 26471831]

[137] Chen Y, Tsai YH, Tseng BJ, Pan HY, Tseng SH. Suppression of miR-19b enhanced the cytotoxic effects of mTOR inhibitors in human neuroblastoma cells. J Pediatr Surg 2016; 51(11): 1818-25.
[http://dx.doi.org/10.1016/j.jpedsurg.2016.07.003] [PMID: 27492819]

[138] Hu M, Huang H, Zhao R, *et al.* AZD8055 induces cell death associated with autophagy and activation of AMPK in hepatocellular carcinoma. Oncol Rep 2014; 31(2): 649-56.
[PMID: 24297300]

[139] Sini P, James D, Chresta C, Guichard S. Simultaneous inhibition of mTORC1 and mTORC2 by mTOR kinase inhibitor AZD8055 induces autophagy and cell death in cancer cells. Autophagy 2010; 6(4): 553-4.
[http://dx.doi.org/10.4161/auto.6.4.11671] [PMID: 20364113]

[140] Sharma S, Yao HP, Zhou YQ, Zhou J, Zhang R, Wang MH. Prevention of BMS-777607-induced polyploidy/senescence by mTOR inhibitor AZD8055 sensitizes breast cancer cells to cytotoxic chemotherapeutics. Mol Oncol 2014; 8(3): 469-82.
[http://dx.doi.org/10.1016/j.molonc.2013.12.014] [PMID: 24444656]

[141] Shen C, Oswald D, Phelps D, *et al.* Regulation of FANCD2 by the mTOR pathway contributes to the resistance of cancer cells to DNA double-strand breaks. Cancer Res 2013; 73(11): 3393-401.
[http://dx.doi.org/10.1158/0008-5472.CAN-12-4282] [PMID: 23633493]

[142] Wei F, Liu Y, Guo Y, *et al.* miR-99b-targeted mTOR induction contributes to irradiation resistance in pancreatic cancer. Mol Cancer 2013; 12: 81.
[http://dx.doi.org/10.1186/1476-4598-12-81] [PMID: 23886294]

[143] Li H, Wang X, Chen T, Qu J. p38 inhibitor SB203580 sensitizes the resveratrol-induced apoptosis in human lung adenocarcinoma (A549) cells. J Biochem Mol Toxicol 2012; 26(7): 251-7.
[http://dx.doi.org/10.1002/jbt.21413] [PMID: 22644961]

[144] Lim SJ, Lee YJ, Lee E. p38MAPK inhibitor SB203580 sensitizes human SNU-C4 colon cancer cells to exisulind-induced apoptosis. Oncol Rep 2006; 16(5): 1131-5.
[PMID: 17016604]

[145] Aroui S, Najlaoui F, Chtourou Y, *et al.* Naringin inhibits the invasion and migration of human glioblastoma cell via downregulation of MMP-2 and MMP-9 expression and inactivation of p38 signaling pathway. Tumour Biol 2016; 37(3): 3831-9.
[http://dx.doi.org/10.1007/s13277-015-4230-4] [PMID: 26474590]

[146] Marengo B, De Ciucis CG, Ricciarelli R, *et al.* p38MAPK inhibition: A new combined approach to reduce neuroblastoma resistance under etoposide treatment. Cell Death Dis 2013; 4: e589.
[http://dx.doi.org/10.1038/cddis.2013.118] [PMID: 23579276]

[147] Tate DJ Jr, Vonderhaar DJ, Caldas YA, *et al.* Effect of arginase II on L-arginine depletion and cell growth in murine cell lines of renal cell carcinoma. J Hematol Oncol 2008; 1: 14.
[http://dx.doi.org/10.1186/1756-8722-1-14] [PMID: 18817562]

[148] Costa H, Xu X, Overbeek G, *et al.* Human cytomegalovirus may promote tumour progression by upregulating arginase-2. Oncotarget 2016; 7(30): 47221-31.
[PMID: 27363017]

[149] Samoilenko OA, Milinevska OA, Karnaushenko OV, Shlyakhovenko VA, Zaletok SP. Effect of polyamine metabolism inhibitors on Lewis lung carcinoma growth and metastasis. Exp Oncol 2015; 37(2): 151-3.
[PMID: 26112945]

[150] Feng PH, Lee KY, Chang YL, *et al.* CD14(+)S100A9(+) monocytic myeloid-derived suppressor cells and their clinical relevance in non-small cell lung cancer. Am J Respir Crit Care Med 2012; 186(10): 1025-36.
[http://dx.doi.org/10.1164/rccm.201204-0636OC] [PMID: 22955317]

[151] Bak SP, Alonso A, Turk MJ, Berwin B. Murine ovarian cancer vascular leukocytes require arginase-1 activity for T cell suppression. Mol Immunol 2008; 46(2): 258-68.
[http://dx.doi.org/10.1016/j.molimm.2008.08.266] [PMID: 18824264]

[152] Yuan C, Zheng Y, Zhang B, *et al.* Thymosin α1 promotes the activation of myeloid-derived suppressor cells in a Lewis lung cancer model by upregulating Arginase 1. Biochem Biophys Res Commun 2015; 464(1): 249-55.
[http://dx.doi.org/10.1016/j.bbrc.2015.06.132] [PMID: 26111447]

[153] Rodriguez PC, Quiceno DG, Zabaleta J, *et al.* Arginase I production in the tumor microenvironment by mature myeloid cells inhibits T-cell receptor expression and antigen-specific T-cell responses. Cancer Res 2004; 64(16): 5839-49.
[http://dx.doi.org/10.1158/0008-5472.CAN-04-0465] [PMID: 15313928]

[154] Narita Y, Kitamura H, Wakita D, *et al.* The key role of IL-6-arginase cascade for inducing dendritic cell-dependent CD4(+) T cell dysfunction in tumor-bearing mice. J Immunol 2013; 190(2): 812-20.
[http://dx.doi.org/10.4049/jimmunol.1103797] [PMID: 23248265]

[155] Bronte V, Kasic T, Gri G, *et al.* Boosting antitumor responses of T lymphocytes infiltrating human prostate cancers. J Exp Med 2005; 201(8): 1257-68.
[http://dx.doi.org/10.1084/jem.20042028] [PMID: 15824085]

[156] Gostner JM, Becker K, Überall F, Fuchs D. The potential of targeting indoleamine 2,3-dioxygenase for cancer treatment. Expert Opin Ther Targets 2015; 19(5): 605-15. [http://dx.doi.org/10.1517/14728222.2014.995092] [PMID: 25684107]

[157] Vacchelli E, Aranda F, Eggermont A, *et al.* Trial watch: IDO inhibitors in cancer therapy. OncoImmunology 2014; 3(10): e957994. [http://dx.doi.org/10.4161/21624011.2014.957994] [PMID: 25941578]

[158] Liu Y, Zhang Y, Zheng X, *et al.* Gene silencing of indoleamine 2,3-dioxygenase 2 in melanoma cells induces apoptosis through the suppression of NAD+ and inhibits *in vivo* tumor growth. Oncotarget 2016; 7(22): 32329-40. [PMID: 27058624]

[159] Sheridan C. IDO inhibitors move center stage in immuno-oncology. Nat Biotechnol 2015; 33(4): 321-2. [http://dx.doi.org/10.1038/nbt0415-321] [PMID: 25850038]

[160] Harrop R, Kelleher M, Shingler W, Kingsman SM, Carroll MW. Chemo-immunotherapy method. US8133681, 2012.

[161] Gabizon AA, Kedar E, Barenholz Y. Combined chemo-immunotherapy with liposomal drugs and cytokines. US6787132, 2004.

[162] Fewell JG, Matar M, Rice J, Lewis DH, Anwer K. Combination of immuno gene therapy and chemotherapy for treatment of cancer and hyperproliferative diseases. US7964571, 2011.

[163] Weichselbaum RR, Kufe DW, Posner M, Mauceri H, Park JO. Activation of Egr-1 promoter by DNA damaging chemotherapeutics. US8034791, 2011.

[164] Salem AK, Geary SM, Weiner GJ, Lemke C, Krishnamachari Y. Biodegradable particulate formulations. US20140127253, 2014.

[165] Rudolph AR, Los AH. Reducing side effects of chemotherapy in cancer patients. EP1357935, 2006.

[166] Gevas PC, Grimes S, Karr SL, Watson SA, Michaeli D. Combination therapy for the treatment of tumors. US8343930, 2013.

[167] Santoli D, Rovera G, Cesano A. Method of treating malignancies. US6022538, 2000.

[168] Santoli D, Rovera G, Cesano A. Use of a combination of TALL-104 cells with adriayamcin or cisplatin in the therapy of malignancies. EP0980205, 2003.

[169] Correale P, Cusi MG, Francini G, Giorgi G. Poly-epitope peptide derived from thymidylate synthase having immunological and anti-tumour activity. US8344100, 2013.

[170] Jure-kunkel M. Combination of anti-CTLA4 antibody with diverse therapeutic regimens for the synergistic treatment of proliferative diseases. US8685394, 2014.

[171] Menrad A, Menssen HD, Wagner K. Combination of an anti-ED-B fibronectin domain antibody-IL-2 fusion protein and gemcitabine. US7851599, 2010.

[172] Vernejoul F, Drocourt D, Romo J, Tiraby G, Lioux T. Combined use of a chemotherapeutic agent and a cyclic dinucleotide for cancer treatment. WO2016096577, 2016.

[173] Schroeder A, Helwig C, Loos A-H, *et al.* Method of treating lung cancer by vaccination with MUC-1 lipopeptide. US20160067322, 2016.

[174] Paterson Y. Combination therapy for use in cancer therapy. WO2016061182, 2016.

[175] Hagemann T. Cancer therapy. US20160074494, 2016.

[176] Ganss R, Johansson A. Treatment of tumours using peptide-protein conjugates. WO2016041014, 2016.

[177] Kim J, Cheung J. Methods of treating cancers using PD-1 axis binding antagonists and taxanes. WO2015095404, 2015.

[178] Tsang TC, Meade-tollin L, Pennington ME. Methods of metabolic targeting cancer cells using chemo- and immunotherapy for treating cancer. US20140056844, 2014.

[179] Schultes BC, Noujaim AA, Nicodemus CF. Evaluating synergy of combinations comprising an antibody in immune suppressive pathways concurrent to immunotherapy. WO2008091643, 2008.

[180] Apetoh L, Ladoire S, Coukos G, Ghiringhelli F. Combining immunotherapy and anticancer agents: The right path to achieve cancer cure? Ann Oncol 2015; 26(9): 1813-23. [http://dx.doi.org/10.1093/annonc/mdv209] [PMID: 25922066]

[181] Cook AM, Lesterhuis WJ, Nowak AK, Lake RA. Chemotherapy and immunotherapy: Mapping the road ahead. Curr Opin Immunol 2016; 39: 23-9. [http://dx.doi.org/10.1016/j.coi.2015.12.003] [PMID: 26724433]

CHAPTER 7

Recent Advances and Challenges in microRNA-Based Cancer Therapeutics

Amjad Ali[*], **Faryal M. Awan**, **Aqsa Ikram** and **Shifa T. Ashraf**

Atta-ur-Rahman School of Applied Biosciences (ASAB), National University of Sciences and Technology (NUST), H-12 Islamabad, Pakistan

Abstract: Despite significant advancements in understanding the cancer-associated signaling cascades, effective treatment strategies remain scarce. This intricacy of cancer enigma highlights a pressing need to develop novel therapeutics. The seminal discovery of microRNAs (miRNAs), a class of natural RNA-interfering agents, provides a new hope for accomplishing this task. Bolstered by a novel mode of action, the ability to function as tiny master regulators of cellular processes, ease of administration and sufficient uptake along with apparent lack of toxicity in normal tissues give miRNAs an extra edge and make them an ideal candidate for emerging therapeutic developments. Genome-wide investigations have shown more than half of the human miRNA genes being located on genomic regions or at fragile sites associated with cancer, unveiling the substantial significance of these small RNAs. Very soon after the discovery of the first miRNA, miRNA-based therapeutics has entered clinical trials and has shown fascinating results in preclinical development. This rapid progress through the discovery pipeline into clinical development imitates the significance of miRNAs as critical regulators in human diseases, and holds the pledge of yielding a novel class of therapeutics that could signify an attractive addition to the existing drug pipeline of Big Pharma. In this chapter, we will give an overview of the recent miRNA-based therapeutic approaches (patents: EP3110951, WO2017005771, EP3126496, EP3106168, WO2017005773, US9399773, EP2217248 and US9469854), and will discuss current translational challenges and further potential developments. These patents describe the potential of different miRNAs inhibitors/mimics for treating various types of cancers, these miRNAs include miR-34 mimic to treat hematologic malignancy/solid tumors; miR-409-5p, miR-379 and miR-154 inhibitors to treat prostate cancer and drug resistant lung cancer; miR-548z, miR-624-5p, let-7i-3p, miR-885-5p, miR-449b-3p to treat hepatoblastoma cancer; pre-miR-302 (an miRNA precursor) for cancer reversion; miR-21, miR-125a-5p, miR-191, miR-210, miR-222, miR-378, miR-423-3p, miR-638 inhibitors to treat hepatocellular carcinoma (HCC); hsa-miR-4510, hsa-miR-548aa, hsa-miR- 548v and hsa-miR-37-b-3p mimics to treat HCC; sorafenib- miR- 34-mimic/ miR-215 mimic combination therapy for treating liver cancer and miR-21-3p mimic for treating liver diseases. The outcome of these patents may hopefully provide exciting opportunities and deeper

[*] **Corresponding author Amjad Ali:** Atta-ur-Rahman School of Applied Biosciences (ASAB), National University of Sciences and Technology (NUST), H-12 Islamabad, Pakistan;
Tel: +92-51-90856138/+92-333-9191903; E-mails: amjaduni@gmail.com, amjad.ali@asab.nust.edu.pk

Atta-ur-Rahman and Khurshid Zaman (Eds.)

insights into novel anti-cancer paradigms. Compared to conventional drug therapies, miRNA-based therapeutics appears to hold great promise to combat cancer, at least for those cancers where other treatment options have plateaued. Further developments in miRNA-based therapeutics are anticipated to translate miRNA-based therapeutic strategies into a clinical reality and may create a paradigm shift in medicine and pharmaceutical industry.

Keywords: Anti-miR oligonucleotides, cancer, cancer therapy, cancerous cells, clinical trials, drug resistance, drug target, *in vivo* studies, miRNA inhibitor, miRNA masking, miRNA mimic, miRNAs sponges, miRNA therapeutics, mouse models, mRNAs, Non-coding RNAs, oncogenic miRNAs, pre-clinical trials, siRNAs, tumor suppressor miRNAs.

1. INTRODUCTION

The genesis of the current non-coding RNAs' (ncRNAs) scientific paradigm can easily be traced to the influential discovery of a microRNA (miRNA) gene in 1993 by a group led by Ambros [1]. Extensive research on these evolutionarily conserved, small, regulatory RNAs in the last decade has shown fascinating breakthroughs of recent times [2]. Concomitantly, experimental confirmation of the results attained by the human genome project further revealed that several transcripts are actually non-coding transcripts, and that miRNAs signify the most important class of ncRNA molecules. The involvement of miRNAs in the development of cancer was initially reported in 2002: since then, the role of miRNAs has been intensively investigated in manifold human disorders [3, 4]. The noteworthy increment in the number of patent application filings over the last 10 years reflects a considerable amount of novelty in this area.

miRNAs are currently considered as master regulators of the human genome [5]. Clinical and functional implications of miRNAs in various disorders have hauled up these tiny cellular components to the ranks of ideal drug targets [6]. In eukaryotes, they serve as significant modulators of gene expression. They influence the transcriptome and proteome by targeting protein coding transcripts, hence aiding in cell fate determination. Furthermore, miRNAs have loomed as vital molecules in cancer research and they have proved to hold potential in cancer. They have the ability to repress stability of protein-coding transcripts and cellular translation by targeting the 3′ untranslated regions (UTRs) in a sequential manner [7, 8]. This nature of selective silencing of gene expression by miRNAs is known to have a significant effect on human health and disease [9]. The therapeutic functioning of miRNA is based upon the catalytic process of the naturally occurring 15-22 nucleotide single stranded RNA, that enters the cytoplasmic multiprotein complex RNA-Induced Silencing Complex (RISC) to pair with mRNAs carrying complementary sequences and, as a result, repress gene expression. Over 500 miRNAs of distinct nature have been identified in humans and more than 1000 have been predicted in total [10, 11]. Furthermore, exploration of the human genome sequences facilitated the discovery of the fact that miRNA genes frequently resides in fragile sites and genomic regions which are hot spots for chromosomal abnormalities [12]. Chromosomal abnormalities have been shown to be important for the etiology of various cancers. Various studies based on genome-wide approaches have reported strong association between various cytogenetic and molecular abnormalities and the location of miRNA genes [13 - 15]. Wey *et al.* investigated the genome-wide miRNA expression profiling in Intraductal papillary mucinous neoplasms (IPMNs) tissue and discovered six miRNAs (miR-100, miR-99b, miR-99a, miR-342-3p, miR-126, miR-130a) that may differentiate 'high-risk' IPMNs from 'low-risk' IPMNs [14]. Faltejskova *et al.* studied genome-wide miRNA expression profiling in colorectal cancer patients in order to discover miRNA signatures (miR-122, miR-122*, miR-885-5p, miR-10b, miR-143, and miR 28-5p) that would enable differentiation between primary tumors and their corresponding matched liver metastases [15, 16].

The ability of miRNAs to target multiple genes may hold the key to therapeutic accomplishment in cancer which is a heterogenic disease and cannot be effectively treated by targeting a single gene of interest. Calin *et al.* first reported the role of miRNAs in cancer through the characterization of chromosome 13q14 done on chronic lymphocytic leukemia [3]. Successively, numerous studies gave strong evidences of deregulated miRNA expression in the hallmarks of cancer [17, 18]. In cancer, various cellular mechanisms are involved in the miRNA dysregulation such as genetic mutations [19], aberrant DNA methylation [20] and histone acetylation [21] along with alternative splicing, changes in the miRNA processing machinery and polyadenylation may cause hindrance in the maturation of miRNA [9, 22]. Abnormal gain or loss of miRNAs plays a role in initiation, progression, and metastasis and drug resistance in a variety of cancers. They can act as either oncogenes or tumor suppressors, depending upon the pathway or genes they impact. For instance, miRNAs of the let-7 family are a class of tumor suppressors. Let-7 expression has been reported to be downregulated in breast, head, neck, ovarian, lung and prostate cancers [23]. Additional miRNAs, namely miR-17/92 cluster, miR-221, miR-222, miR-21, miR-155 and miR-9 are upregulated in various cancers [24]. The therapeutic and diagnostic significance of miRNAs is remarkable since they have unique profiles and high stability in biological samples. For cancer therapy, miRNA expression modulation is under investigation but therapeutic tempering is attained by oncogenic inhibition of miRNAs, or by altering tumor suppressor miRNAs [9]. Furthermore, Phytonutrients that modulate expression and action of miRNA which are functionally involved in cancer pathobiology may have a potential to consider as a candidate for cancer treatment, overcome drug resistance or improve drug sensitivity [25].

Moreover, there is an emerging role of miRNAs in pharmacogenomics and cumulating evidences have demonstrated that miRNA levels can be a major determinant of drug resistance/sensitivity [26]. MiR-24 was the first miRNA associated with drug resistance and several investigations on other miRNAs have highlighted their significance in chemo-resistance [27]. Studies have shown that miRNAs hamper the growth of gefitinib-resistant cancerous cells both *in vitro* and *in vivo* [28]. miR-34a was shown to reverse gefitinib resistance in HCC827 and PC-9 cells by targeting MET and restoring apoptosis [29]. Awan *et al.* exploited hybrid Petri net based computational model to study the harmonious effect of modulators of miR-17-92 cluster to overcome sorafenib resistance in HCC. The authors suggested that synergistic effect of four inhibitors (miR-17-5p, miR-19a, miR-92 and miR-18a) and three mimics (miR-17-3p, miR-19b and miR-20a) of miR-17-92 cluster may overcome sorafenib resistance [30]. Similarly, targeting miRNAs have been shown to regulate chemoresistance in colorectal cancer and have been revealed to be a novel strategy for re-sensitizing drug-resistant cells for improving colorectal cancer treatment [31]. The study conducted by Gan *et al.* revealed that miR-339-5p sensitized lung carcinoma cells to Taxol by influencing FUT1. The authors also reported that the effect of miR-339-5p depletion on Taxol resistance was restored after FUT1 knockdown [32].

The aim of this chapter is to provide a comprehensive review of the miRNA based therapeutic strategies against various cancers (Fig. **1**), recent patents regarding miRNA based therapeutics currently undergoing clinical/pre-clinical trials (Table **1**) to treat various cancers as well as the challenges for developing miRNA-based drugs. A brief account of promising miRNA based drugs in various stages of clinical development and some strategies for overcoming the problem of drug resistance have also been discussed.

2. miRNA BIOGENESIS

In miRNA biogenesis pathway, primary miRNAs also known as pri-miRNA are handled by Drosha in the nucleus and by Dicer in the cytoplasm. The pri-miRNA which consists of 7-methylguanosine cap (m^7Gppp) in the start and ends with a 3′ poly (A) tail is transcribed by RNA polymerase II (Pol II). The pri-miRNA contains a stem-loop structure that is cleaved by the endonuclease Drosha together with its double-stranded RNA (dsRNA)-binding protein partner DGCR8 (in mammals) in the nucleus. The resulting precursor miRNA (pre-miRNA) is distributed from the nucleus to cytoplasm by exportin 5. It is further cleaved by the endonuclease Dicer together with its companion TRBP (Transactivation-

Response RNA-Binding Protein; in mammals). This results in miRNA-miRNA* duplex formation and is supported by the HSC70-HSP90 chaperone machinery and is loaded into an Argonaute (AGO) protein as a dsRNA. Subsequent maturation steps expel the miRNA*, producing a mature RNA-induced silencing complex (RISC) [33]. Mature miRNAs then guide the RNA-induced silencing complex to related target genes and suppress target gene expression by either repressing their translation or destabilizing target mRNAs.

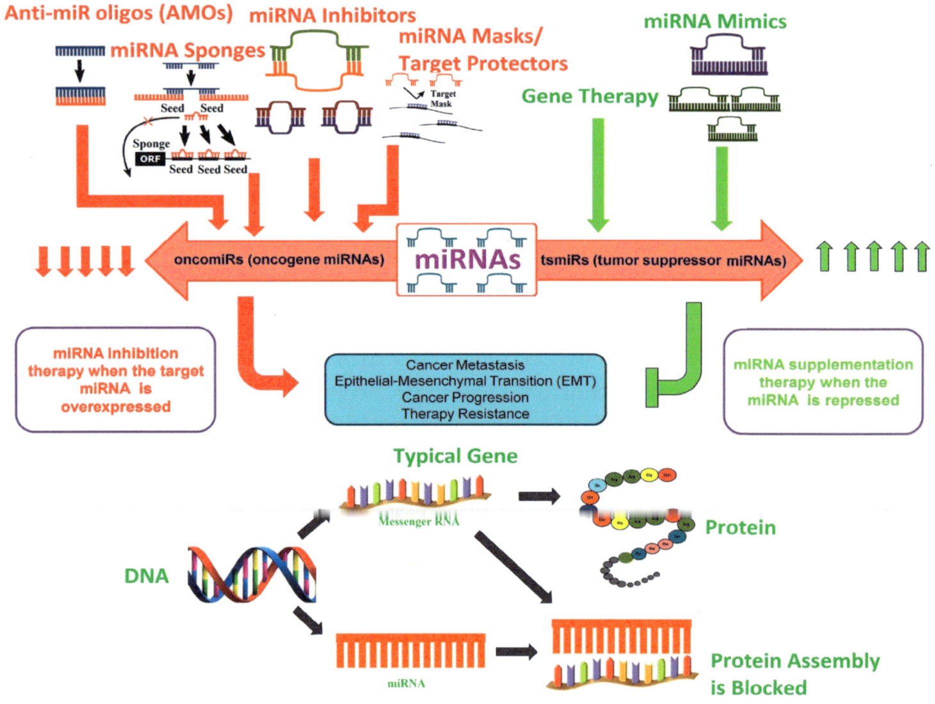

Fig. (1). miRNA-based cancer therapeutics. The function of tumor promoter/ oncogenic miRNAs (oncomiRs) could be stopped by miRNA inhibitors, anti-miR oligonucleotides (AMOs), miRNAs masking/ target protectors or miRNAs sponges. Tumor suppressor miRNAs either through gene therapy or through miRNA mimics.

Table 1. List of miRNA Therapeutics in Preclinical and Clinical Trials Stage.

Name	Company	Therapeutic Components	Delivery System/ Carrier	Target Diseases	Preclinical/ Clinical Trial Particulars
MGN-1374	miRagen Therapeutics	nti-miRNA-15	LNA-modified ASO	Post-myocardial infarction remodeling	Preclinical stage

(Table 1) contd

Name	**Company**	**Therapeutic Components**	**Delivery System/ Carrier**	**Target Diseases**	**Preclinical/ Clinical Trial Particulars**
Mirvirasen	Santaris Pharma A/S and Hoffmann-La Roche	antimiR-122	LNA-modified antisense inhibitor	Hepatitis C	Single-centre Phase I, completed
					Multicentre Phase II, completed
					Multicentre Phase II, ongoing
					Single-centre Phase II, ongoing
					Single-centre Phase II, ongoing
RG-101	Regulus Therapeutics	antimiR-122	GalNAc-conjugated antimiRs	Hepatitis C	Phase I, completed
					Multiple Phase II, ongoing
RG-012	Regulus Therapeutics	anti-miRNA-21	-	Alport syndrome	In the pipeline to initiate clinical trial Phase II
RG-125/ AZD4076	Regulus Therapeutics	AntimiR-103/107	GalNAc-conjugated antimiRs	Type 2 diabetes and non-alcoholic fatty liver diseases	Single-centre Phase I, ongoing
					Single-centre Phase I/IIa, ongoing
MRG-106	miRagen Therapeutics	antimiR-155	LNA-modified antisense inhibitor	Cutaneous T cell lymphoma and mycosis fungoides	Multicentre Phase I, ongoing
MRG-201	miRagen Therapeutics	miR-29 mimic	Cholesterol-conjugated miRNA duplex	Scleroderma	Single-centre Phase I, ongoing
MesomiR-1	EnGeneIC	miR-16 mimic	EnGeneIC delivery vehicle	Mesothelioma, non-small cell lung cancer	Multi-centre Phase I, ongoing

(Table 1) contd

Name	Company	Therapeutic Components	Delivery System/ Carrier	Target Diseases	Preclinical/ Clinical Trial Particulars
MRX34	Mirna Therapeutics	miR-34 mimic	LNPs (Smarticles)	Multiple solid tumours	Multicentre Phase I, halted following multiple immune-related severe adverse events observed in patients dosed with MRX34 over the course of the trial

3. STRATEGIES FOR miRNA MANIPULATION

With advances in knowledge on expression of miRNA along with its function, this field of study stands as prime target for exploiting disease therapeutics. MiRNAs are emerging as attractive therapeutic targets since they are involved in gene silencing and are part of various pathological states, but efficient delivery mechanisms to tumor sites are a roadblock to utility [34]. In the state of cancer, miRNAs are present as either a tumor suppressor or an oncogene. miRNAs have been reported to have pathological roles in tumor progression and metastasis. In addition, loss or gain function of miRNAs has been the highlight in almost every cancer type [35, 36]. MiRNA manipulation in cancer cell lines is proven to have potential therapeutic effects [37]. Following are the strategies used for miRNA manipulation (see Fig. **2**).

3.1. Sandwich RNAi Inhibition Strategy

This strategy involves the usage of several agents for specific targeting of a molecular defect during pathogenesis [38]. This was shown by Nishimura *et al.*, where they targeted EphA2, an oncogene involved in ovarian cancer, by combining EphA2-targeting siRNAs and miR-520d-3p mimics [39]. Combination targeting revealed efficient anti-tumor properties rather than monotherapy. This cocktail therapy leads to a decrease in EphA2 levels, tumor suppression, and inhibition of invasion. RNAi-based therapeutics will serve as an outstanding therapeutic tool to target dominant oncogenes in human cancers.

3.2. Multiplex RNAi Inhibition Strategy

A 'multiplex RNAi inhibition' strategy targets the various molecular defects found in the cancer pathway [38]. It was exemplified by using sensor siRNAs to target the RAF node (KRAS + PIK3CA/B) in order to treat colorectal cancer with a KRAS mutation [40]. Using *in vivo* and *in vitro* models they revealed that siRNA-mediated inhibition of KRAS as well as RAF or PI3K combinations could impair *KRAS*-mutant colorectal cancer in xenograft models. These studies highlight the effectiveness of RNAi-based therapeutic strategies in cancer management.

3.3. Small Molecules Inhibitors of miRNAs

These inhibitors are small molecules that largely function by actively obstructing interaction between miRNA and the target or by inhibiting miRNA biogenesis [41]. The SMIR-strategy is a way of reducing production time, time of approval and the cost of it. Gumireddy *et al.* [42], reported a cellular screen for miRNA-pathway inhibitors and found the first small-molecule inhibitor of miRNA function. The mode of action of the small molecules is primarily through the transcriptional regulation of miR-21 rather than inhibition of target recognition by miR-21. It was reported that the small molecule enoxacin, an antibacterial fluoroquinolone, binds to the miRNA biosynthesis protein TAR RNA-binding protein 2 (TRBP) and enhances the production of tumor suppressor miRNAs [43]. Thus, small molecule modulators of miRNAs signify a distinctive approach for restoring defective miRNAs in cancer.

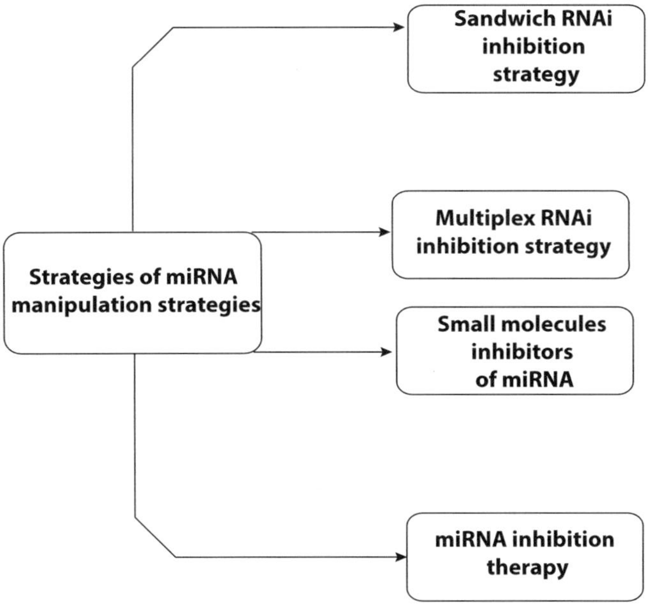

Fig. (2). Flow chart of the strategies used for miRNA manipulation.

4. THE POTENTIAL OF miRNAs IN CANCER THERAPY: SAFETY AND TOXICITY

Targeting manifold genes implicated in human disease at once is considered as a dominant ability of therapeutic miRNAs (in the form of miRNA mimics) or as targets of therapeutics (in the form of antimiRs) [44]. Various experimental studies indicated that targeting miRNA expression can bring the cancer cells back to its normal phenotype [45]. Nevertheless, it also raises concerns about possible toxicity in normal tissues - particularly under conditions where the therapeutic delivery of miRNA mimics will also lead to potential off-target effects, can cause supraphysiological levels of the miRNA, affect the normal functions of cells by accumulation of exogenous miRNA and susceptibility to nuclease degradation [46]. These noxious effects might be the consequence of exogenous miRNAs competing with endogenous miRNAs which are indispensable for normal cellular wellbeing, or hyperactivating inherently oncogenic pathways that will also lessen the viability of normal cells [47]. On the contrary, several studies have also revealed non-toxic effect in normal tissues after the administration of tumor suppressor miRNA mimics in mouse models, and therefore suggest that the delivery of miRNA to normal tissues was well endured [48 - 50]. While these assumptions are well-founded, in vivo facts for mimics-induced toxicity is still lacking. Furthermore, sequences of miRNAs used in these studies were identical between the mouse and human species and, thus, differences in homology will not account for the lack of toxicity in normal tissues. Detailed *in vivo* experiments remain to be done to assess the dose and long-term toxicity. The reason that therapeutic miRNA mimics may be better endured by normal cells than cancer cells might include:

i. Pathways repressed or activated by the miRNA mimic are already repressed or activated by the endogenous miRNA
ii. Administration is only an inconsequential incremental increase of what is already present in normal cells
iii. Normal cells tries to recover from the therapeutic dose used
iv. Normal cells can regulate the activity or presence of the miRNA mimic while cancer cells do not.

Limitations and advantages of miRNA therapy are given in Table **2**.

5. miRNAs IN TUMOR GROWTH AND METASTASIS

According to various studies, miRNAs are evolving as significant therapeutic targets to treat diseases like cancer. Their role in cancer progression has been described through various discoveries. They can either work as tumor suppressors or oncogenes, depending upon their targets. miRNAs play important roles in invasion, metastasis, cell cycle regulation and proliferation. Several functions of miRNA are studied trough *in vitro* and *in vivo* studies by either knocking out or overexpression of cell lines through experiments in mouse models. Cell invasion is the primary step towards metastasis and progression of cancer, as it requires the degradation of extracellular matrix proteins. miR-21 is known to be overexpressed in various cancers, such as, prostate cancer, leukemia, liver cancer, lung cancer, gastric carcinoma, glioma and prostate cancer [51]. A recent study highlighted the role of miR-21 in glioma malignancy by downregulating inhibitors of matrix metalloproteinases (MMPs) such as TIMP3 and RECK [52]. Furthermore, miR-205 is overexpressed in prostate cancer, by upregulating E-cadherin, leading the cancer cells towards mesenchymal epithelial transition (MET) [53]. miR-182 has been recognized as the most perilous miRNA in the case of melanoma. It promotes cell migration and metastasis, according to experimental evidences. miR-182 overexpression promotes survival by repressing FOXO3 and microphthalmia-associated transcription factor-M [54]. In lung cancer, miR-126 is overexpressed by increasing Crk (v-crk sarcoma virus CT10 oncogene homolog) levels and causing adhesion and invasion of lung cancer cells [55]. Studies involving miRNAs may lead to outstanding therapeutic interventions by serving as biomarkers for cancer therapy.

Table 2. Overview of the Limitations and Advantages of miRNA based Therapeutics.

miRNA Therapeutics	Advantages	Limitations
miRNA mimics	• Improve biological effect by Increasing the levels of a miRNA that is decreased during disease progression	• Potential off-target effects as a result of uptake by non-target tissues • Can potentially induce a nonspecific interferon response through Toll-like receptors
Anti-miRNAs	• Competitive inhibition • Successfully applied in cell culture and animal models • Efficient delivery	• Off target effects • Cannot cross blood brain barrier

6. SIGNIFICANCE AND CONTRIBUTION OF BIOINFORMATICS PREDICTION IN miRNA-BASED CANCER THERAPEUTICS

In recent years, bioinformatics and next-generation sequencing (NGS) have emerged as tools that led towards the identification of additional miRNAs across various organisms. Even though, a great amount of human miRNAs (about 2500) have been identified, however, the process of miRNA identification is still a complex procedure including the integrative approach using experimental and computational techniques [56]. The timely prognosis, diagnosis, and treatment of cancer stands as a substantial challenge for the research community [57].

Bioinformatics provides insights in cancer biology through the application of clever systems. A considerable amount of bioinformatics potential is observed in cancer research. Systems biology is considered to be the most reliable path in cancer research for developing diagnostic therapies [58]. Integrative approaches that combine the knowledge of cancer biology with bioinformatics approaches have shown great potential in identifying the miRNAs as novel biomarkers for detection of cancer [59]. Analysis of miRNA and gene expression data collectively with computational methods has led to understand the role of miRNAs in progression and metastasis during cancer. This has also led towards the identification of their role as therapeutic agents in diagnosis and cure of cancer [60]. An overview of the methods can be seen in Fig. (**3**).

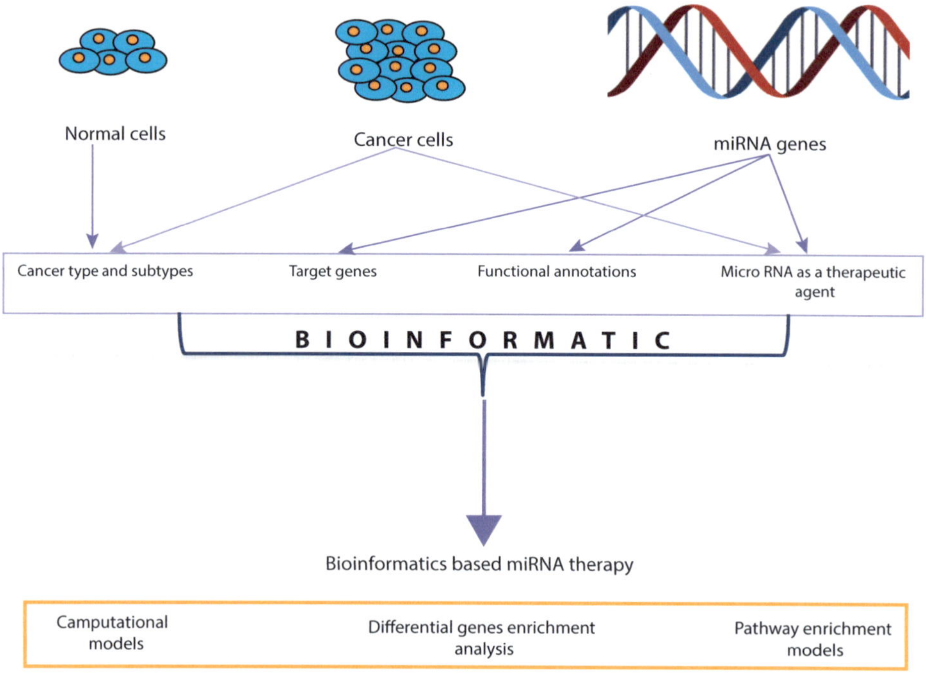

Fig. (3). Significance of bioinformatic tools in miRNA based therapeutics.

Various techniques like RNASeq, microarray and northern blots have been used to study the impending role of miRNAs in cancer development and metastasis, in order to provide valuable insights in cancer research. Moreover, their expression can either be upregulated or downregulated to act as therapeutic agents. Similarly, interference in the miRNA-mRNA regulatory interaction can be used for therapeutic purposes [57]. Later, researchers made an attempt to recognize miRNAs based on the structure, sequence and thermodynamic data in the nucleic acid sequence. MiRNAs have been identified by both approaches i.e.

experimental and computational. The experimental approach consumes a handsome amount of time and resources, hence, researchers have now moved on to use the computational methods for the predictions based on the genomic sequence information [57]. The following computational based approaches are used for predicting miRNAs:

i. Sequence- or structure-based approaches
ii. Machine learning-based approaches
iii. Expression data-based approaches
iv. Integrated approaches

Currently available bioinformatics tools aids in the identification of miRNA regulatory networks (including mirConnX http://www.benoslab.pitt.edu/mirconnx, CoMeTa http://cometa.tigem.it/), miRNA detection (including miRDeep http://www.australianprostatecentre.org/research/software/mirdeep-star, miRanalyzer http://bioinfo2.ugr.es/miRanalyzer/standalone.html), miRNA target prediction (including TargetScan http://www.targetscan.org/vert_71/, PicTar http://pictar.mdc-berlin.de/), miRNA expression analysis (including miRGator http://mirgator.kobic.re.kr/, MiRonTop http://www.microarray.fr:8080/miRon Top/index), analysis of miRNA signaling and metabolic pathways (including DIANA-mirPath http://snf-515788.vm.okeanos.grnet.gr/, miRNApath http://lgmb.fmrp.usp.br/mirnapath/) study of transcription factor-miRNA interplay (including PuTmiR http://www.isical.ac.in/~bioinfo_miu/TF- miRNA/TF-miRNA.html, TranmiR http://www.cuilab.cn/transmir) and linking miRNAs to diseases (including PhenomiR http://mips.helmholtz-muenchen.de/phenomir/, miR2Disease http://www.mir2disease.org/).

7. APPROACHES USED IN miRNA BASED THERAPIES

miRNAs have been recognized as important regulators of many cellular and developmental processes [61]. The mounting evidences also infer that miRNAs play significant roles in the pathogenesis of many cancers. In general, there are two methods in developing miRNA-based therapeutics: miRNA mimics and miRNA antagonists and they have rapidly appeared as a hopeful targets for cancer therapeutics [62]. The first methodology is based on reinstating the activity of tumor suppressor miRNAs by using miRNA mimics, whereas pharmacological inhibition of oncogenic miRNAs has been accomplished by using, antimiR oligonucleotides (Fig. **4**). Both of these strategies have been highlighted in this chapter.

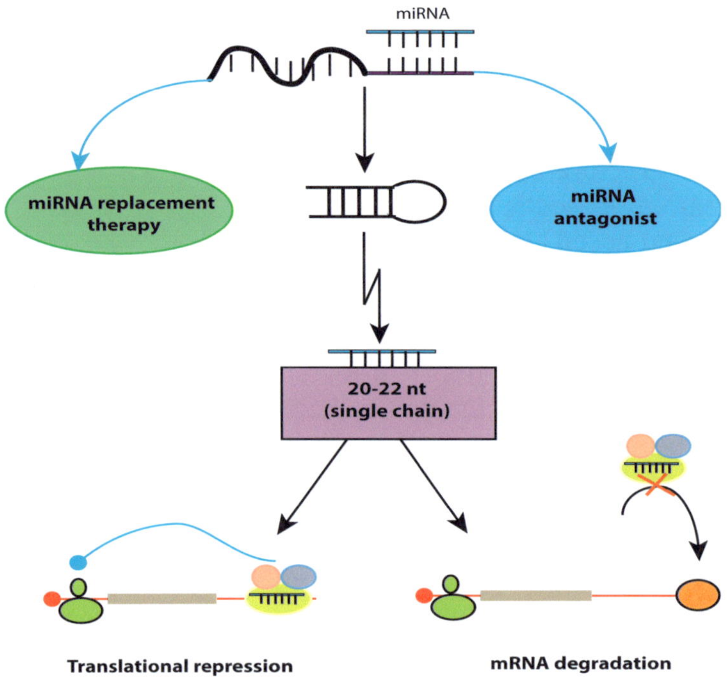

Fig. (4). The two main approaches to control cancer-associated miRNAs *in vivo* are based on double-stranded miRNA mimics, single-stranded antimiR oligonucleotides. Both approaches lead to inducing translational repression or targeted mRNA degradation.

8. miRNA MIMIC THERAPY

miRNA mimics are synthetic double-stranded small RNA molecules that match the corresponding miRNA sequence and functionally intends to re-introduce miRNAs into diseased cells to recover loss of function [44]. The loss or down-regulation of miRNAs is predominant in many cancers whereas numerous miRNAs have been categorized as tumor suppressors based on their role in neoplastic transformation and reduced expression level in tumors. The careful selection of miRNAs mimics to target multiple mRNAs that are known to be altered in cancers makes these molecules interesting therapeutic candidates. This approach is also recognized as 'miRNA replacement therapy [47]. In various cases, the replacement of these miRNAs leads to a re-activation of important pathways that are vital for normal cellular functions and block those responsible for the cancer progression. Perception for miRNA replacement therapy has been verified by mimics of tumour suppressor miRNAs that stimulate anti-oncogenic pathways, apoptosis and eventually lead to eradication of cancerous cells. Many experimental suggestions demonstrates that by modifying specific miRNA variations using miRNA mimics can stabilize the signaling pathways, gene regulatory networks and reverse the phenotype in various cancerous cells conferring the importance of miRNA replacement therapy [48, 50, 63]. Observing that most targeted cancer therapeutics that are developed to date results in recovery of a specific function has increased the anticipation about miRNA replenish therapy as it can provides a new vision to exploit tumour suppressors. miRNA mimics can be delivered by using same technologies as used for therapeutic siRNAs. Therefore, it is believed miRNA mimics will face less of a delivery hurdle compared to methods being used in gene therapy. Also, miRNA mimics are likely to be well tolerated and highly specific in normal tissues grounded on the fact that miRNA mimics carry the same naturally occurring sequences and are expected to target the same set of genes [61].

Various strategies have also been investigated to replenish miRNAs with tumour suppressive function by using miRNA mimics. The most considered and studied tumor suppressor miRNAs are the members of the miR-34 and let-7 families [64]. The let-7 family of miRNAs is well known suppressor of oncogenes, such as RAS, HMGA2, and MYC in lungs [49]. Recent studies reported that by restoring let-7 function in mouse models of lung cancer by using different delivery methods results in induced necrosis, reduced tumor growth,, and de-repression of the let-7 targets such as CDK6 and N-Ras [34, 65]. Furthermore, a 64% to 75% reduction of tumor burden compared with control animals was observed with intranasal delivery of a lentiviral construct expressing let-7 in K-Ras G12D mice with lung tumors [65]. These findings suggest the therapeutic potential of restoring let-7 activity in the treatment of lung cancer.

Among the miR-34 family three members, miR-34a, miR-34b and miR-34c are downregulated in lung, breast, colon, pancreatic, kidney, bladder cancers and melanomas [66]. During the DNA damage response all these members are transcriptionally regulated by the tumour suppressor p53. miR-34a plays a part in p53-mediated apoptosis upon DNA damage by directly targeting the anti-apoptotic protein sirtuin 1 (SIRT1) (Fig. **5**).

The tumour suppressive role of miR-34 is also evidenced by its target mRNA network, affecting the expression of cell cycle proteins such as cyclin-dependent kinase 4 (CDK4) and CDK6, anti-apoptotic proteins such as BCL-2 and metastasis-related proteins such as MET, Notch, MYC and AXL (Fig. **5**). Several preclinical studies using miR-34 mimics have validated their potential as anticancer therapeutics. Systemic delivery of miR-34 in an orthotopic model of pancreatic cancer using MiaPaca-2 cells resulted in increased tumor cell apoptosis and decreased tumor growth and the number of metastatic cells [67]. Delivery of miR-34 in a prostate cancer mouse model achieved a modest decrease in tumour growth but significant increase in survival times was observed due to a reduction in metastatic spread [68]. A liposomal formulation of miR-34 mimics was delivered. In mice models of NSCLC results in significant inhibition of tumour growth and lower level of oncogenic proteins expression such as MET and BCL-2 was observed. In the (KrasLSL-G12D/+;Trp53LSL−R172H/+) model of NSCLC, miR-34 mimics induction results in a decrease levels of the miR-34-regulated anti-apoptotic protein BCL 2 was observed, and the animals experienced a significant reduction in tumour burden [69]. Another following study showed that treatment with a miR-34 mimic (MRX34) in the aggressive Kras; Trp53 NSCLC mouse model consequences in significant tumor reduction [34]. Furthermore, a combination approach of co-provision of let-7 and miR-34 results in a significant reduction in tumour nodules and extended survival benefit [70]. In addition, combination treatment with the EGFR inhibitor Erlotinib and miR-34 and let-7 showed synergistic effects in inhibiting the growth of NSCLC cell lines *in vitro* [70].

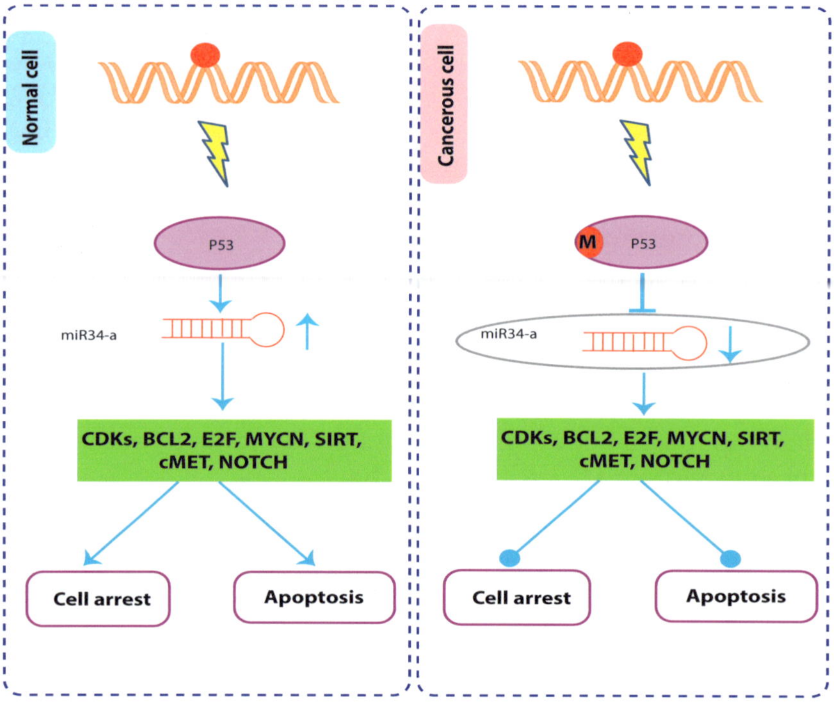

Fig. (5). Mechanistic role of miR-34a in normal and cancerous cells.

In addition to let-7 and miR-34 many other miRNAs mimics are also investigated in preclinical analysis in many cancers which are mentioned in Fig. (**6**).

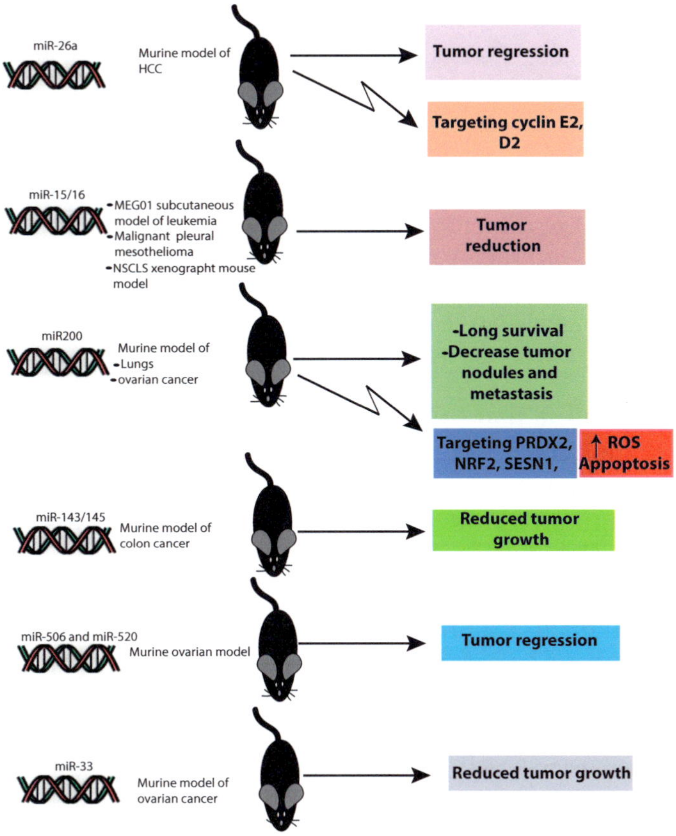

Fig. (6). Recent in vivo studies involving potential use of mimic miRNA in cancer therapy.

9. ANTI-miRNA THERAPY

AntimiRs are single stranded antisense oligonucleotides that target to their corresponding mRNAs. They have a corresponding sequence to the miRNA and result in hampering the function of the targeted miRNA (Fig. **3**). Since binding is often unchangeable, the new miRNA duplex is incapable to be processed or degraded by RISC. A likely concern about anti-miRNA is its ability to bind non-specifically to other RNAs that could result in many side effects. Anti-miRNA, also called as miRNA antagonists possess different subtypes. Some of them are mentioned in Table **3** [71 - 73].

Table 3. Different Subtypes of Anti-miRs.

Anti-MicroRNA	Functions	References
Antisense oligonucleotide (AMO)	Locked nucleic acid possesses stronger affinity to targeted miRNA, more resistant to nucleases, and have lower toxicity	[71, 72]

(Table 3) contd

Anti-MicroRNA	Functions	References
Peptide nucleic acid (PNA)	Binds the targeted nucleotide more tightly than the nucleotide/nucleotide binding, are relatively stable, have low toxicity, and could be administered systematically	[71, 72]
miRNA sponge	Down regulates the targeted miRNA and possesses multiple complementary sites to the targeted miRNA	[73]
miRNA masking	Complimentary to miRNA binding site in the 3′ UTR of the target mRNA to inhibit competitively and decreases the activity of endogenous miRNA	[73]

Emerging evidence infers that miRNAs are often dysregulated and overexpressed in many cancers, thus may function as oncogenes [74]. Different molecular and cellular pathways participate in cancer development including migration, cellular proliferation and apoptosis are regulated by miRNAs [75]. Pharmacological inhibition of such miRNAs in vivo is of great interest and holds promises in the development of novel anti miRNA based cancer therapy. miR-122 restricted to the liver, has also been established to be necessary for the replication and infectious production of hepatitis C virus (HCV). Binding of miR-122 to the 5′ noncoding region of the HCV genome, results in upregulated expression and accumulation of viral RNA in liver cells. Miravirsen, which is an antimiR inhibitor of the liver-expressed miR-122 is the first miRNA-based therapeutic that has led to the clinical development. miR-122 inhibition by antimiR oligonucleotides leads to rapid loss of HCV RNA in cultured liver cells, suggesting that miR-122 as a therapeutic target for the HCV treatment. miR221 is highly expressed in HCC and involved in down regulation of key tumor suppressors like p27KIP1, PTEN and TIMP3. antimiR-221, delivered intravenously to HCC mice model results in down regulated miR-221 and increase levels of its mRNA targets. The inhibition also results in tumor shrinkage and long survival of mice. miR-630 is another oncomiRNA that is upregulated was observed in the tumour environment. antimiR against miR-630 in an orthotopic model of ovarian cancer results in a noteworthy reduction in metastasis and tumour growth. In miR-155 model of lymphoma delivery of antimiR-155 results in reduce burden of tumor. In another approach where the mice were treated with pHLIP-antimiR-155, also results in a significant reduction in tumour burden. Further approaches for treating antimiR as a therapeutic target are briefly discussed in Fig. (**7**).

A number of strategies i.e. pharmacological and molecular have been applied to exploit this potential. Oncogenic miRNAs can be silenced or deactivated through a number of strategies involving RNA-interference, such as, specific miRNA knockdown by anti-miRNA oligonucleotides (AMOs), miRNA masking and miRNA sponges [37]. AMOs are antisense oligonucleotides that are synthetic in nature. They hinder the interaction between miRNAs and their target mRNAs and the most used are locked nucleic acids (LNAs), 2′-*O*-methoxyethyl AMOs and 2′-*O*-methyl AMOs [76]. Among them, locked nucleic acids are being utilized in current in vivo therapies due to their advantage over the other two AMOs.

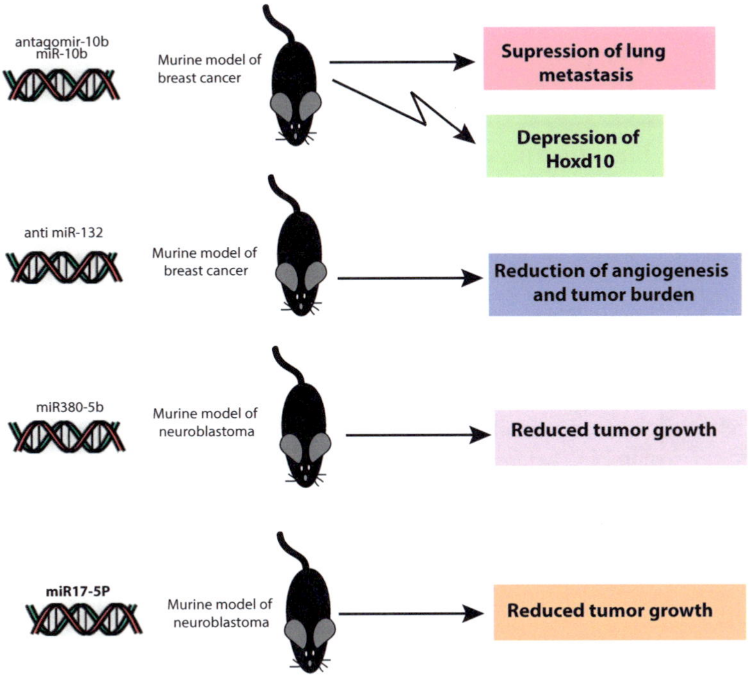

Fig. (7). Recent *in vivo* studies involving potential use of anti miRNA in cancer therapy.

Since, miRNAs have been detected to function in clusters in various processes of the pathological nature, the concept of "miRNA sponges" holds great potential. MiRNA sponges are competitive inhibitors that are expressed as transcripts from promoters that display binding sites for miRNAs. "Ebert *et al.* confirmed the efficacy of these miRNA inhibitors *in vitro* by transiently transfecting cultured cells with vectors encoding miRNA sponges" [37]. A sole sponge bears a heptameric seed sequence and it targets over-expressed miRNAs shared by this seed. Hence, the sponge can manipulate the anomalous levels of expression, effectively, thus causing hindrance in their binding with mRNA targets [77].

MiRNA knockdown can be performed through an approach alternative to the AMO method called "miRNA masking". The benefit it holds over AMOs is that it can target miRNAs in a gene-specific manner [78]. An miRmask is synthesized as a single-stranded 2′-*O*-methyl modified oligonucleotide, that is highly complementary to a miRNA binding site present endogenously in a protein coding gene at the 3′ UTR [37]. AMOs bind to a specific target miRNA, whereas the miR-mask causes binding to the 3′ UTR of target miRNAs binding site. This mechanism prevents off-target binding. This technology has high clinical potential since it has been validated *in vivo*.

10. RECENT PATENTS AND CLINICAL TRIAL STATUS OF miRNA THERAPEUTICS IN VARIOUS CANCERS

Table **4** [79 - 93] has discussed recent patents related to miRNA based cancer therapeutics in the year 2005 and 2010-2017.

Table 4. Patents Related to miRNA Based Cancer Therapeutics 2005/2010-2017.

Sr. No.	Patent Number	Patent Title	Publication Date	References
1	EP3126496	MicroRNA dosing regimens	February 8, 2017	[79]
2	EP3106168	Targeting microRNAs mir-409-5p, mir-379 and mir-154* to treat prostate cancer bone metastasis and drug resistant lung cancer	February 22, 2017	[80]
3	EP3110951	Sorafenib-microRNA combination therapy for liver cancer	January 4, 2017	[81]
4	WO2017005771	Use of glypican-3-targeting microRNAs for treating liver cancer	January 12, 2017	[82]
5	WO2017005773	Use of catenin- beta 1-targeting microRNAs for treating liver cancer	January 12, 2017	[83]
6	US9399773	Production and extraction of microRNA precursor as drug for cancer therapy	July 26, 2016	[84]
7	EP2217248	Targeting microRNAs for the treatment of liver cancer	November 30, 2016	[85]
8	US9469854	A pharmaceutical composition comprising a microRNA (miRNA) mimic containing a single-strand RNA molecule of hsa-miR-21-3p, which can be used to treat liver diseases through regulating the expression of methionine adenosyltransferase 2A and 2B (MAT2A and MAT2B), acetyl-CoA carboxylase 1 and 2 (ACACA and ACACB), diglyceride acyltransferase 2 (DGAT2)	October 18, 2016	[86]
9	US9365852	Compositions and methods related to miRNA modulation of neovascularization or angiogenesis	June 14, 2016	[87]
10	US20150080244	Biomarkers useful for detection of types, grades and stages of human breast cancer	March 19, 2015	[88]
11	WO2014140797	MicroRNA-based approach to treating malignant pleural mesothelioma	September 18, 2014	[89]

(Table 4) contd

Sr. No.	Patent Number	Patent Title	Publication Date	References
12	US8658370	MicroRNA-based methods and compositions for the diagnosis, prognosis and treatment of breast cancer	February 25, 2014	[90]
13	US20140309278	Combination cancer treatments utilizing micrornas and EGFR-TKI inhibitors	October 16, 2014	[91]
14	US7960359	Methods and compositions involving miRNA and miRNA inhibitor molecules	June 14, 2011	[92]
15	US20100179213	Methods and compositions involving miRNAs in cancer stem cells	July 15, 2010	[93]

10.1. Targeting miRNAs miR-409-5p, miR-379 and miR-154* to Treat Prostate Cancer Bone Metastasis and Drug Resistant Lung Cancer

This invention involves the use of short oligonucleotides that target and inhibit miRNAs *in vivo*, along with their use in therapeutic compositions. This study is based on the fact that short oligonucleotides that target miRNAs with a great proportion of analogue nucleotides, such a LNA nucleotides, are significantly effective in enhancing the repression of RNAs by targeted miRNAs, *in vivo*.

Furthermore, this invention provides an oligomer a contiguous sequence of 7-10 nucleotide units in length, to decrease the amount of a miRNA target in an organism or in a cell, where at least eighty percent of the nucleotides of the oligomer are selected from the LNA units and 2′ are substituted analogues of the nucleotide. Also, this invention provides an oligomer a contiguous sequence of 7-10 nucleotide units in length, to decrease the amount of a miRNA target in an organism or in a cell, where at least seventy percent of the nucleotide units of the oligomer are carefully chosen from LNA units and 2′ substituted analogues of the nucleotide, and at least sixty to seventy percent of the oligomer nucleotide units are nucleic acid (LNA) units.

This invention provides oligomers with length between 7-10 nucleotides which comprises a contiguous nucleotide sequence between these nucleotides, such as 7, 8, and 9, nucleotide units, where fifty percent of the oligomer nucleotide units are analogues of nucleotides.

Furthermore, this invention focuses on the treatment of a disease or medical disorder related with the overexpression or mere presence of the miRNA, comprising the step of administering a pharmaceutical composition including an oligomer or conjugate according to the invention to a patient suffering from or likely to suffer from said disease or medical disorder. The inventors provide for a method for decreasing the amount of a miRNA target effectively in an organism or a cell, containing the administration of oligomer, or a pharmaceutical composition including the oligomer or conjugate.

This invention also introduces a method for reversing the repression of one or more target mRNA in an organism or a cell, containing the administration of an oligomer or conjugate conferring to the discovery, or a therapeutic composition including the mentioned oligomer or conjugate, to the mentioned organism. Also, this discovery uses an oligomer or a conjugate, for inhibiting the miRNA in a cell which comprises a human cell. This might be employed *in vitro* or *in vivo* .

10.2. Use of Catenin- Beta 1-Targeting miRNAs for Treating Liver Cancer

Hepatoblastoma is a rare liver neoplasm that mostly occurred in newborns and children. Numerous therapeutic approaches are available while the most effective is the surgical removal of the tumor or liver transplantation. However, this strategy is possible only in about 70% of hepatoblastoma. In the present study, it has been observed that Hsa-miR-548z, hsa-miR-624-5p, hsa-let-7i-3p, miR-88--5p and miR-449b-3p are down-regulated in hepatoblastoma tumors and causes inhibition of hepatoblastoma cell growth *in vitro*. In this study, the inventors identified that by replacing these 5 miRNAs (i.e., hsa-miR-548z, hsa-miR-624-5p, hsa-let-7i-3p, miR-885-5p, miR-449b-3p) results in the decrease level of the oncoprotein catenin beta 1 (CTNNB1) in hepatoblastoma cell lines. It is proposed that these molecules can be optionally used in combination with one or more preferred therapeutic agents, drug lowering the side effects and toxicity of the antitumor therapy and immunotherapeutic agents. The present invention relates that the molecule selected from the group consisting of hsa-miR-624-5p, hsa-mi--548z, hsa-let-7i-3p, hsa-miR-885-5p, hsa-miR-449b-3p or any combination of DNA or RNA encoding for said miRNA, or in combination of various anti tumor drugs can be used for treating a hepatoblastoma cancer. Also, these molecules identified in this study can be used as a marker for the diagnosis of patients having a hepatoblastoma. This invention is related to the designing of a kit for detecting a hepatoblastoma or a vulnerability of a subject to develop a hepatoblastoma cancer in near future.

10.3. Production and Extraction of MiRNA Precursor as Drug for Cancer Therapy

The present study normally is related to a composition and its production method that are useful for developing vaccines or drugs therapies against human cancers. It identifies essential steps of production and purification methods necessary for extracting natural non-coding RNA (ncRNA) such as miRNA precursors (pre-miRNA) and small hairpin RNAs (shRNA), which can be used for treating human cancers. The principle of the present invention is relied on the unlike and mismatched properties of transcription systems of prokaryotes and eukaryotes, as prokaryotic RNA polymerases do not recognize eukaryotic promoters and vice versa. However, the present invention has identified chemical agents that can serve as transcriptional inducers to trigger and/or enhance eukaryotic promoter-driven RNA transcription in prokaryotes. The novelty of this procedure is creation of an artificially enhanced environment for prokaryotic cells to adopt eukaryotic pol-2 and/or pol-2-like promoters in order to transcribe desired ncRNAs or their precursors without going through error-prone prokaryotic promoters. Preferably, the prokaryotic cells used for the present study are *Escherichia coli* (*E. coli*), and the chemical inducers are MOPS, ethanol, or glycerin, or a mixture thereof. The resulting ncRNAs, preferably pre-miRNAs and shRNAs, are potential therapeutic drug targets against human cancers, in particular liver cancers. The use of novel prokaryote-produced miRNA precursor (pro-miRNA) is capable of being delivered into human cells and are treated by the cells into miRNA-like effectors to provoke specific silencing effects on certain oncogenic targets that subsequently leads to a therapeutic result of tumor suppression . The present study includes inducing an expression of the pre-miRNA/pro-miRNAs, particularly human pre-miR-302, in prokaryotes through pol-2 or pol-2-like RNA promoter. This composition is further confirmed as a novel pre-miRNA-based drug that is capable of a mechanism called “Cancer Reversion”, i.e. reprogramming high-grade human liver cancers malignant properties into a low-grade benign or even relatively normal stage.

10.4. Targeting miRNAs for the Treatment of Liver Cancer

Liver cancer including hepatocellular carcinoma (HCC) is the most common cause of deaths in both men and women worldwide. Certain changes in miRNA expression patterns in liver cancer cells comparative to non-cancerous cells have been reported. Accordingly there exists a need for methods of treating liver cancer, such as HCC, by administering a pharmaceutical agent capable of inhibiting a dysregulated miRNA identified in connection with liver cancer, such as HCC. In this invention, different methods are provided that are useful for the treatment of liver cancer, such as HCC. These methods may result in one or more clinically desirable outcomes such as reduction in tumor size, reduced metastatic progression and prolonged survival time. Also, administration of a invented compound reduces serum alpha-fetoprotein and/or serum des-gamm--carboxyprothrombin in a subject having liver cancer. The levels of serum alpha-fetoprotein and/or serum des-gamma-carboxyprothrombin are important measures to assess therapeutic efficacy of the treatment and demonstrate the improvement of liver function of the subject. In this study, microarrays containing probes were designed to about 700 miRNAs, liver samples from HCC tumors and were compared to normal liver tissue samples. Out of 700 miRNAs, approximately 90 were found to be upregulated in HCC samples relative to normal liver tissue samples. 8 miRNAs were further selected as candidate miRNAs to be targeted for HCC therapy: miR-21, miR-125a-5p, miR-191, miR-210, miR-222, miR-378, miR-423-3p, and miR-638. Following the inhibition of 8 of these miRNAs in liver cancer cell lines using modified oligonucleotides complementary to the miRNAs resulted in reduction in cell proliferation and increased apoptosis of liver cancer cells. Also in a mouse subcutaneous tumor model, the administration of a modified oligonucleotide resulted in tumor volume reduction. Also in a mouse tumor model (subcutaneous xenograft mouse model, an orthotopic liver xenograft mouse model, an SV40 t/T transgenic mouse model, a TGF-α/c-myc transgenic mouse model and a chemically induced carcinogenic (diethylnitrosamine) mouse model.), the administration of a modified oligonucleotide resulted in tumor volume reduction.

10.5. Pharmaceutical Composition for Treating Liver Diseases

Nonalcoholic fatty liver disease (NAFLD) is now emerging as one of the most common liver diseases due to the increasing rate of obesity. Generally, NAFLD is referred as triglycerides accumulation in hepatocytes that exceeds 5% of liver weight. During the progression of NAFLD, growth of lipid droplets and intrahepatic lipid accumulation results in inflammation and liver fibrosis. This stage may progress towards advanced cirrhosis, hepatocellular carcinoma and hepatic decompensation. However, there is no specific drug regimen to reverse fatty liver associated diseases. Currently, researchers are intended to uncover the novel strategies that may activate fatty liver development.

Methionine adenosyltransferase (MAT) is known enzyme that speed up the production of S-adenosyl methionine (SAM) and is a important regulator of hepatocyte proliferation, differentiation and death. Two catalytic MAT isoforms are generated by two genes, MAT1A and MAT2A while a MAT2A regulatory subunit is encoded by a third gene MAT2B. MAT1A is expressed in the adult liver but MAT2A is widely distributed within the liver. Because of the difference in regulatory properties and catalytic kinetics, MAT1A-expressing cells have considerably higher SAM levels as compared to MAT2A-expressing cells. In HCC, there is a down-regulation of MAT1A and up-regulation of MAT2A. This phenomenon is known as the MAT1A:MAT2A switch and is accompanied with lower S-adenosyl methionine (SAM) contents that provide additional developmental advantage to hepatoma cells [94 - 97]. Increased expression of MAT2B in HCC is also related to decrease SAM levels and facilitates the growth of cancer cells [98]. As MAT2A and MAT2B play critical role in facilitating the hepatoma cells growth, they are potential targets for antineoplastic therapy.

In this invention, it was observed that the miR-21-3p (mature miRNAs of miR21 gene) mimic reduces the expression of EEF2K, MAT2B and MAT2A in hepatocellular carcinoma cells and increases concentration of intracellular SAM. This results in growth inhibition of cancer cells and induces apoptosis in hepatoma. In addition, the lipid droplet contents in primary human hepatocytes were also decreased. It was caused by the inhibition of ACACA, ACACB and DGAT2 expression that finally reduces the expression level of lipid biosynthesis-related genes, including HLCS, MTOR, RPTOR, in primary human hepatocytes.

In this invention, it was observed that the miR-21-3p (mature miRNAs of miR21 gene) mimic reduces the expression of EEF2K, MAT2B and MAT2A in hepatocellular carcinoma cells and increases concentration of intracellular SAM. This results in growth inhibition of cancer cells and induces apoptosis in hepatocytes. In addition, the lipid droplet contents in primary human hepatocytes were also decreased by reducing the lipid biosynthesis in liver, and finally improving fatty liver status. It was caused by the inhibiting the expression of DGAT2, ACACA, ACACB that finally reduces the lipid biosynthesis-related genes (HLCS, MTOR, RPTOR) expression level in primary human hepatocytes. One of the key inventions of this study was to provide a method for decreasing the expression of MAT2A and MAT2B that played a key role in liver cancers.

10.6. Use of Glypican-3-Targeting miRNAs for Treating Liver Cancer

Glypican-3 (GPC3) is a cell surface heparan-sulfate proteoglycan that is known to be overexpressed in HCC, but is absent from normal adult human tissues [99]. The ability of miRNAs to target multiple genes within a signaling cascade engenders a novel way of thinking about modulating pathways. Instead of relying on a one-inhibitor-one-target model, multiple components in a signaling network can be modulated by a miRNA resulting in a potent impact on the respective pathway. Based on this hypothesis, a patent entitled "Use of glypican-3-targeting miRNAs for treating liver cancer" (2017) was submitted which describes the potential of using tumor suppressor miRNAs (hsa-miR-4510, hsa-miR-548aa, hsa-miR- 548v and hsa-miR-376b-3p) through negatively regulating GPC3 for the treatment of HCC and hepatoblastoma. The inventors identified 5 novel miRNAs decreasing the level of the GPC3 in liver cancer cells. These miRNAs were found to be down-regulated in liver tumors and were capable of inhibiting HCC cell growth and inducing HCC cell cycle arrest *in vitro*. Some of them are even capable of inducing tumor cell apoptosis. Furthermore, the inventors revealed that miR-4510 is more effective *in vitro* than miR-34a for inhibiting the growth of HCC and hepatoblastoma cells and for inducing their apoptosis. The authors utilized chick chorioallantoic membrane in order to determine the ability of miR-4510 to inhibit the growth of a HCC *in vivo*. The authors also employed various bioinformatics algorithms for the scrutinization of miRNA: mRNA interactions including miRanda, RNA Hybrid, TargetScan, miRDB, TargetMiner, PICTAR5, Diana lab and DIANAmt. Moreover, Ingenuity Pathways Analysis tool was used for the investigation of the molecular pathways and cellular functions of miRNA target genes. Through computational analysis, the inventors also found a key role of miR- 4510 as a tumor suppressor in liver by finding out association of its predicted targets with cancerous processes and liver tumorigenesis. The inventors also considered the use of these miRNAs in combination with sorafenib for the treatment of HCC and in combination with cisplatin and/or doxorubicin for the treatment of hepatoblastoma cells. Their patent also relates to a kit for detecting a liver cancer by determining the level of GPC3 targeting miRNAs.

10.7. Sorafenib-miRNA Combination Therapy for Liver Cancer

The invention unveils combination therapy (sorafenib- miRNA mimic) for liver cancer. This invention includes the use of sorafenib tosylate as well as other pharmaceutically acceptable forms, esters and salts of sorafenib. Sorafenib (marketed as NEXAVAR®) is currently the only FDA-approved drug for patients with advanced primary liver cancer. It is a small molecule interacting with multiple intracellular and cell surface kinases and unique in targeting the Raf/Mek/Erk pathway. By inhibiting these kinases, genetic transcription involving cell proliferation and angiogenesis is inhibited. However, even with the development of drugs like sorafenib, the current treatment options for liver cancer are insufficient due to its limited effectiveness and severe toxicity. The results illustrate the *in vivo* efficacy of the miR- 34-mimic or miR-215 mimic in combination with sorafenib in orthotopic human Hep3b xenografts. The invention is based on the discovery that sorafenib can effectively act synergistically in combination with miRNA to inhibit and prevent the proliferation of liver cancer cells. The inventors further reported that synergism is not a common property of tumor suppressor miRNAs. While miR-215 mimic and miR-34 mimic showed synergistic effects in combination with sorafenib, none of miR-101, miR-124a, miR-101 or miR-26a mimics showed any such effects. Moreover, the authors stated that synergism only exists within a certain therapeutically effective range and ratios above a certain point can cause antagonism. The inventors also stated that this combination therapy can include additional therapies and can be used as concomitant, concurrent, adjuvant, neoadjuvant or palliative therapy as well as first line therapy, second line therapy, or crossover therapy. Furthermore, the invention provides methods and compositions for treating liver cancer. The authors stated that the nature of drug-drug interactions (synergism, addition, antagonism) can vary depending on drug ratios, drug concentrations and the desired potency. In this model, combination index (CI) values are calculated that are derived from dose-response curves of the single agents alone when used alone and in combination. CI < 1, CI = 1, and CI > 1 indicate synergistic, additive and antagonistic interactions, respectively.

CHALLENGES & FUTURE PERSPECTIVES

The challenges for developing miRNA-based therapeutics are not different from siRNA therapeutics and comprise of efficient delivery of antimiRs and miRNA mimics, low bioavailability, poor cellular uptake, long term safety concerns in humans, potential off-target effects and instability in biological fluids or tissues. Biological instability of these compounds in biological fluids or tissues is due to the rapid degradation of unmodified 'naked' oligonucleotides by cellular and serum nucleases. Furthermore, poor cellular uptake is due to their size and negative charge, which could prevent them from crossing through cell membranes. Another major problem for the use of *in vivo* miRNA-based therapeutics is related to tissue-specific delivery and cellular up-take of sufficient amounts of synthetic oligonucleotides to achieve sustained target inhibition. Novel miRNA-formulations including nanoparticles and polymers as well as virus-based approaches could be employed to overcome these problems. Recently, a patent describes that miRNA dosing regimens provide beneficial and superior therapies with properties like decreased toxicity, increased efficacy and decreased side effects. This invention provides better methods for miRNA treatment in solid and hematologic tumors [79]. It has been mentioned that "The invention provides therapeutic miRNA dosing regimens for hematologic malignancies and/or solid tumors where the miRNAs are mimics of miRNAs involved in the hematologic malignancy and/or solid tumors being treated. For example, the miRNA can be a mimic of a miR-34 family member, a miRNA downregulated in a hematologic malignancy and/or solid tumors. The miRNA mimic is administered in more than one treatment cycles in which the miRNA is administered daily for a certain number of consecutive days, followed by a number of consecutive days without miRNA administration" [79]. This invention can be used in therapies involving adjuvants or as a part of therapy used in accordance with another therapy for cancer also known as combination therapy. This invention can also include a combination of additional therapies to improve the mimic's efficacy.

CURRENT & FUTURE DEVELOPMENTS

Currently, miRNA function is focused on post-transcriptional silencing of genes in the targeted mRNA 3′ untranslated (UTR) region. There is a lot more room for future work and developments as this represents only one aspect of miRNA function. More recent studies suggest that miRNAs have key roles in transcriptional regulation through several epigenetic mechanisms, translational regulation and in the regulation of long RNAs. Hence, it will be significant to further explore the roles of miRNAs in post-transcriptional modifications such as methylation. In future developments, there is a need to study the probable drug resistance tools for anti-miR therapeutics. Three mechanisms can be observed. First, a change in the ADME (absorption, distribution, metabolism and excretion) of miRNA-inhibiting oligonucleotides. This could involve enzymes responsible for metabolism that work to remove the drug from cells along with the addition of neutralizing antibodies that help with clearing the drug. The second tool is to upregulate the expression of miRNAs or by enhancing miRNA biogenesis in order to counteract the effect of inhibition. The third approach focuses specific upregulation of miRNAs that can target the same set of genes, thus offsetting the anti-miR effect. A trend towards the function and expression of specific miRNA and related target genes can be perceived. However, challenges with respect to the use of miRNA-based therapeutics such as low bioavailability or poor cellular uptake as well as off-target effects or long-term safety concerns in humans remain to be further explored. Therefore, future developments in miRNA-based treatment will require further adjustments to maximize miRNAs potency while minimizing off target toxicity and immunogenicity. Exploring the mechanisms of drug resistance could open more options for the understanding of miRNA-targeting strategies for the development of future therapies.

CONSENT FOR PUBLICATION

Not applicable.

CONFLICT OF INTEREST

The authors declare no conflict of interest, financial or otherwise.

ACKNOWLEDGEMENTS

All authors sincerely extend their thanks to Atta-ur-Rahman School of Applied Biosciences (ASAB), National University of Sciences and Technology (NUST), Islamabad for their administrative support.

REFERENCES

[1] Lee RC, Feinbaum RL, Ambros V. The *C. elegans* heterochronic gene lin-4 encodes small RNAs with antisense complementarity to lin-14. Cell 1993; 75(5): 843-54. [http://dx.doi.org/10.1016/0092-8674(93)90529-Y] [PMID: 8252621]

[2] Shah MY, Calin GA. MicroRNAs as therapeutic targets in human cancers. Wiley Interdiscip Rev RNA 2014; 5(4): 537-48. [http://dx.doi.org/10.1002/wrna.1229] [PMID: 24687772]

[3] Calin GA, Dumitru CD, Shimizu M, *et al.* Frequent deletions and down-regulation of micro- RNA genes miR15 and miR16 at 13q14 in chronic lymphocytic leukemia. Proc Natl Acad Sci USA 2002; 99(24): 15524-9. [http://dx.doi.org/10.1073/pnas.242606799] [PMID: 12434020]

[4] Mendell JT, Olson EN. MicroRNAs in stress signaling and human disease. Cell 2012; 148(6): 1172-87.
[http://dx.doi.org/10.1016/j.cell.2012.02.005] [PMID: 22424228]

[5] Felekkis K, Touvana E, Stefanou Ch, Deltas C. microRNAs: A newly described class of encoded molecules that play a role in health and disease. Hippokratia 2010; 14(4): 236-40.
[PMID: 21311629]

[6] Bader AG, Brown D, Stoudemire J, Lammers P. Developing therapeutic microRNAs for cancer. Gene Ther 2011; 18(12): 1121-6.
[http://dx.doi.org/10.1038/gt.2011.79] [PMID: 21633392]

[7] Bartel DP. MicroRNAs: Target recognition and regulatory functions. Cell 2009; 136(2): 215-33.
[http://dx.doi.org/10.1016/j.cell.2009.01.002] [PMID: 19167326]

[8] Djuranovic S, Nahvi A, Green R. A parsimonious model for gene regulation by miRNAs. Science 2011; 331(6017): 550-3.
[http://dx.doi.org/10.1126/science.1191138] [PMID: 21292970]

[9] Naidu S, Magee P, Garofalo M. MiRNA-based therapeutic intervention of cancer. J Hematol Oncol 2015; 8: 68.
[http://dx.doi.org/10.1186/s13045-015-0162-0] [PMID: 26062952]

[10] Bentwich I, Avniel A, Karov Y, *et al.* Identification of hundreds of conserved and nonconserved human microRNAs. Nat Genet 2005; 37(7): 766-70.
[http://dx.doi.org/10.1038/ng1590] [PMID: 15965474]

[11] Griffiths-Jones S, Saini HK, van Dongen S, Enright AJ. miRBase: Tools for microRNA genomics. Nucleic Acids Res 2008; 36(Database issue): D154-8.
[PMID: 17991681]

[12] Calin GA, Sevignani C, Dumitru CD, *et al.* Human microRNA genes are frequently located at fragile sites and genomic regions involved in cancers. Proc Natl Acad Sci USA 2004; 101(9): 2999-3004.
[http://dx.doi.org/10.1073/pnas.0307323101] [PMID: 14973191]

[13] Calin GA, Croce CM. MicroRNAs and chromosomal abnormalities in cancer cells. Oncogene 2006; 25(46): 6202-10.
[http://dx.doi.org/10.1038/sj.onc.1209910] [PMID: 17028600]

[14] Permuth-Wey J, Chen YA, Fisher K, *et al.* A genome-wide investigation of microRNA expression identifies biologically-meaningful microRNAs that distinguish between high-risk and low-risk intraductal papillary mucinous neoplasms of the pancreas. PLoS One 2015; 10(1): e0116869.
[http://dx.doi.org/10.1371/journal.pone.0116869] [PMID: 25607660]

[15] Vychytilova-Faltejskova P, Pesta M, Radova L, *et al.* Genome-wide microRNA expression profiling in primary tumors and matched liver metastasis of patients with colorectal cancer. Cancer Genomics Proteomics 2016; 13(4): 311-6.
[PMID: 27365381]

[16] Shah MY, Ferrajoli A, Sood AK, Lopez-Berestein G, Calin GA. MicroRNA therapeutics in cancer-An emerging concept. EBioMedicine 2016; 12: 34-42.
[http://dx.doi.org/10.1016/j.ebiom.2016.09.017] [PMID: 27720213]

[17] Di Leva G, Garofalo M, Croce CM. MicroRNAs in cancer. Annu Rev Pathol 2014; 9: 287-314.
[http://dx.doi.org/10.1146/annurev-pathol-012513-104715] [PMID: 24079833]

[18] Xue J, Yang J, Luo M, Cho WC, Liu X. MicroRNA-targeted therapeutics for lung cancer treatment. Expert Opin Drug Discov 2017; 12(2): 141-57.
[http://dx.doi.org/10.1080/17460441.2017.1263298] [PMID: 27866431]

[19] Laganà A, Russo F, Sismeiro C, Giugno R, Pulvirenti A, Ferro A. Variability in the incidence of miRNAs and genes in fragile sites and the role of repeats and CpG islands in the distribution of genetic

material. PLoS One 2010; 5(6): e11166.
[http://dx.doi.org/10.1371/journal.pone.0011166] [PMID: 20567512]

[20] Weber B, Stresemann C, Brueckner B, Lyko F. Methylation of human microRNA genes in normal and neoplastic cells. Cell Cycle 2007; 6(9): 1001-5.
[http://dx.doi.org/10.4161/cc.6.9.4209] [PMID: 17457051]

[21] Saito Y, Liang G, Egger G, *et al.* Specific activation of microRNA-127 with downregulation of the proto-oncogene BCL6 by chromatin-modifying drugs in human cancer cells. Cancer Cell 2006; 9(6): 435-43.
[http://dx.doi.org/10.1016/j.ccr.2006.04.020] [PMID: 16766263]

[22] Jansson MD, Lund AH. MicroRNA and cancer. Mol Oncol 2012; 6(6): 590-610.
[http://dx.doi.org/10.1016/j.molonc.2012.09.006] [PMID: 23102669]

[23] Boyerinas B, Park S-M, Hau A, Murmann AE, Peter ME. The role of let-7 in cell differentiation and cancer. Endocr Relat Cancer 2010; 17(1): F19-36.
[http://dx.doi.org/10.1677/ERC-09-0184] [PMID: 19779035]

[24] Esquela-Kerscher A, Slack FJ. Oncomirs - microRNAs with a role in cancer. Nat Rev Cancer 2006; 6(4): 259-69.
[http://dx.doi.org/10.1038/nrc1840] [PMID: 16557279]

[25] Nosrati N, Bakovic M, Paliyath G. Molecular mechanisms and pathways as targets for cancer prevention and progression with dietary compounds. Int J Mol Sci 2017; 18(10): 2050.
[http://dx.doi.org/10.3390/ijms18102050] [PMID: 28946660]

[26] Mishra PJ. The miRNA-drug resistance connection: A new era of personalized medicine using noncoding RNA begins. Pharmacogenomics 2012; 13(12): 1321-4.
[http://dx.doi.org/10.2217/pgs.12.121] [PMID: 22966880]

[27] Mishra PJ, Humeniuk R, Mishra PJ, Longo-Sorbello GS, Banerjee D, Bertino JR. A miR-24 microRNA binding-site polymorphism in dihydrofolate reductase gene leads to methotrexate resistance. Proc Natl Acad Sci USA 2007; 104(33): 13513-8.
[http://dx.doi.org/10.1073/pnas.0706217104] [PMID: 17686970]

[28] Sin TK, Wang F, Meng F, *et al.* Implications of MicroRNAs in the treatment of gefitinib-resistant non-small cell lung cancer. Int J Mol Sci 2016; 17(2): 237.
[http://dx.doi.org/10.3390/ijms17020237] [PMID: 26891293]

[29] Zhou J-Y, Chen X, Zhao J, *et al.* MicroRNA-34a overcomes HGF-mediated gefitinib resistance in EGFR mutant lung cancer cells partly by targeting MET. Cancer Lett 2014; 351(2): 265-71.
[http://dx.doi.org/10.1016/j.canlet.2014.06.010] [PMID: 24983493]

[30] Awan FM, Naz A, Obaid A, *et al.* MicroRNA pharmacogenomics based integrated model of miR-1--92 cluster in sorafenib resistant HCC cells reveals a strategy to forestall drug resistance. Sci Rep 2017; 7(1): 11448.
[http://dx.doi.org/10.1038/s41598-017-11943-1] [PMID: 28904393]

[31] Liu X, Fu Q, Du Y, Yang Y, Cho WC. C Cho W. MicroRNA as regulators of cancer stem cells and chemoresistance in colorectal cancer. Curr Cancer Drug Targets 2016; 16(9): 738-54.
[http://dx.doi.org/10.2174/1568009616666151118114759] [PMID: 26577538]

[32] Gan CZ, Li G, Luo QS, Li HM. miR-339-5p downregulation contributes to Taxol resistance in small-cell lung cancer by targeting α1,2-fucosyltransferase 1. IUBMB Life 2017; 69(11): 841-9.
[http://dx.doi.org/10.1002/iub.1679] [PMID: 28940895]

[33] Ameres SL, Zamore PD. Diversifying microRNA sequence and function. Nat Rev Mol Cell Biol 2013; 14(8): 475-88.
[http://dx.doi.org/10.1038/nrm3611] [PMID: 23800994]

[34] Trang P, Wiggins JF, Daige CL, *et al.* Systemic delivery of tumor suppressor microRNA mimics using a neutral lipid emulsion inhibits lung tumors in mice. Mol Ther 2011; 19(6): 1116-22.

[http://dx.doi.org/10.1038/mt.2011.48] [PMID: 21427705]

[35] Calin GA, Croce CM. MicroRNA signatures in human cancers. Nat Rev Cancer 2006; 6(11): 857-66. [http://dx.doi.org/10.1038/nrc1997] [PMID: 17060945]

[36] Spizzo R, Nicoloso MS, Croce CM, Calin GA. SnapShot: MicroRNAs in cancer. Cell 2009; 137(3): 586-586.e1. [http://dx.doi.org/10.1016/j.cell.2009.04.040] [PMID: 19410551]

[37] McDermott AM, Heneghan HM, Miller N, Kerin MJ. The therapeutic potential of microRNAs: Disease modulators and drug targets. Pharm Res 2011; 28(12): 3016-29. [http://dx.doi.org/10.1007/s11095-011-0550-2] [PMID: 21818713]

[38] Calin GA, Croce CM. Chronic lymphocytic leukemia: Interplay between noncoding RNAs and protein-coding genes. Blood 2009; 114(23): 4761-70. [http://dx.doi.org/10.1182/blood-2009-07-192740] [PMID: 19745066]

[39] Nishimura M, Jung EJ, Shah MY, *et al.* Therapeutic synergy between microRNA and siRNA in ovarian cancer treatment. Cancer Discov 2013; 3(11): 1302-15. [http://dx.doi.org/10.1158/2159-8290.CD-13-0159] [PMID: 24002999]

[40] Yuan TL, Fellmann C, Lee C-S, *et al.* Development of siRNA payloads to target KRAS-mutant cancer. Cancer Discov 2014; 4(10): 1182-97. [http://dx.doi.org/10.1158/2159-8290.CD-13-0900] [PMID: 25100204]

[41] Monroig PdelC, Chen L, Zhang S, Calin GA. Small molecule compounds targeting miRNAs for cancer therapy. Adv Drug Deliv Rev 2015; 81: 104-16. [http://dx.doi.org/10.1016/j.addr.2014.09.002] [PMID: 25239236]

[42] Gumireddy K, Young DD, Xiong X, Hogenesch JB, Huang Q, Deiters A. Small-molecule inhibitors of microrna miR-21 function. Angew Chem Int Ed Engl 2008; 47(39): 7482-4. [http://dx.doi.org/10.1002/anie.200801555] [PMID: 18712719]

[43] Melo S, Villanueva A, Moutinho C, *et al.* Small molecule enoxacin is a cancer-specific growth inhibitor that acts by enhancing TAR RNA-binding protein 2-mediated microRNA processing. Proc Natl Acad Sci USA 2011; 108(11): 4394-9. [http://dx.doi.org/10.1073/pnas.1014720108] [PMID: 21368194]

[44] Rupaimoole R, Slack FJ. MicroRNA therapeutics: Towards a new era for the management of cancer and other diseases. Nat Rev Drug Discov 2017; 16(3): 203-22. [http://dx.doi.org/10.1038/nrd.2016.246] [PMID: 28209991]

[45] Garzon R, Marcucci G, Croce CM. Targeting microRNAs in cancer: Rationale, strategies and challenges. Nat Rev Drug Discov 2010; 9(10): 775-89. [http://dx.doi.org/10.1038/nrd3179] [PMID: 20885409]

[46] Jing Z, Han W, Sui X, Xie J, Pan H. Interaction of autophagy with microRNAs and their potential therapeutic implications in human cancers. Cancer Lett 2015; 356(2 Pt B): 332-8. [http://dx.doi.org/10.1016/j.canlet.2014.09.039] [PMID: 25304373]

[47] Bader AG, Brown D, Winkler M. The promise of microRNA replacement therapy. Cancer Res 2010; 70(18): 7027-30. [http://dx.doi.org/10.1158/0008-5472.CAN-10-2010] [PMID: 20807816]

[48] Kota J, Chivukula RR, O'Donnell KA, *et al.* Therapeutic microRNA delivery suppresses tumorigenesis in a murine liver cancer model. Cell 2009; 137(6): 1005-17. [http://dx.doi.org/10.1016/j.cell.2009.04.021] [PMID: 19524505]

[49] Esquela-Kerscher A, Trang P, Wiggins JF, *et al.* The let-7 microRNA reduces tumor growth in mouse models of lung cancer. Cell Cycle 2008; 7(6): 759-64. [http://dx.doi.org/10.4161/cc.7.6.5834] [PMID: 18344688]

[50] Takeshita F, Patrawala L, Osaki M, *et al.* Systemic delivery of synthetic microRNA-16 inhibits the

growth of metastatic prostate tumors via downregulation of multiple cell-cycle genes. Mol Ther 2010; 18(1): 181-7.
[http://dx.doi.org/10.1038/mt.2009.207] [PMID: 19738602]

[51] Krichevsky AM, Gabriely G. miR-21: A small multi-faceted RNA. J Cell Mol Med 2009; 13(1): 39-53.
[http://dx.doi.org/10.1111/j.1582-4934.2008.00556.x] [PMID: 19175699]

[52] Gabriely G, Wurdinger T, Kesari S, *et al.* MicroRNA 21 promotes glioma invasion by targeting matrix metalloproteinase regulators. Mol Cell Biol 2008; 28(17): 5369-80.
[http://dx.doi.org/10.1128/MCB.00479-08] [PMID: 18591254]

[53] Gandellini P, Folini M, Longoni N, *et al.* miR-205 Exerts tumor-suppressive functions in human prostate through down-regulation of protein kinase Cepsilon. Cancer Res 2009; 69(6): 2287-95.
[http://dx.doi.org/10.1158/0008-5472.CAN-08-2894] [PMID: 19244118]

[54] Segura MF, Hanniford D, Menendez S, *et al.* Aberrant miR-182 expression promotes melanoma metastasis by repressing FOXO3 and microphthalmia-associated transcription factor. Proc Natl Acad Sci USA 2009; 106(6): 1814-9.
[http://dx.doi.org/10.1073/pnas.0808263106] [PMID: 19188590]

[55] Crawford M, Brawner E, Batte K, *et al.* MicroRNA-126 inhibits invasion in non-small cell lung carcinoma cell lines. Biochem Biophys Res Commun 2008; 373(4): 607-12.
[http://dx.doi.org/10.1016/j.bbrc.2008.06.090] [PMID: 18602365]

[56] Gomes CP, Cho JH, Hood L, Franco OL, Pereira RW, Wang K. A review of computational tools in microRNA discovery. Front Genet 2013; 4: 81.
[http://dx.doi.org/10.3389/fgene.2013.00081] [PMID: 23720668]

[57] Banwait JK, Bastola DR. Contribution of bioinformatics prediction in microRNA-based cancer therapeutics. Adv Drug Deliv Rev 2015; 81: 94-103.
[http://dx.doi.org/10.1016/j.addr.2014.10.030] [PMID: 25450261]

[58] Blair RH, Trichler DL, Gaille DP. Mathematical and statistical modeling in cancer systems biology. Front Physiol 2012; 3: 227.
[http://dx.doi.org/10.3389/fphys.2012.00227] [PMID: 22754537]

[59] Lu J, Getz G, Miska EA, *et al.* MicroRNA expression profiles classify human cancers. Nature 2005; 435(7043): 834-8.
[http://dx.doi.org/10.1038/nature03702] [PMID: 15944708]

[60] Edelman LB, Eddy JA, Price ND. *In silico* models of cancer. Wiley Interdiscip Rev Syst Biol Med 2010; 2(4): 438-59.
[http://dx.doi.org/10.1002/wsbm.75] [PMID: 20836040]

[61] Bader AG, Lammers P. The therapeutic potential of microRNAs. IPT 2011; pp. 52-5.

[62] Thorsen SB, Obad S, Jensen NF, Stenvang J, Kauppinen S. The therapeutic potential of microRNAs in cancer. Cancer J 2012; 18(3): 275-84.
[http://dx.doi.org/10.1097/PPO.0b013e318258b5d6] [PMID: 22647365]

[63] Wiggins JF, Ruffino L, Kelnar K, *et al.* Development of a lung cancer therapeutic based on the tumor suppressor microRNA-34. Cancer Res 2010; 70(14): 5923-30.
[http://dx.doi.org/10.1158/0008-5472.CAN-10-0655] [PMID: 20570894]

[64] He L, Thomson JM, Hemann MT, *et al.* A microRNA polycistron as a potential human oncogene. Nature 2005; 435(7043): 828-33.
[http://dx.doi.org/10.1038/nature03552] [PMID: 15944707]

[65] Trang P, Medina PP, Wiggins JF, *et al.* Regression of murine lung tumors by the let-7 microRNA. Oncogene 2010; 29(11): 1580-7.
[http://dx.doi.org/10.1038/onc.2009.445] [PMID: 19966857]

[66] Lodygin D, Tarasov V, Epanchintsev A, *et al.* Inactivation of miR-34a by aberrant CpG methylation in multiple types of cancer. Cell Cycle 2008; 7(16): 2591-600.
[http://dx.doi.org/10.4161/cc.7.16.6533] [PMID: 18719384]

[67] Pramanik D, Campbell NR, Karikari C, *et al.* Restitution of tumor suppressor microRNAs using a systemic nanovector inhibits pancreatic cancer growth in mice. Mol Cancer Ther 2011; 10(8): 1470-80.
[http://dx.doi.org/10.1158/1535-7163.MCT-11-0152] [PMID: 21622730]

[68] Liu C, Kelnar K, Liu B, *et al.* The microRNA miR-34a inhibits prostate cancer stem cells and metastasis by directly repressing CD44. Nat Med 2011; 17(2): 211-5.
[http://dx.doi.org/10.1038/nm.2284] [PMID: 21240262]

[69] Kasinski AL, Slack FJ. miRNA-34 prevents cancer initiation and progression in a therapeutically resistant K-ras and p53-induced mouse model of lung adenocarcinoma. Cancer Res 2012; 72(21): 5576-87.
[http://dx.doi.org/10.1158/0008-5472.CAN-12-2001] [PMID: 22964582]

[70] Stahlhut C, Slack FJ. Combinatorial action of microRNAs let-7 and miR-34 effectively synergizes with erlotinib to suppress non-small cell lung cancer cell proliferation. Cell Cycle 2015; 14(13): 2171-80.
[http://dx.doi.org/10.1080/15384101.2014.1003008] [PMID: 25714397]

[71] Czech MP. MicroRNAs as therapeutic targets. N Engl J Med 2006; 354(11): 1194-5.
[http://dx.doi.org/10.1056/NEJMcibr060065] [PMID: 16540623]

[72] Fabani MM, Abreu-Goodger C, Williams D, *et al.* Efficient inhibition of miR-155 function *in vivo* by peptide nucleic acids. Nucleic Acids Res 2010; 38(13): 4466-75.
[http://dx.doi.org/10.1093/nar/gkq160] [PMID: 20223773]

[73] Lee JB, Hong J, Bonner DK, Poon Z, Hammond PT. Self-assembled RNA interference microsponges for efficient siRNA delivery. Nat Mater 2012; 11(4): 316-22.
[http://dx.doi.org/10.1038/nmat3253] [PMID: 22367004]

[74] Ventura A, Jacks T. MicroRNAs and cancer: Short RNAs go a long way. Cell 2009; 136(4): 586-91.
[http://dx.doi.org/10.1016/j.cell.2009.02.005] [PMID: 19239879]

[75] Kaboli PJ, Rahmat A, Ismail P, Ling K-H. MicroRNA-based therapy and breast cancer: A comprehensive review of novel therapeutic strategies from diagnosis to treatment. Pharmacol Res 2015; 97: 104-21.
[http://dx.doi.org/10.1016/j.phrs.2015.04.015] [PMID: 25958353]

[76] Weiler J, Hunziker J, Hall J. Anti-miRNA oligonucleotides (AMOs): Ammunition to target miRNAs implicated in human disease? Gene Ther 2006; 13(6): 496-502.
[http://dx.doi.org/10.1038/sj.gt.3302654] [PMID: 16195701]

[77] Ebert MS, Neilson JR, Sharp PA. MicroRNA sponges: Competitive inhibitors of small RNAs in mammalian cells. Nat Methods 2007; 4(9): 721-6.
[http://dx.doi.org/10.1038/nmeth1079] [PMID: 17694064]

[78] Wang Z. The principles of MiRNA-masking antisense oligonucleotides technology. Methods Mol Biol 2011; 676: 43-9.
[http://dx.doi.org/10.1007/978-1-60761-863-8_3] [PMID: 20931388]

[79] Kim S. MicroRNA dosing regimens. EP3126496, 2015.

[80] Chung LWK, Josson S, Gururajan M, Jain A. Targeting microRNAs miR-409-5p, miR-379 and miR-154* to treat prostate cancer bone metastasis and drug resistant lung cancer. EP3106168, 2017.

[81] Bader A, Zhao J. Sorafenib-microRNA combination therapy for liver cancer. EP3110951, 2017.

[82] Grosset C, Cartier F, Lesjean S, Sagliocco F. Use of glypican-3-targeting microRNAs for treating liver cancer. WO2017005771, 2017.

[83] Grosset C, Lesjean S, Sagliocco F, Buendia M, Indersie E. Use of catenin- beta 1-targeting microRNAs for treating liver cancer. WO2017005773, 2017.

[84] Lin SL, Chang D, Wu DTS. Production and extraction of MicroRNA precursor as drug for cancer therapy. US9399773, 2016.

[85] Bennett CF, Chajut A, Esau C, Marcusson EG, Yerushalmi N. Targeting microRNAs for the treatment of liver cancer. EP2217248, 2016.

[86] Chen ST, Lo TF, Tsai WC. Pharmaceutical composition for treating liver diseases. US9469854, 2016.

[87] Shen J, Kelnar K, Shelton J, Brown D, Campochiaro P. Compositions and methods related to miRNA modulation of neovascularization or angiogenesis. US9365852, 2016.

[88] Kumar LD, Verma VK, Nair RA, Prabhakar J, Kattoor J. Biomarkers useful for detection of types, grades and stages of human breast cancer. US20150080244, 2015.

[89] Reid G, Van ZN. MicroRNA-based approach to treating malignant pleural mesothelioma. US20140275223, 2014.

[90] Croce CM, Calin GA. MicroRNA-based methods and compositions for the diagnosis, prognosis and treatment of breast cancer. US8658370, 2014.

[91] Bader A, Zhao J, Kelnar K. Combination cancer treatments utilizing microRNAs and EGFR-TKI inhibitors. WO2014143855, 2014.

[92] Brown D, Ford L, Cheng A, *et al.* Methods and compositions involving miRNA and miRNA inhibitor molecules. US7960359, 2011.

[93] Patrawala L, Tang DG, Kelnar K, *et al.* Methods and compositions involving miRNAs in cancer stem cells. WO2010056737, 2010.

[94] Mato JM, Lu SC. Role of S-adenosyl-L-methionine in liver health and injury. Hepatology 2007; 45(5): 1306-12.
[http://dx.doi.org/10.1002/hep.21650] [PMID: 17464973]

[95] Mato JM, Alvarez L, Ortiz P, Pajares MA. S-adenosylmethionine synthesis: Molecular mechanisms and clinical implications. Pharmacol Ther 1997; 73(3): 265-80.
[http://dx.doi.org/10.1016/S0163-7258(96)00197-0] [PMID: 9175157]

[96] Cai J, Mao Z, Hwang J-J, Lu SC. Differential expression of methionine adenosyltransferase genes influences the rate of growth of human hepatocellular carcinoma cells. Cancer Res 1998; 58(7): 1444-50.
[PMID: 9537246]

[97] Garcea R, Daino L, Pascale R, *et al.* Inhibition of promotion and persistent nodule growth by S-adenosyl-L-methionine in rat liver carcinogenesis: role of remodeling and apoptosis. Cancer Res 1989; 49(7): 1850-6.
[PMID: 2564313]

[98] Martínez-Chantar ML, García-Trevijano ER, Latasa MU, *et al.* Methionine adenosyltransferase II β subunit gene expression provides a proliferative advantage in human hepatoma. Gastroenterology 2003; 124(4): 940-8.
[http://dx.doi.org/10.1053/gast.2003.50151] [PMID: 12671891]

[99] Fleming BD, Ho M. Glypican-3 targeting immunotoxins for the treatment of liver cancer. Toxins (Basel) 2016; 8(10): 274.
[http://dx.doi.org/10.3390/toxins8100274] [PMID: 27669301]

Author Index

SUBJECT INDEX

A

B

C

D

E

F

G

H

I

J

K

L

M

N

O

P

Q

R

S

T

U

V

W

X

Made in the USA
Monee, IL
01 May 2026

49334983R00140